Atlas o

Amputations *and* Limb Deficiencies

Surgical, Prosthetic, and Rehabilitation Principles

Fourth Edition

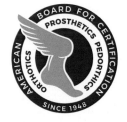

This book belongs to:

_____

This book is a special gift from the American Board for Certification in Orthotics, Prosthetics & Pedorthics, Inc. (ABC), the premier certifying and accrediting body for the orthotic and prosthetic profession.

As the future of this profession, we would like to congratulate you on choosing such an inspiring and rewarding career. We hope that this book becomes a useful tool and career-long resource, helping guide you through your studies and professional journey. We wish you continued success and hope that you look to ABC not only for your practitioner certification but guidance throughout your career.

ABCop.org

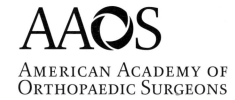

Atlas of Amputations and Limb Deficiencies

Surgical, Prosthetic, and Rehabilitation Principles

Fourth Edition

Volume 3
Pediatrics

Editors

Joseph Ivan Krajbich, MD

Michael S. Pinzur, MD

LTC Benjamin K. Potter, MD

Phillip M. Stevens, MEd, CPO

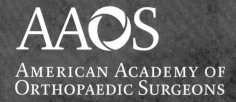

AAOS

AMERICAN ACADEMY OF
ORTHOPAEDIC SURGEONS

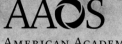
The material presented in the fourth edition of the *Atlas of Amputations and Limb Deficiencies: Surgical, Prosthetic, and Rehabilitation Principles* has been made available by the American Academy of Orthopaedic Surgeons for educational purposes only. This material is not intended to present the only, or necessarily best, methods or procedures for the medical situations discussed, but rather is intended to represent an approach, view, statement, or opinion of the author(s) or producer(s), which may be helpful to others who face similar situations.

Some drugs or medical devices demonstrated in Academy courses or described in Academy print or electronic publications have not been cleared by the Food and Drug Administration (FDA) or have been cleared for specific uses only. The FDA has stated that it is the responsibility of the physician to determine the FDA clearance status of each drug or device he or she wishes to use in clinical practice.

Furthermore, any statements about commercial products are solely the opinion(s) of the author(s) and do not represent an Academy endorsement or evaluation of these products. These statements may not be used in advertising or for any commercial purpose.

Published 2016 by the
American Academy of Orthopaedic Surgeons
9400 West Higgins Road
Rosemont, IL 60018

Copyright 2016
by the American Academy of Orthopaedic Surgeons

Library of Congress Control Number: 2015959857

ISBN 978-1-62552-437-9

Printed in Canada

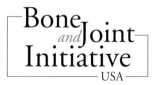

Editors

**American Academy of Orthopaedic Surgeons
Atlas of Amputations and Limb Deficiencies:
Surgical, Prosthetic, and Rehabilitation Principles
Fourth Edition**

Joseph Ivan Krajbich, MD, FRCS(C)
Staff Orthopaedic Surgeon
Shriners Hospital for Children
Portland, Oregon

Michael S. Pinzur, MD
Professor of Orthopaedic Surgery and Rehabilitation
Department of Orthopaedic Surgery and Rehabilitation
Loyola University Health System
Maywood, Illinois

LTC Benjamin K. Potter, MD
Chief Orthopaedic Surgeon, Amputee Care Program
Deputy Chief, Orthopaedic Surgery
Vice Chair (Research) and Associate Professor
Uniformed Services University-Walter Reed
    Department of Surgery
Bethesda, Maryland

Phillip M. Stevens, MEd, CPO, FAAOP
Prosthetist/Orthotist
Hanger Clinic
Adjunct Assistant Professor
Division of Physical Medicine and Rehabilitation
University of Utah
Salt Lake City, Utah

Explore the full portfolio of AAOS educational programs and publications across the orthopaedic spectrum for every stage of an orthopaedic surgeon's career, at www.aaos.org/store. The AAOS, in partnership with Jones & Bartlett Learning, also offers a comprehensive collection of educational and training resources for emergency medical providers, from first responders to critical care transport paramedics. Learn more at www.aaos.org/ems.

Contributors

Joseph F. Alderete Jr, MD
Chief, Orthopaedic Oncology Section
Associate Program Director, Orthopaedic Residency
Department of Orthopaedic Surgery
San Antonio Military Medical Center (formerly Brooke
    Army Medical Center)
San Antonio, Texas

Motasem A. Al Maaieh, MD
Instructor
Department of Orthopaedic Surgery
University of Miami
Miami, Florida

Edward A. Athanasian, MD
Associate Professor of Clinical Orthopedics
Chief, Hand Surgery Service
Hospital for Special Surgery
New York, New York

M. David Beachler, CP
Lead Clinical Prosthetist
Orthotic and Prosthetic Services
Walter Reed National Military Medical Center
Bethesda, Maryland

Christopher Bibbo, DO, FACS
Department of Surgery
Division of Plastic and Reconstructive Surgery
Hospital of the University of Pennsylvania
Philadelphia, Pennsylvania

John H. Bowker, MD
Professor Emeritus
Department of Orthopaedics
Miller School of Medicine
University of Miami
Miami, Florida

Mihai Bragaru, PhD
Chelmsford, United Kingdom

Rickard Brånemark, MD, MSc, PhD
Orthopaedic Surgeon
Department of Orthopaedics
Sahlgrenska University Hospital
Gothenburg, Sweden

Joseph Karl Brenner, BSc/Biology, CP, FAAOP
Director of Clinical Prosthetics
Hanger Clinic
Michigan Institute for Electronic Limb Development
Livonia, Michigan

John T. Brinkmann, MA, CPO/L, FAAOP
Assistant Professor and Research Prosthetist
Department of Physical Medicine and Rehabilitation
Northwestern University
Chicago, Illinois

Helena Burger, MD, PhD
Medical Director
University Rehabilitation Institute
Ljubljana, Slovenia

Greg Bush, BA, CP(C)
Research Prosthetist
Institute of Biomedical Engineering
University of New Brunswick
Fredericton, New Brunswick, Canada

Federico Canavese, MD, PhD
Head, Department of Pediatric Surgery
University Hospital Estaing
Clermont-Ferrand, France

Kevin Carroll, MS, CP, FAAOP
Vice President, Prosthetics
Department of Prosthetics
Hanger Clinic
Orlando, Florida

Min Ho Chang, MD
Staff Physician
Interdisciplinary Pain Management Center
Womack Army Medical Center
Fort Bragg, North Carolina
Assistant Professor, Department of Physical Medicine
    and Rehabilitation
Uniformed Services University of the Health Sciences
Bethesda, Maryland

Ee Ming Chew, MBBS
Consultant
Department of Hand Surgery
Singapore General Hospital
Singapore

Benjamin B. Chi, MD
Orthopaedic Surgery Resident
Department of Orthopaedic Surgery
Walter Reed National Military Medical Center
Bethesda, Maryland

W. Lee Childers, PhD, MSPO, CP
Assistant Professor
Department of Prosthetics and Orthotics
Alabama State University
Montgomery, Alabama

Mickey S. Cho, MD
Attending Hand Surgeon
Department of Orthopaedics and Rehabilitation
San Antonio Military Medical Center (formerly
    Brooke Army Medical Center)
San Antonio, Texas

Helen Cochrane, CPO(c), MSc
Project Director
College of Allied Rehabilitation Sciences
University of the East Ramon Magsaysay Memorial
    Center
Manila, Philippines

Sheila A. Conway, MD
Associate Professor
Department of Orthopaedic Surgery
University of Miami Miller School of Medicine
Miami, Florida

Colleen P. Coulter, PT, DPT, PhD, PCS
Physical Therapist IV
Department of Orthotics and Prosthetics
Children's Healthcare of Atlanta
Atlanta, Georgia

Robin C. Crandall, MD
Orthopaedic Surgeon
Limb Deficiency Clinic
Twin Cities Shriners Hospitals for Children
Minneapolis, Minnesota

Donald R. Cummings, CP, LP
Director
Department of Prosthetics
Texas Scottish Rite Hospital for Children
Dallas, Texas

Anna Cuomo, MD
Pediatric Orthopaedic Surgeon
Department of Orthopaedics
University of North Carolina
Chapel Hill, North Carolina

Charles d'Amato, MD, FRCSC
Orthopaedic Surgeon
Shriners Hospital for Children
Portland, Oregon

Todd DeWees, BS, CPO
Prosthetist/Orthotist
Pediatric Orthotic and Prosthetic Services
Shriners Hospital for Children
Portland, Oregon

Michael P. Dillon, PhD
Senior Lecturer in Prosthetics and Orthotics
Department of Prosthetics and Orthotics
La Trobe University
Bundoora, Victoria, Australia

Kim Doolan, BA, CPV
Clinical Coordinator
Allen Orthotics and Prosthetics
Midland, Texas

Paul J. Dougherty, MD
Professor
Department of Orthopaedic Surgery
Wayne State University
Detroit, Michigan

Gregory A. Dumanian, MD, FACS
Chief, Division of Plastic and Reconstructive Surgery
Northwestern University, Feinberg School of Medicine
Chicago, Illinois

Tobin T. Eckel, MD
Orthopaedic Foot and Ankle Surgeon
Department of Orthopaedic Surgery
Walter Reed National Military Medical Center
Bethesda, Maryland

Mark Edwards, MHPE, CP
Director
Professional and Clinical Services
Ottobock
Austin, Texas

Jorge A. Fabregas, MD
Residency Director
Department of Orthopaedics
Children's Orthopaedics of Atlanta
Atlanta, Georgia

Stefania Fatone, BPO(Hons), PhD
Associate Professor
Northwestern University Prosthetics-Orthotics Center
Northwestern University
Chicago, Illinois

James R. Ficke, MD
Chairman and Professor
Department of Orthopaedic Surgery
Johns Hopkins Hospital
Baltimore, Maryland

Sandra Fletchall OTR/L, CHT, MPA, FAOTA
Manager, Department of Burn Rehabilitation
Firefighters' Regional Burn Center
Memphis, Tennessee

Michael J. Forness, DO
Director, Limb Differences Clinic
Department of Pediatric Orthopaedics
Helen Devos Children's Hospital/Spectrum Health
Grand Rapids, Michigan

Johnathan A. Forsberg, MD, PhD
Orthopaedic Oncologist
National Institutes of Health and John P. Murtha
    Cancer Center
Naval Medical Research Center
Silver Spring, Maryland

Robert S. Gailey, PhD, PT
Professor
Department of Physical Therapy
University of Miami Miller School of Medicine
Coral Gables, Florida

Donald A. Gajewski, MD
Director
Center for the Intrepid
San Antonio Military Medical Center (formerly Brooke
    Army Medical Center)
San Antonio, Texas

Ignacio A. Gaunaurd, PhD, MSPT
Research Physical Therapist
Department of Research
Miami Veterans Affairs Healthcare System
Miami, Florida

Brian J. Giavedoni, MBA, CP, LP
Senior Prosthetist
Department of Orthotics and Prosthetics
Children's Healthcare of Atlanta
Atlanta, Georgia

Frank A. Gottschalk, MD
Professor
Department of Orthopaedic Surgery
University of Texas Southwestern Medical Center
Dallas, Texas

James A. Harder, BSc, MD, FRCS(C)
Pediatric Orthopaedic Surgeon
Department of Pediatric Orthopaedics
Alberta Children's Hospital
Calgary, Alberta, Canada

Carson Harte, CEO
Exceed
Lisburn, Northern Ireland

Bradford D. Hendershot, PhD
Lead Scientist
Center for Rehabilitation Sciences Research
Uniformed Services University of the Health Sciences
Bethesda, Maryland

Andrea Hess, CP
Upper Limb Clinical Specialist
Ottobock Healthcare
San Jose, California

James T. Highsmith, MD, MS
Dermatologist
Fellowship, Private Practice
Total Skin and Beauty Dermatology Center
Birmingham, Alabama

M. Jason Highsmith, PhD, DPT, CP, FAAOP
Associate Professor
University of Southern Florida School of Physical
    Therapy and Rehabilitation Sciences
Tampa, Florida

Wendy Hill, BScOT
Occupational Therapist
Atlantic Clinic for Upper Limb Prosthetics
University of New Brunswick
Fredericton, New Brunswick, Canada

Ali Hussaini, BASc, MScE
Engineer
Institute of Biomedical Engineering
University of New Brunswick
Fredericton, New Brunswick, Canada

Sabrina Jakobson Huston, CPO
Prosthetist/Orthotist
Department of Pediatric Orthotic Prosthetic Services
Shriners Hospital for Children
Portland, Oregon

Brad M. Isaacson, PhD, MBA, MSF
Program Manager/Lead Scientist
Center for Rehabilitation Sciences Research
The Henry M. Jackson Foundation for the
    Advancement of Military Medicine
Bethesda, Maryland

Michelle A. James, MD
Chief of Orthopaedic Surgery
Shriners Hospital for Children, Northern California
Sacramento, California

Brian Kaluf, BSE, CP
Clinical Outcome and Research Director
Ability Prosthetics and Orthotics
Greenville, South Carolina

JoAnne L. Kanas, PT, CPO, DPT
Corporate Director of Orthotics and Prosthetics
Department of Orthotics and Prosthetics
Shriners Hospital for Children
Tampa, Florida

Stephen J. Kovach III, MD
Assistant Professor of Surgery, Division of Plastic Surgery
Department of Orthopaedic Surgery
University of Pennsylvania Health System
Philadelphia, Pennsylvania

Joseph Ivan Krajbich, MD, FRCS(C)
Staff Orthopaedic Surgeon
Shriners Hospital for Children
Portland, Oregon

Peter Kyberd, BSc, MSc, PhD
Vice President's Research Chair in Rehabilitation
    Cybernetics
Institute of Biomedical Engineering
University of New Brunswick
Fredericton, New Brunswick, Canada

Justin Z. Laferrier, PT, PhD, OCS, SCS, ATP, CSCS
Assistant Professor
Department of Physical Therapy
University of Connecticut
Storrs, Connecticut

Chris Lake, L/CPO, FAAOP
Owner, Clinical Director
Department of Upper Limb Prosthetics
Lake Prosthetics and Research
Euless, Texas

Jakub Stuart Langer, MD
Orthopaedic and Hand Surgeon
Shriners Hospital for Children – Consultant Hand Surgeon
Portland, Oregon

John F. Lawrence, MD
Senior Physician
Department of Orthopaedic Surgery
University of California, Los Angeles
Los Angeles, California

L. Scott Levin, MD, FACS
Chair, Department of Orthopaedic Surgery
Penn Medicine
Philadelphia, Pennsylvania

Robert D. Lipschutz, CP, BSME
Assistant Professor
Department of Physical Medicine and Rehabilitation,
    Feinberg School of Medicine
Northwestern University
Clinical Practice Leader
Department of Prosthetics and Orthotics
Rehabilitation Institute of Chicago
Chicago, Illinois

Ellen J. MacKenzie, MSc, PhD
Professor and Chair
Department of Health Policy and Management
Johns Hopkins Bloomberg School of Public Health
Baltimore, Maryland

Samir Mehta, MD
Chief, Orthopaedic Trauma and Fracture Service
Department of Orthopaedic Surgery
University of Pennsylvania
Philadelphia, Pennsylvania

John W. Michael, MEd, CPO, FAAOP
Assistant Professor and Director
Department of Physical Medicine and Rehabilitation
Northwestern University Prosthetics–Orthotics Center
Chicago, Illinois

Laura A. Miller, PhD, CP
Research Prosthetist
Center for Bionic Medicine
Rehabilitation Institute of Chicago
Chicago, Illinois

Mark David Muller, CPO, MS, FAAOP
Instructor
Department of Health Science, Prosthetics and
  Orthotics Program
California State University, Dominguez Hills
Carson, California

George Peter Nanos III, MD
Navy Orthopaedic Surgery Specialty Leader
Department of Orthopaedic Surgery
Walter Reed National Military Medical Center
Bethesda, Maryland

LeRoy H. Oddie, CP
Research Prosthetist
Department of Extremity Trauma and Amputation
  Center of Excellence
Walter Reed National Military Medical Center
Bethesda, Maryland

Ramona M. Okumura, BS, CP
Senior Lecturer
Department of Rehabilitation Medicine
University of Washington
Seattle, Washington

Michael Orendurff, PhD
Director
Biomechanics Laboratory
Orthocare Innovations
Mountlake Terrace, Washington

Paul F. Pasquina, MD
Chair, Department of Physical Medicine and Rehabilitation
Uniformed Services University of the Health Sciences
Bethesda, Maryland

Thomas Passero, CP, AS
Clinical Director
Department of Upper Limb Prosthetics
Handspring Rehabilitation, LLC
Middletown, New York

Kathryn M. Peck, MD
Hand and Upper Extremity Surgeon
The Indiana Hand to Shoulder Center
Indianapolis, Indiana

Branden Petersen, BS, CP
Upper Extremity Prosthetic Specialist
National Upper Extremity Prosthetic Program
Hanger Clinic
Watertown, New York

Terrence M. Philbin, DO
Foot and Ankle Orthopedic Surgeon
Orthopedic Foot and Ankle Center
Westerville, Ohio

Michael S. Pinzur, MD
Professor of Orthopaedic Surgery and Rehabilitation
Department of Orthopaedic Surgery and Rehabilitation
Loyola University Health System
Maywood, Illinois

David J. Polga, MD
Orthopaedic Surgeon
Department of Orthopaedic Surgery
Marshfield Clinic
Marshfield, Wisconsin

LTC Benjamin K. Potter, MD
Chief Orthopaedic Surgeon, Amputee Care Program
Deputy Chief, Orthopaedic Surgery
Vice Chair (Research) and Associate Professor
Uniformed Services University-Walter Reed
  Department of Surgery
Bethesda, Maryland

Charles H. Pritham, CPO
Supervisor, Orthotic and Prosthetic Services
Prosthetics and Sensory Aids Service
North Florida/South Georgia Veterans Health System
Gainesville, Florida

Alison L. Pruziner, PD, DPT
Research Physical Therapist
Department of Rehabilitation
Department of Defense and Veterans Affairs Extremity
  Trauma and Amputation Center of Excellence
Bethesda, Maryland

Mark Edward Puhaindran, MBBS, MMED (Surg), MRCS (Edin)
Senior Consultant
Department of Hand and Reconstructive Microsurgery
National University Hospital of Singapore
Singapore

Robin M. Queen, PhD, FACSM
Associate Professor
Director, Kevin P. Granata Biomechanics Lab
Biomedical Engineering and Mechanics
Virginia Tech
Blacksburg, Virginia

Robert Radocy, MSc
CEO/President
TRS Inc.
Boulder, Colorado

Peter Charles Rhee, DO, MS
Hand and Microvascular Surgeon
Department of Orthopaedics and Rehabilitation
San Antonio Military Medical Center (formerly Brooke
    Army Medical Center)
San Antonio, Texas

John Rheinstein, CP
Lower/Upper Extremity Specialist
Hanger Clinic
New York, New York

Randall W. Richardson, ABC-CPA, RPA
Hanger Clinic
Oklahoma City, Oklahoma

Aimee J. Riley, DO
Orthopedic Surgery Resident
Department of Orthopedic Surgery
OhioHealth Doctors Hospital
Columbus, Ohio

Bradley M. Ritland, PT, DPT
Chief, Amputee Section
Department of Physical Therapy
Walter Reed National Military Medical Center
Bethesda, Maryland

David B. Rotter, CPO
Clinical Manager
Department of Prosthetics
Scheck & Siress
Chicago, Illinois

Michael Schmitz, MD
Chief of Orthopedics/Children's Healthcare of Atlanta
Department of Orthopaedics
Children's Orthopedics of Atlanta
Atlanta, Georgia

Phoebe Scott-Wyard, DO, FAAP, FAAPMR
Medical Director
Child Amputee Prosthetics Project
Shriners Hospital for Children
Los Angeles, California

Charles R. Scoville, PT, MEd, DPT
Department Head
Department of Rehabilitation
Walter Reed National Military Medical Center
Bethesda, Maryland

Scott B. Shawen, MD
Chief, General and Foot and Ankle Surgery
Department of Orthopaedic Surgery
Walter Reed National Military Medical Center
Bethesda, Maryland

Alexander Yong Shik Shin, MD
Consultant and Professor of Orthopedic Surgery
Department of Orthopedic Surgery, Division of Hand
    and Microvascular Surgery
Mayo Clinic
Rochester, Minnesota

Jaime T. Shores, MD, FACS
Clinical Director of Hand and Upper Extremity
    Transplant Program
Department of Plastic and Reconstructive Surgery
The Johns Hopkins University School of Medicine
Baltimore, Maryland

Jason M. Souza, MD
Department of Plastic and Reconstructive Surgery
Northwestern University
Feinberg School of Medicine
Chicago, Illinois

Gerald E. Stark, MSEM, CPO/L, FAAOP
Senior Upper Limb Clinical Specialist
Department of Professional Clinical Services
Ottobock
Austin, Texas

Phillip M. Stevens, MEd, CPO, FAAOP
Prosthetist/Orthotist
Hanger Clinic
Adjunct Assistant Professor
Division of Physical Medicine and Rehabilitation
University of Utah
Salt Lake City, Utah

John Sullivan MSc, HCPC, Registered Prosthetist
Clinical Specialist, Prosthetics
Prosthetic Rehabilitation Unit
Royal National Orthopaedic Hospital
Stanmore, London, UK

LCDR Scott M. Tintle, MD, MC, USN
Hand and Microsurgeon, Director of Research
Department of Orthopaedics
Walter Reed National Military Medical Center
Bethesda, Maryland

Ian P. Torode, MD, FRACS
Director of Orthopaedics
Department of Orthopaedics
The Royal Children's Hospital
Melbourne, Victoria, Australia

Jack W. Tsao, MD, DPhil
Professor
Department of Neurology
University of Tennessee Health Science Center
Memphis, Tennessee

Elaine N. Uellendahl, BA, CP
Certified Prosthetist
Department of Prosthetics
New Touch Prosthetics
Cave Creek, Arizona

Jack E. Uellendahl, CPO
Prosthetist
Hanger Clinic
Phoenix, Arizona

Francois Van Der Watt, CPO, LPO
Director
Department of Sports Prosthetics and Development
Horton's Orthotics and Prosthetics
Fort Smith, Arizona

Hugh G. Watts, MD
Department of Pediatric Orthopedic Surgery
Shriners Hospital for Children
Clinical Professor of Orthopedic Surgery
Department of Orthopedics
University of California at Los Angeles
Los Angeles, California

Stephen T. Wegener, MA, PhD
Director, Division of Rehabilitation Psychology and
    Neuropsychology
Professor of Physical Medicine and Rehabilitation
Johns Hopkins University School of Medicine
Baltimore, Maryland

Rebecca C. Whitesell, MD, MPH
Pediatric Orthopedic Surgeon
Department of Pediatric Orthopedics
Mary Bridge Children's Hospital
Tacoma, Washington

Shane R. Wurdeman, PhD, MSPO, CP
Research Scientist–Certified Prosthetist
Biomechanics Research Building
University of Nebraska at Omaha
Omaha, Nebraska

Vivian J. Yip, OTD, OTR/L
Occupational Therapist
Child Amputee Prosthetics Project
Shriners Hospital for Children-Los Angeles
Los Angeles, California

Preface

The fourth edition of the *Atlas of Amputations and Limb Deficiencies: Surgical, Prosthetic, and Rehabilitation Principles* represents the continued commitment of the American Academy of Orthopaedic Surgeons to patients with congenital or acquired limb loss and the medical professionals who dedicate their lives to optimizing the functional independence of this patient population. This new edition is divided into three volumes: Volume 1–General Topics, Upper Limb; Volume 2–Lower Limb, Management Issues; Volume 3–Pediatrics. We hope that this presentation makes the book more user-friendly compared with a single volume.

The recent conflicts in the Middle East have served to bring amputees and the challenges that they face to the front pages of our newspapers and magazines. We have leaned heavily on our military colleagues to bring together in one text the latest surgical, prosthetic, and rehabilitation methodologies, many of which were developed or refined over the past decade. In addition to the need to meet simple, daily functional requirements, this very motivated and demanding group of patients has inspired the recognition of newly evolving techniques and tools to promote sports participation and advanced rehabilitation. There is a new and expanded focus on such rehabilitation, which is now viewed as a continuous, integrated process.

The sections on osseointegration and transplantation have been expanded because the science of these techniques has evolved since the publication of the last edition of this text. An expanded section on pediatrics focuses on current approaches and considerations for treating this special group of patients.

Although all of the chapters in this fourth edition have been revised, we hope, in particular, that the new and expanded chapters will enhance the book's usefulness to all members of the treatment team, including surgeons (whether general, vascular, pediatric, plastic, or orthopaedic); prosthetists; physiatrists; physical, occupational, and recreational therapists; biomedical engineers; rehabilitation nurses; social workers; and individuals with limb loss and their families. The goals of this comprehensive text are, ultimately, to enhance and advance the care of those living with congenital or acquired limb loss. The dedicated involvement of all members of the treatment team is essential to the success of this process.

The support of the Board of Directors of the American Academy of Orthopaedic Surgeons has made this volume possible and is gratefully acknowledged. The contributions of the authors and editors has been enhanced by the work and commitment of the Academy's publications staff. We trust that the reader will find this volume a valuable educational resource.

Joseph Ivan Krajbich, MD
Michael S. Pinzur, MD
LTC Benjamin K. Potter, MD
Phillip M. Stevens, MEd, CPO

Table of Contents

Volume 2

Section 3: Lower Limb

Volume 3

Section 5: Pediatrics

Section 5

Pediatrics

Chapter 62

The Child With a Limb Deficiency

James A. Harder, BSc, MD, FRCS(C)   Joseph Ivan Krajbich, MD, FRCS(C)

Abstract

Limb deficiencies in children caused by failure of formation or amputation are challenging to treat and differ from amputations in adult patients. When caring for an infant or child, it is important to be knowledgeable about limb development in utero and to be aware of specific pediatric considerations, including etiology, associated medical conditions, and the effects of growth plate preservation, angular deformities, and bony overgrowth. Familiarity with the International Organization for Standardization (ISO) classification system allows for better understanding and communication in treating pediatric patients with limb deficiencies present at birth.

Keywords: amputation; bony overgrowth; congenital deficiency; embryology; growth plate; longitudinal deficiency; transverse deficiency

Introduction

Limb deficiencies in children present unique challenges that are very different from limb deficiencies in the adult population. This chapter highlights these differences and introduces a rational approach to treating the child with a limb deficiency that is based on knowledge and understanding of the unique issues affecting these children. The main differences between adults and children with limb loss are based on the etiology of the deficit; the presence of a growing skeleton; and physiologic, psychological, and lifestyle issues.

More than 50% of the children seen in practices that treat children with limb deficiencies have deficiencies with a congenital etiology. These congenital limb deficiencies are frequently more complex than the usual transverse amputations seen in the adult population. Entirely different classification systems are required for these congenital deficiencies to enhance communication among practitioners and provide treatment guidance. A basic understanding of limb development allows for a logical explanation of some of these deficiencies, and it is a good starting point for understanding limb deficiencies.

Brief Outline of Embryology

Limb development occurs very early in fetal life, with upper limb development beginning 1 to 2 days before lower limb development. Limb buds start as a local thickening of lateral plate mesoderm in the region where the limb will develop. This leads to hypertrophy of the overlying ectoderm (called the apical ectodermal ridge), which occurs in the fourth week of gestation. Thereafter, limb development progresses at a rapid rate. By the end of the eighth week of gestation, both the upper and the lower limbs are in place, fully formed, and rotated into their normal postnatal anatomic positions.

The limb growth along the three spatial planes is controlled by different groups of cells. The growth along the proximal-distal axis is controlled by the apical ectodermal ridge, whereas radial-ulnar plane development is controlled by the zone of polarizing activity. Development in the dorsoventral plane (the palm of the hand or sole of the foot) is controlled by the dorsal ectoderm. By the seventh week of gestation, toward the end of the limb formation process, the limbs rotate to their normal anatomic locations. The forelimbs rotate laterally, which places the thumb laterally in the anatomic plane, and the hind limbs rotate medially, which places the big toe medially in the anatomic plane[1] (**Figures 1** and **2**).

Many animal experiments have shown that interference with any of the controlling cell groups (apical ectodermal ridge, zone of polarizing activity, or dorsal ectoderm) will produce either limb absence or a substantial malformation.[2] The earlier the insult occurs during gestation, the more dramatic the effect.

Etiology

Although all new amputations in adults are acquired, usually secondary to vascular disease or trauma, in the pediatric population most limb deficiencies have a congenital etiology, and only a small number have acquired causes such as traumatic injury, neoplasm, or infection. A congenital etiology frequently results in a complex deficiency that is not easily

Dr. Harder or an immediate family member has stock or stock options held in Medtronic. Dr. Krajbich or an immediate family member is a member of a speakers' bureau or has made paid presentations on behalf of K2m and serves as a board member, owner, officer, or committee member of the Association of Children's Prosthetic and Orthotic Clinics and the Scoliosis Research Society.

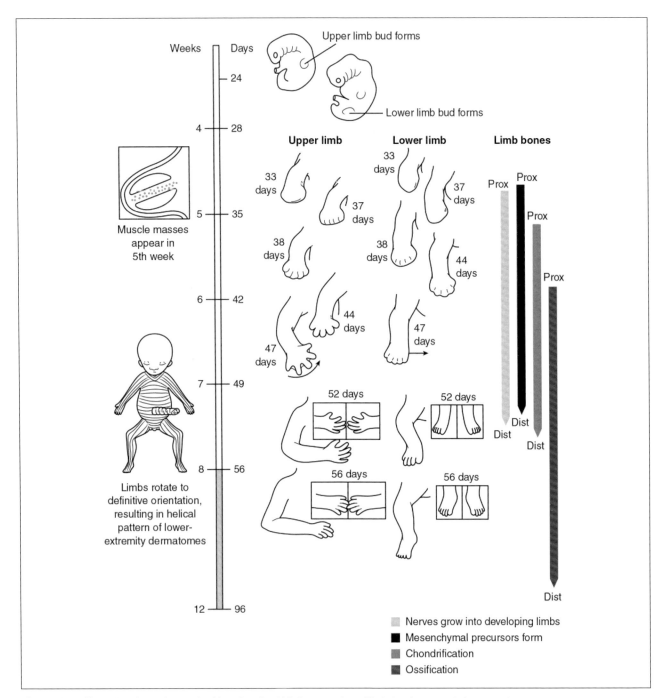

Figure 1 Illustration shows the proximal (prox) to distal (dist) progression of limb development during gestation.

described in the terms commonly used to characterize transverse deficiencies in adults. Congenital etiologies often result in multimembral deficiencies with other organ involvement.[3] In most congenital limb deficiencies, no clear mechanism or causative factor has been identified. Based on the limb defect and knowledge of embryology, an educated estimate can be made regarding the timing of the intrauterine insult that caused the limb deficiency. Clearly, in most patients, the insult occurs in the first trimester. Several factors have been identified that can influence early skeletal development, including drugs (for example, thalidomide), environmental toxins (for example, mercury), ionizing radiation (for example, x-rays), genetic defects, trauma, and poor intrauterine environmental maternal health (for example, maternal diabetes).

Maternal nutritional deficiencies (particularly insufficient folic acid) have

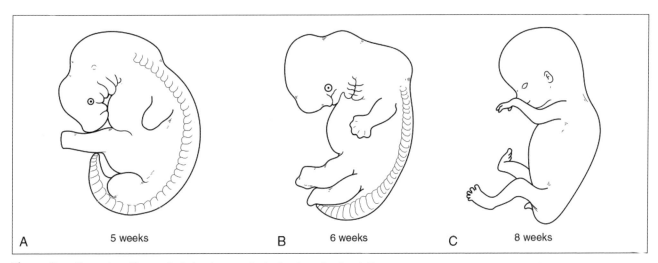

Figure 2   Illustration of human limb development in the first 8 weeks of gestation.

been identified as a causative factor in neural tube defects (such as spina bifida with meningomyelocele); however, poor nutrition has not been conclusively linked to congenital limb deficiencies. Because all major organ development occurs early in gestation, it is often complete before the mother realizes that she is pregnant. Nutritional supplements, which are thought to promote healthy organ development, should be part of a good antepartum diet. Some conditions occur later in pregnancy and are usually caused by mechanical factors or abnormalities in the later stages of fetal development. A classic example is Streeter dysplasia, which is also known as intrauterine constriction band syndrome. This condition frequently leads to multimembral amputations, deep constriction bands in the limbs, and tissue defects on the trunk and face.

Early recognition of congenital limb deficiencies associated with medical conditions is important because lifesaving medical management may be required. In patients with thrombocytopenia with absent radius (TAR) syndrome, the multimembral limb deficiency is associated with substantial thrombocytopenia. This condition is autosomal recessive. A platelet count should be obtained and treatment instituted if there is danger of bleeding. The risks for intracranial hemorrhage and neurologic damage may be minimized with platelet transfusion. Fanconi pancytopenia syndrome, which is an autosomal recessive condition, is associated with bleeding, pallor, recurrent infections, and reduction limb deformities or dislocated hips. Holt-Oram (handheart) syndrome is associated with upper limb reduction deformities and heart defects. It is autosomal dominant with variable penetrance.[4] In these situations, genetics counseling is a mandatory part of the discussion with the child's family.

Other than etiologic factors, acquired deficiencies in children follow more standard patterns seen in transverse terminal deficiencies in adults. Traumatic causes of amputation include burns, neoplasms, and infections. Lawnmower injuries, pedestrian motor vehicle collisions, and thermal and electrical burns account for most acquired amputations in children in the Western world. The Pediatric Orthopaedic Society of North America has worked to raise public and manufacturer awareness of the danger of lawnmower injuries in young children. Injuries in war zones, such as landmine explosions, are the most common cause of acquired childhood amputations throughout much of the world, with the incidence likely to rise because of the increasing number of conflicts in the Middle East. Although rare, frostbite is a possible cause of acquired amputation in countries in the most northern latitudes.

In the past, malignant tumors of the limbs such as osteosarcoma and Ewing sarcoma were treated with amputation, but most of these neoplasms are now treated with limb salvage. However, amputation may be necessary if the lesion precludes efforts at limb salvage or limb salvage fails because of complications. Limb amputation may be the treatment of choice or a lifesaving procedure in some patients with massive benign lesions seen in Klippel-Trenaunay syndrome, neurofibromatosis type 1, Proteus syndrome, or other forms of limb gigantism.

Septicemia associated with purpura fulminans is the most common infectious cause of amputation in infants and children. Purpura fulminans, which can be rapidly fatal and may result in multiple limb amputations in survivors, is most commonly associated with meningococcal infection, but it is also caused by other infectious agents such as *Pneumococcus* and *Streptococcus* bacterial species[5] (**Figure 3**). The development and wide use of the meningococcemia vaccine has diminished but not eliminated the incidence of purpura fulminans. Limb gangrene caused by *Staphylococcus* bacteria (flesh-eating bacteria) is

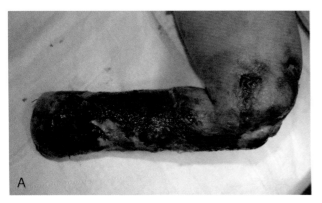 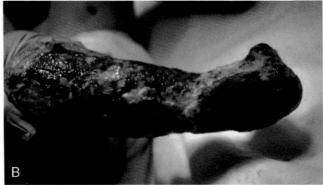

Figure 3   **A** and **B,** Clinical photographs of multimembral limb loss secondary to purpura fulminans septicemia.

another cause of limb loss.

Rarely, a vascular injury, which is usually iatrogenic, can be a cause of amputation. These injuries typically occur in premature infants in a neonatal intensive care unit secondary to attempts by the medical staff to gain vascular access to the patient's cardiovascular system.

The Growing Skeleton

The growing skeleton of a child presents several challenges to the treatment team in the management of both congenital and acquired limb deficiencies. These challenges are associated with the growth potential of the various growth plates and their presence or absence in the residual limb, magnification of some angular deformities near the joints caused by growth, and the tendency for bony overgrowth to form at the terminal end of the residual limb after transosseous amputation.

The potential growth of any residual limb must be carefully assessed before a planned intervention. The growing limb has growth plates at each end of the bone and a thick periosteum surrounding the cortical bone. In contrast, the growth plates in an adult are closed and the periosteum is thin. In a child, the bone will grow at different rates at each of the physes. For example, for every 10 mm the humerus grows, 8 mm of growth will occur at the proximal physis and 2 mm at the distal physis. In the radius, the opposite growth

pattern occurs, with most of the growth of the radius occurring at the distal end. Knowledge of these differential growth rates is important when estimating the final length of the residual limb in a child or predicting the progression of a longitudinal deficiency with growth.

The importance of preserving the major growth plates in a young child or infant who will be treated with a lower limb amputation is best illustrated by the differing outcomes that can result from preservation or loss of the distal femoral growth plate. If the growth plate is preserved in an infant undergoing a lower limb amputation, when that patient becomes a skeletally mature teenager, he or she can be fitted with a transfemoral or knee disarticulation prosthesis and function as an above-knee amputee. In contrast, loss of the distal femoral growth plate in infancy will result in a very short residual limb, likely requiring a hip disarticulation–like prosthesis, which will require greater energy consumption during ambulation and limit the patient's functional ability.

Angular limb deformities also can be magnified as the child grows. This is particularly true in congenital longitudinal deficiencies in which a worsening valgus deformity may occur at the knee in children with a congenital fibular deficiency, or a worsening joint deformity may occur in children with hip dysplasia and some types of femoral deficiencies.

Terminal bony overgrowth is a poorly understood phenomenon associated with transosseous amputations of the growing bone. It is an appositional growth on the end of the bone, producing a pointed end that irritates and traumatizes the overlying soft tissue, causing pain, fluid filled bursae, and even complete erosion through the skin (**Figures 4** and **5**). Terminal bony overgrowth is the most common cause of revision surgery in pediatric amputees. Multiple procedures have been designed to treat this complication, including simple excision of the offending part of the bone, osteotomy, various peritoneal and soft-tissue reconstructions, and metal or plastic cap implants to transfer or transplant cartilage-covered epiphyses or apophyses. At best, many of these techniques have been partially successful. It appears that the greatest success has been achieved with a procedure in which the proximal fibular metaphysis with its epiphysis is inserted into the transected diaphysis of the tibia (**Figure 6**).

As is the case in many other conditions, the best treatment for bony overgrowth is prevention. If possible, transosseous amputations should be avoided in children. The overgrowth phenomenon does not occur in the natural ends of bones covered by articular cartilage. Therefore, a Syme ankle disarticulation or a Boyd amputation is preferable to a transtibial amputation, and a knee disarticulation is preferable to a transfemoral amputation. The preferred procedure can usually be accomplished even if intercalary shortening of the affected bone is required.

The final length of the residual limb and the type of amputation will greatly influence function. The closer the residual limb is to the prosthetic terminal device, the more effectively the child will be able to control his or her prosthesis. A longer residual limb will provide a longer lever arm; therefore, the weight of the prosthesis will be distributed over a greater surface area and the contact area will be larger, improving proprioception. The residual limb, however, should allow enough space to accommodate a terminal device. For example, an energy-storing foot requires a minimum space of 3 inches and a knee joint requires approximately 2.5 to 3 inches of space to allow femurs of equal length. These considerations are not a justification to amputate through the bone in a patient with a traumatic injury, but they

provide an opportunity to plan for the necessary joint. Epiphysiodesis can be considered at the proper time, or elective shortening of the bone in the diaphyseal

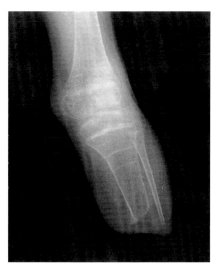

Figure 4 Radiograph of a traumatic left lower limb amputation, with a long fibula and bony overgrowth forming a spur of bone at both sites. (Courtesy of M. Fong, Alberta Children's Hospital, Juvenile Amputee Clinic, Alberta, Canada.)

region may be undertaken in a more mature patient while still preserving the distal end of the bone in its normal state. Preservation of the original distal bone end will allow effective end bearing, improve proprioception, and prevent the bony overgrowth that occurs when an amputation takes place through bone in a patient with an immature skeleton.

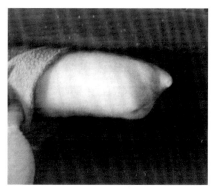

Figure 5 Photograph of a residual fibula, with overgrowth and bursae about to erode through the skin. (Courtesy of M. Fong, Alberta Children's Hospital, Juvenile Amputee Clinic, Alberta, Canada.)

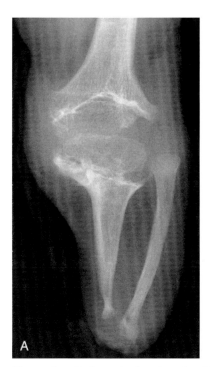
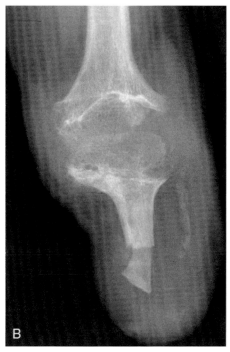
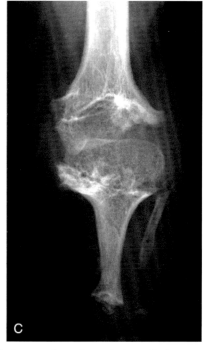

Figure 6 Radiographs show transfer of the proximal fibula into the terminal end of the tibia. **A,** Preoperative radiograph shows fibular overgrowth. **B,** Radiograph taken 6 weeks after surgery to transfer the proximal fibular metaphysis and epiphysis into the tibial diaphysis. **C,** Radiograph taken 2.5 years after the index procedure shows preservation of the fibular epiphysis.

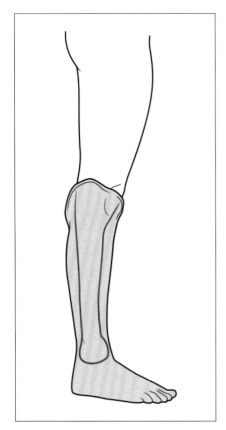

Figure 7   Illustration of a long residual lower limb that is close to the terminal device (foot).

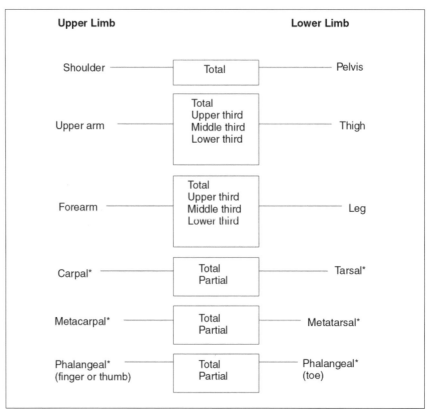

Figure 8   Illustration shows the International Organization for Standardization (ISO) designation of levels of transverse deficiencies of upper and lower limbs. The skeletal elements marked with an asterisk are used as adjectives in describing transverse deficiencies (for example, transverse carpal total deficiency). A total absence of the shoulder or hemipelvis (and all distal elements) is a transverse deficiency. If only a portion of the shoulder or hemipelvis is absent, the deficiency is of the longitudinal type. (Adapted with permission from Day HJ: The ISO/ISPO classification of congenital limb deficiency. *Prosthet Orthot Int* 1991;15[2]:67-69.)

Suspension of the prosthesis also will be simplified with a longer and properly contoured residual limb. The contour of the limb is used to provide suspension. The best examples of this principle are seen in Syme ankle disarticulations or Boyd amputations where the distal end of the limb is larger than the proximal tibial shaft (**Figure 7**). This contour allows the prosthesis to be mainly self-suspended on the distal, more bulbous end of the residual limb.

Physiology

Generally, children have healthy, growing tissue that heals rapidly with relatively few complications. This physiology allows the use of a more aggressive approach in surgical preservation of limb components along with innovative and unorthodox techniques to accomplish goals that would likely be unsuccessful in adults. In addition, the sequela of acquired amputations in children are generally not as severe as in adults. Phantom limb sensation, although common in children, is rarely associated with disabling pain or the need for medication or treatment.

Psychological and Lifestyle Issues

The psychological development of children is very dependent on their environmental interactions and their successful integration into peer groups. The level of energy, natural curiosity, and adaptability of children allow most children to achieve a mainstream education and lifestyle. It is the task and goal of the treatment team to help the child in achieving a smooth and successful transition into as normal a lifestyle as possible.

The child's rapid growth necessitates more frequent prosthetic evaluations and fittings. In addition, the active lifestyle of children can place more wear and tear on prostheses, and several types of prostheses may be needed to accommodate participation in sports and recreational activities.

Classification of Congenital Deficiencies

In 1961, Frantz and O'Rahilly[6] published the first consistent classification of congenital limb deficiencies. This classification system introduced important terminology that was later

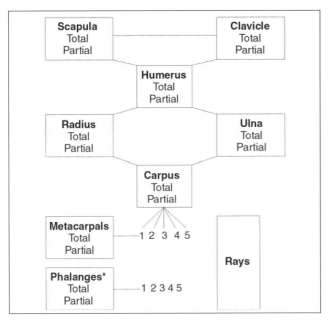

Figure 9 Illustration describes longitudinal deficiencies of the upper limb using the International Organization for Standardization (ISO) classification system. The asterisk indicated that the digits of the hand are sometimes referred to by name: 1 = thumb; 2 = index; 3 = middle; 4 = ring; 5 = little (or small). For the purpose of this classification, such naming is depreciated because it is not equally applicable to the foot. (Adapted with permission from Day HJ: The ISO/ISPO classification of congenital limb deficiency. *Prosthet Orthot Int* 1991;15[2]:67-69.)

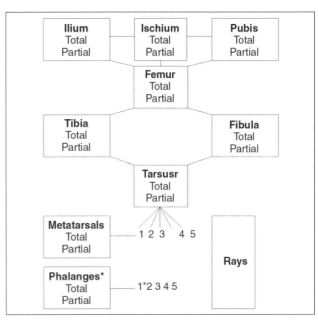

Figure 10 Illustration describes longitudinal deficiencies of the lower limb using the International Organization for Standardization (ISO) system. The asterisk indicates the great toe, or hallux. (Adapted with permission from Day HJ: The ISO/ISPO classification of congenital limb deficiency. *Prosthet Orthot Int* 1991;15[2]:67-69.)

incorporated into current classification systems. Deficiencies were described as transverse, longitudinal, terminal, and intercalary. However, the authors' use of various Greek or Latin names with Latin prefixes were frequently inaccurate and poorly descriptive of many of the congenital conditions. Much of the terminology of Frantz and O'Rahilly[6] is still quite widely used, particularly in informal communications. Terms such as fibular hemimelia, tibial hemimelia, phocomelia, and amelia are still frequently encountered.

In the early 1970s, the International Society for Prosthetics and Orthotics (ISPO) established a committee under the leadership of Hector W. Kay to formulate a more rational classification system. This ISPO system, with some minor modifications, became the widely recognized International Organization for Standardization (ISO) classification of congenital limb deficiencies, and it

is now the most accepted worldwide classification.[7,8] The ISO classification is limited to failures of formation and describes the amputation anatomically, which prevents misinterpretation or confusion. It is simple, precise, and based on anatomic and radiologic observations. The ISO classification does not address etiology or angular or rotational deformities of the bones or joints.

When describing a limb deficiency, the terms longitudinal or transverse are used (**Figures 8**, **9**, and **10**). The individual bone involvement is described as total or partial absence. Partial absence may be described as absence of the proximal one-third, middle one-third, or distal one-third of the involved bone. Complete bone absence would be described as complete absence of the missing bone or bones. Absence of the carpus, tarsals, metacarpals, metatarsals, and phalanges may be total or partial. In some instances, the phalanges

will be described by stating the missing parts.

Longitudinal deficiencies may be total or partial and may have normal elements distally. For example, when describing a fibular deficiency, there might be absence of all or part of the fibula, with a relatively normal ankle and foot. HJB Day, a member of the Kay committee of the ISPO, developed a stylized illustrative system of recording deficiencies (**Figures 11** and **12**), which incorporated a skeletal drawing of the affected part; the deficient areas were shaded. The Day diagrams are not part of the ISPO classification but are useful in clinical situations for quick recall of a deficiency.

Summary

The child with a limb deficiency presents a unique challenge to the treatment team. To adequately care for this patient population, it is important to

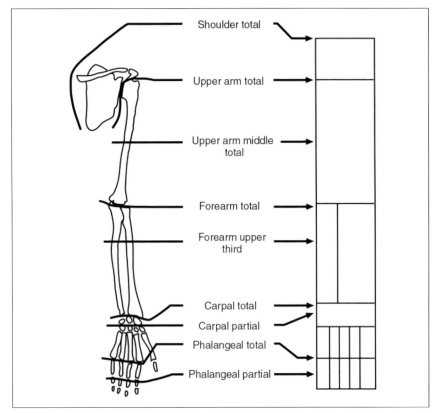

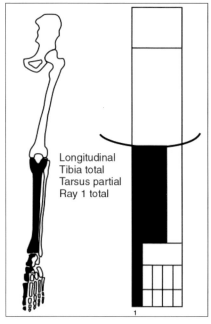

Figure 11 Illustration of the Day system of recording deficiencies. Transverse upper limb deficiencies at various levels are shown on the skeleton and in Day's stylized version on the right. (Adapted with permission from Day HJ: The ISO/ISPO classification of congenital limb deficiency. *Prosthet Orthot Int* 1991;15[2]:67-69.)

Figure 12 Illustration of a longitudinal deficiency shown on the skeleton (left) and in Day's stylized representation (right), which shows the original deficiency and treatment by knee disarticulation. (Adapted with permission from Day HJ: The ISO/ISPO classification of congenital limb deficiency. *Prosthet Orthot Int* 1991;15[2]:67-69.)

be cognizant of the etiology of the limb deficiency, the unique characteristics of a growing skeleton, and physiologic and psychological issues involved. The ISO classification allows for better understanding and communications in treating children with congenital limb deficiencies.

References

1. Sadler TW: *Embryology and Gene Regulation of Limb Development: The Child With a Limb Deficiency.* Rosemont, Illinois, American Academy of Orthopaedic Surgeons, 1998, pp 3-12.

2. Saunders JW Jr: Developmental control of three-dimensional polarity in the avian limb. *Ann N Y Acad Sci* 1972;193:29-42.

3. Smith D: *Recognizable Patterns of Human Malformation, ed 5.* Philadelphia, PA, WB Saunders, 1997.

4. Setoguchi Y: *Medical Conditions Associated With Congenital Limb Deficiency.* Rosemont, Illinois, American Academy of Orthopaedic Surgeons, 1998, pp 51-58.

5. Canavese F, Krajbich JI, LaFleur BJ: Orthopaedic sequelae of childhood meningococcemia: Management considerations and outcome. *J Bone Joint Surg Am* 2010;92(12):2196-2203.

6. Frantz CH, O'Rahilly R: Congenital skeletal limb deficiencies. *J Bone Joint Surg Am* 1961;43:1202-1204.

7. Kay HW, Day HJ, Henkel HL, et al: The proposed international terminology for the classification of congenital limb deficiencies. *Dev Med Child Neurol Suppl* 1975;34(34):1-12.

8. Day HJ: The ISO/ISPO classification of congenital limb deficiency. *Prosthet Orthot Int* 1991;15(2):67-69.

Chapter 63

Development of Locomotor Systems

Phoebe Scott-Wyard, DO, FAAP, FAAPMR

Abstract

An understanding of typical embryologic limb development and the disturbances that can result in limb deficiencies is important for treatment and aids in counseling parents regarding causation. It is helpful to be familiar with the process of limb development and the current theories surrounding the causes of congenital limb deformity. Childhood motor development has a considerable effect on the success or failure of prosthetic fitting. Aspects of motor and psychological development can influence prosthetic fitting in children with limb deficiencies.

Keywords: developmental milestones; embryology; limb deficiency

Introduction

The development of the limbs and motor systems is a complex and orchestrated process, the interruption or disturbance of which can result in limb deficiency or deformity and subsequent disability. This chapter provides a brief review of embryologic limb development and how it relates to limb deficiency. Following birth, the developmental processes of the growing child are integral to motor capabilities and should be considered when fitting prosthetic devices. Therefore, this chapter also reviews the childhood stages of motor development.

Embryologic Limb Development

Limb development occurs via multiple signaling pathways, each responsible for its own differentiation, yet working in concert with complex interactions, including signaling, regulation, feedback loops, and maintaining the additional axes of development.[1,2] The limbs start to appear at the end of the fourth week and continue to develop through the eighth week after fertilization. The limbs

begin as small growths on the ventrolateral body wall, directed caudally. The upper limb buds appear at the level of the pericardial swelling and precede those of the lower limb (just caudal to the umbilical cord) by approximately 2 days. The limb bud tissue is composed of a mass of mesoderm tissue, covered with ectoderm. The apical ectodermal ridge (AER) is an ectodermal thickening that forms at the tip of each limb bud. Three axes of development occur: proximal-distal (controlled by the AER), anterior-posterior (radioulnar), and dorsal-ventral (back of hand to palm). The AER secretes fibroblast growth factors that stimulate the underlying mesenchymal cells to differentiate and promote proximal-to-distal growth of the limb bud. Defects of the AER and its signaling center can result in anomalies such as transverse deficiencies and syndactyly.[2] A collection of cells along the posterior aspect of the limb bud, called the zone of polarizing activity, secrete the sonic hedgehog protein, which promotes development along the anterior-posterior axis of the limb.

The zone of polarizing activity also contributes to the AER feedback loop. The Wingless-type (Wnt) signaling pathway regulates dorsal-ventral development within the ectoderm, as well as regulation of sonic hedgehog protein.

Chondrification centers appear in the fifth week, and, by the end of the sixth week, the limb skeleton exists in a cartilaginous form. Subsequently, the distal ends of the limb buds begin to flatten into hand and foot plates that are paddle-like in appearance. Near the end of the sixth week, the mesenchymal tissue condenses into the hand plates to form the digital rays; in the seventh week, the same process occurs in the foot plates. At the tip of each ray, the AER induces development of the bony phalanges. Notches form between the rays, and programmed cell death, or apoptosis, breaks down the tissue between the rays, causing separation of the digits by the end of the eighth week. In the beginning of the seventh week, the limbs grow ventrally, then begin to rotate. The upper and lower limbs rotate in opposite directions, according to their function: the upper limbs rotate 90° laterally, such that the elbows point dorsally; the lower limbs rotate medially almost 90°, causing the knees to point ventrally. Limb muscles originate from mesenchymal cells that migrate from the somatic layer of the lateral mesoderm during the fifth week. These split into dorsal and ventral groups, subsequently becoming the extensor and flexor musculature. Nerves develop in the limb buds after the muscle masses form. By the seventh week, the limb buds have innervated muscles and cutaneous tissue in the adult pattern.

Dr. Scott-Wyard serves as a board member, owner, officer, or committee member of the Association of Children's Prosthetic and Orthotic Clinics.

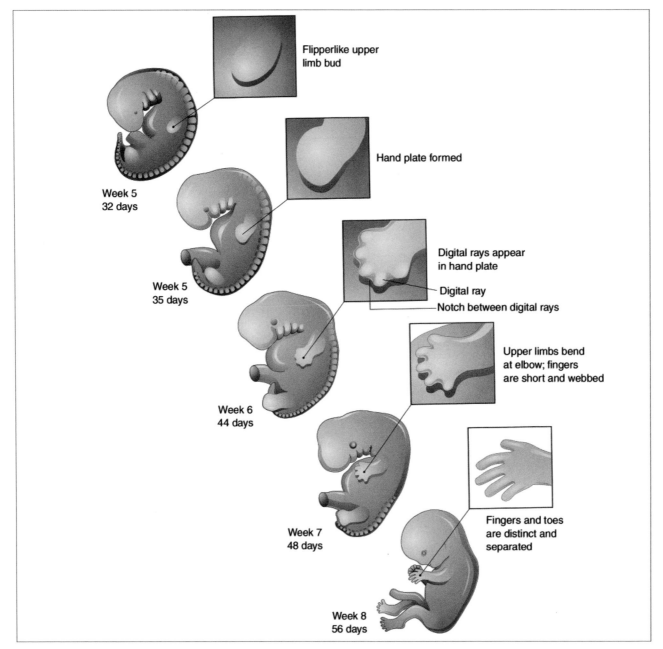

Figure 1 Illustration of embryonic limb development (32 to 56 days). (Reproduced with permission from Moore KL, Persaud TV: *The Developing Human: Clinically Oriented Embryology,* ed 6. Philadelphia, PA, WB Saunders, 1998, p 436.)

Most blood vessels of the limbs are buds from the aorta and cardinal veins. Synovial joints begin to develop during the sixth week from a collection of cells that develop at the joint area called the interzone. These cells differentiate into intra-articular structures, articular cartilage, and synovial cells. Apoptosis again plays a role in development, this time in the formation of the joint space.

Subsequent limb movement becomes critical to normal development of the joints. By the end of the eighth week, limbs are in their final positions and all segments are complete. Ossification also begins at this time, with ossification centers present in all long bones by the 12th week[1,3,4] (**Figure 1**).

The most critical period of limb development is 24 to 36 days after fertilization (during weeks 4 to 6), when the embryo undergoes rapid tissue proliferation.[3] Often, the mother is not aware of her pregnancy; therefore, exposure to teratogenic agents is difficult to prevent. Inhibition of limb bud development in the fourth week can result in complete absence of the limb, whereas interruption of the growth or development in the fifth week can result in partial absence.

Teratogenic factors affecting limb development include drug use during pregnancy, infections, chorionic villus sampling, or exposure to toxins.[5] Some medications affect limb development, including thalidomide, retinoic acid, and misoprostol. The most famous of these is thalidomide, which was marketed in the 1950s to mothers for treatment of nausea and vomiting during pregnancy. Thalidomide was available in most European countries and Canada, and it could be obtained without a prescription in Germany. In 1961, Widukind Lenz, a German pediatric geneticist, began investigating an increasing number of children born with severe limb anomalies; his findings resulted in a withdrawal of thalidomide from the market.[6] Thousands of exposed children exhibited phocomelic limb anomalies, facial malformations, and often, internal organ involvement.

Teratogenic causes are often difficult to study, particularly because prenatal history can be complicated by maternal recall bias.[7] Limb deficiencies also can be caused by vascular disruption (for example, amniotic band syndrome, in which fibrous bands constrict the vascular supply to the limbs), vascular malformations (such as Poland syndrome [subclavian artery disruption sequence]), or genetic factors (often a spontaneous point mutation in an otherwise normal family). In most cases, however, the cause is unknown.[8] Many limb deficiencies are likely the result of an interaction of genetic and environmental factors (multifactorial inheritance). No racial predilection has been observed. Recent data indicate a possible relationship between paternal occupation and an increased prevalence of limb deficiencies in the offspring of artists.[9]

Amniotic band syndrome (also known by more than 30 other names, including congenital constriction band syndrome, amniotic constriction band, and amnion rupture sequence) is a

Table 1 Stages of Motor Development

Average Age of Achievement	Developmental Milestone
2 months	Able to control head in prone position
4 months	Brings hands to midline, rolls prone to supine
6-8 months	Sits independently, transfers objects hand-to-hand
10 months	Crawls, stands with support
12 months	Walks independently
2 years	Jumps
3 years	Climbs stairs by alternating feet, stands on one foot
4 years	Hops on one foot, throws ball overhand
5 years	Skips, dresses independently

very heterogenous group of clinical anomalies, which can include congenital limb deformities, cleft lip and palate, constriction rings, and talipes equinovarus. There is no unanimously accepted etiology for this constellation of findings.[2] Animal studies have suggested that the incidents leading to limb deficiency in amniotic band syndrome may be caused by a cascade of hypoxia, cell damage, hemorrhage, tissue loss, and reperfusion.[5]

Childhood Development

In childhood, development occurs in discontinuous bursts, with complex skills building on simpler skills. A proper understanding of developmental motor milestones (**Table 1**) is important when considering prosthetic prescription in the child with a limb deficiency. Prosthetic fitting should reflect the child's functional needs, not the rather arbitrary chronologic age.[6] Most children with a limb deficiency experience normal development. Those with bilateral upper limb deficiencies can experience a delay in reaching some milestones or miss them completely because of mechanical problems. Parents should be encouraged to treat a child with a limb deficiency in the same manner as they would treat any child.

Early Development

By 2 months of age, a child may be able to hold his or her head steady when sitting, allowing for more visual interaction. However, object permanence is still lacking: if an object is removed from sight, the child will continue to stare at the same spot. The child will also smile in response to a face or voice, resulting in more functional social participation.[10]

At 3 to 4 months, a child will be able to bring hands together in midline, grasping objects and allowing for self-discovery and visual-motor coordination. Palmar and asymmetric tonic neck reflexes are extinguished by this age. The child will stare at his or her own hand, beginning to understand cause and effect.

When the child is approximately 6 months old, he or she can sit without support and roll from supine to prone, allowing increased exploration of the environment. The child can transfer objects from hand to hand and begins learning to compare objects. Monosyllabic babbling is also noted at this age. A child this age with an upper limb deficiency could be fitted with a passive prosthesis to free the contralateral limb for manual activities when sitting. However, substantial controversy exists regarding the timing of prosthetic fitting for children with a unilateral deficiency. Recommendations vary from early fitting to fitting only at the age and time that the child demonstrates a functional or an emotional need for a prosthesis. Some practitioners prefer prosthetic fitting closer to 3 months of age, before the infant develops visually guided reaching.[3] The first prosthesis equalizes the lengths of the upper limbs, provides support when leaned on and during crawling, establishes an early wearing pattern, reduces sensory dependence on the residual limb, and helps in holding large objects.[6,11] A parent can position the prosthesis for optimal use and place objects in the terminal device to help the child become aware of how it can be used. The child does not yet have adequate skills or musculoskeletal excursion to control an activated prosthesis.

By 7 to 8 months of age, the child will begin to exhibit a thumb-finger (pincer) grasp and respond to nonverbal communication (one-step commands with gesture). Cognitively, he or she will start to have object permanence (for example, finding a hidden toy after seeing it hidden) and will actively compare objects (such as banging two cubes together).

At 10 to 12 months of age, the child will crawl, begin to pull himself or herself to a standing position, cruise along furniture, and, ultimately, walk independently, allowing for exploration and control of proximity to his or her parents. The child can follow one-step commands without need for gestures, showing development of verbal receptive language skills. The child with a unilateral lower limb deficiency is ready for prosthetic fitting at this age, with the goals of promoting two-legged standing, reciprocating gait development, and achieving a normal appearance.[12] The prosthesis should be aligned for maximum stability, mimicking the toddler's wide base of support (socket flexion, abduction, and external rotation). For a child with an above-knee limb deficiency, the first prosthesis should not include a mechanical knee unit because of the need for increased function and

stability. The practitioner should be aware that the child with a lower limb deficiency may still be transitioning from crawling to walking; therefore, the first prosthetic suspension should be substantial enough to prevent loss or falling off while crawling. Children often do not require any formal gait training or assistive devices. They often can transition to independent walking as do able-bodied children of the same-age, using push-toys or hand-held assistance from parents.

The child should start to run at approximately 15 to 17 months of age. He or she can use objects in combination (such as building a tower of three cubes), begins acquisition of object and personal names, and can link actions to solve problems. If considered appropriate by the family and the practitioner, this is the approximate age when the child with an upper limb deficiency is ready for fitting with a myoelectric, single-site, voluntary-opening, automatic closing prosthesis, also known as the "cookie cruncher."[3]

By age 2 years, the child should be able to run well, walk up and down stairs (nonreciprocating), and jump. He or she can build a tower of seven cubes, perform circular scribbling, help in undressing, and speak in three-word sentences. At this time, the child with a unilateral upper limb deficiency may be ready for activation of a terminal device for a body-powered prosthesis. The skills needed are the ability to follow two-step commands, interest in two-handed activities, awareness of the holding functionality of a terminal device, ability to tolerate hand-over-hand therapy, and an attention span of at least 5 minutes. However, this is also the age at which behavior may impede prosthetic training, so individual differences are important to consider prior to cable-activation.

Reciprocating stair climbing usually is attained by 2.5 years of age. Hopping on one foot and climbing occurs

closer to 4 years of age. For the child with a limb deficiency above the elbow or with a shoulder disarticulation, a dual-control cable system and elbow lock can be introduced at this age. At 5 years of age, a child is able to skip, copy a triangle, name four colors, dress, and undress. Typically, a child with a unilateral above-knee limb deficiency is fit with a prosthetic knee joint between the ages of 3 and 5 years. By age 5 to 6 years, the prosthetic alignment more closely reflects that of an adult. Because this is the age of school initiation, a child's awareness of his or her limb difference can become acutely apparent, and parents should be encouraged to work closely with the child's school for a smooth transition and introduction of the child to prevent teasing or bullying. Questions about the limb difference are to be expected, and children should be encouraged to provide honest, direct answers.

Development in Middle Childhood and Adolescence
Fine motor abilities continue to progress during middle childhood and adolescence, and psychosocial issues (such as separation from parents) and self-esteem challenges (relationships with peers) become more important. It has been said that a teenager is part child and part adult.[6] Teenagers with a lower limb deficiency may prefer to be fit with cosmetic endoskeletal prostheses so that their peers are less aware of their prosthetic use. Concern about perception of a prosthetic hook or terminal device can compel a teenager with an upper limb deficiency to request changing to a cosmetic or mechanical hand. It is important to provide education regarding function of a cosmetic or mechanical hand. The addition of a cosmetic glove over a mechanical hand reduces efficacy by up to 40%.[12] In addition, it is common for the teenager who does not wear an upper limb prosthesis to request one at this age. Often, the teenager is

looking for a replacement for his or her missing limb and may have unrealistic expectations of the function a prosthetic limb can provide. Psychological support through formal counseling or peer and family support systems can benefit the teenager before initiating prosthetic fitting. This is also the time when adolescents obtain a driver's license, and practitioners should consider referral to a driving clinic for necessary adaptive equipment.

Task-specific prostheses may be beneficial at any age to aid in peer group activity involvement, depending on the child's interest and participation level. Examples include prostheses that aid in playing an instrument (for example, a bow-holding violin terminal device or a guitar pick holder) and sports participation (for example, an upper limb mitt terminal device for catching, a carbon-fiber "running leg" with a dynamic energy-storing foot, or a handlebar terminal device for cycling).

Summary

Children are not simply small adults. With the proper understanding of their growth and development along with timely application of prosthetic principles, children with limb deficiencies can be encouraged and supported to achieve a healthy and fulfilling childhood and successful adulthood.

References

1. Moore KL, Persaud TV: *The Developing Human: Clinically Oriented Embryology*, ed 6. Philadelphia, PA, WB Saunders, 1998.

2. Dy CJ, Swarup I, Daluiski A: Embryology, diagnosis, and evaluation of congenital hand anomalies. *Curr Rev Musculoskelet Med* 2014;7(1):60-67.

3. Herring JA, Birch JG: *The Child With a Limb Deficiency*. Rosemont, IL, American Academy of Orthopaedic Surgeons, 1998.

4. Lovell WW, Winter RB, Weinstein SL, Flynn JM, eds: *Lovell and Winter's Pediatric Orthopaedics*, ed 7. Philadelphia, PA, Lippincott Williams & Wilkins, 2014, pp 1526-1595.

5. McGuirk CK, Westgate MN, Holmes LB: Limb deficiencies in newborn infants. *Pediatrics* 2001;108(4):E64.

6. Setoguchi Y, Rosenfelder R: *The Limb Deficient Child*. Springfield, IL, Charles C. Thomas Publisher, 1982.

7. Werler MM, Pober BR, Nelson K, Holmes LB: Reporting accuracy among mothers of malformed and nonmalformed infants. *Am J Epidemiol* 1989;129(2):415-421.

8. Canfield MA, Honein MA, Yuskiv N, et al: National estimates and race/ethnic-specific variation of selected birth defects in the United States, 1999-2001. *Birth Defects Res A Clin Mol Teratol* 2006;76(11):747-756.

9. Desrosiers TA, Herring AH, Shapira SK, et al: Paternal occupation and birth defects: Findings from the National Birth Defects Prevention Study. *Occup Environ Med* 2012;69(8):534-542.

10. Behrman RE, Kliegman RM, Jenson HB: *Nelson Textbook of Pediatrics*, ed 17. Philadelphia, PA, WB Saunders, 2004.

11. Crandall RC, Tomhave W: Pediatric unilateral below-elbow amputees: Retrospective analysis of 34 patients given multiple prosthetic options. *J Pediatr Orthop* 2002;22(3):380-383.

12. Alexander MA, Matthews DJ: *Pediatric Rehabilitation: Principles and Practice*, ed 4. New York, NY, Demos Medical, 2010, pp 335-360.

Chapter 64

Principles of Amputation Surgery in Children

Anna Cuomo, MD

Abstract

Amputations in children require special considerations. Both acquired amputations and congenital limb anomalies often have unique presentations and require an individualized treatment approach. Knowledge of basic principles will aid the surgeon in the initial patient evaluation and surgical planning. It is also helpful to be aware of the common etiologies of amputations and the nomenclature regarding limb reductions.

Keywords: amputation; child; congenital limb deformity; limb deficiency; pediatric; surgery; traumatic amputation; Van Nes rotationplasty

Introduction

Major differences exist between amputation in adults and children. If a good outcome is expected, orthopaedic surgeons must understand that knowledge about adult amputation does not correlate directly with amputation in children. This chapter discusses the differences between amputations in these two populations and provides a practical approach to surgical planning of limb salvage or amputation that will improve the use of prostheses in children.

Background

The major and most obvious difference between children and adults is that children are still growing. Children have needs specific to their development and underlying diagnoses. Predictions of future growth and limb-length discrepancies are essential to guide (1) whether a child should have an amputation versus a limb equalizing or salvage surgery, (2) the most appropriate level and type of amputation, and (3) the timing of surgical intervention. Cognitive and motor skills will change with age and also may

be abnormal. Both skills will affect the appropriate timing of surgery and which prosthetic components are most appropriate. Because children tend to be more active, the increased physical demands on the residual limb and prosthesis need to be considered. Other issues specific to children include problems with terminal residual limb overgrowth, the presence and morbidity of associated organ anomalies, and the psychological effect of an amputation on both the child and his or her family.

Most pediatric amputations are the result of either trauma or congenital deficiencies; only a limited number result from neoplastic lesions or infections. Traumatic pediatric amputations are often treated in the community or at trauma centers, where greater experience with adult amputations often exists. Most adult amputations are a result of microvascular compromise from diabetes and peripheral artery disease (54%) and trauma (45%); less than 2% result from cancer.[1] Therefore, it is important for the orthopaedic surgeon to recognize that many wound-healing issues and

surgical strategies for adult amputations do not apply in the pediatric population. Also, children may experience phantom limb sensation, but they do not have the same problems with phantom pain as adults. Congenital limb anomalies often are treated at specialized pediatric amputation centers, where the ratio of congenital to traumatic amputations is approximately 2:1.[2] These centers often afford a multidisciplinary approach to surgical planning and rehabilitation for complex limb anomalies.

To recognize the vast differences between pediatric and adult amputations, the Association of Child Prosthetic and Orthotic Clinics was formed to encourage a multidisciplinary approach for pediatric amputations. Children with congenital limb anomalies often have unique morphology, and their treatment plans will be unique. Understanding the basic principles of pediatric amputations and working with a creative team will provide the best opportunity for a good result.

Etiology

The two major etiologies for limb deficiencies in children are acquired amputations and congenital ones caused by the lack of formation of a limb or a limb segment. Evaluation and management vary substantially between these categories.

Acquired amputations are most often from trauma, and the most common mechanisms of injury are dependent on the region. In the United States, the incidence is approximately 1.3 per 100,000 children with a bimodal distribution of 0 to 4 years and 15 to 17 years of age.[3] The most

Dr. Cuomo or an immediate family member serves as a board member, owner, officer, or committee member of the Pediatric Orthopaedic Society of North America.

Table 1 Congenital Longitudinal Lower Limb Deficiencies

Deficiency	Features	Treatment Options
Femoral		
Congenital short femur	Femoral length greater than 50% of normal side; no other bone or soft-tissue abnormalities	Equalize limb lengths: Lengthen short limb, shorten long limb, or a combination of both; shoe lift.
Proximal femoral focal deficiency	Stable hip (coxa vara ± pseudarthrosis, acetabular dysplasia)	If length greater than 50% of the normal side, optimize hip stability and function and equalize limb lengths with proximal femoral valgus osteotomy (to treat coxa vara) and possible soft-tissue release or acute shortening of the femur; acetabular osteotomy (to treat acetabular dysplasia); staged lengthening of short limb, shortening of long limb, or a combination of both (to treat limb-length difference).
		If length less than 50% of the normal side, optimize hip stability and function as described previously and then three options: (1) If knee function is good and the femur is approximately 50% length of the normal side, preserve knee, amputate foot, and make up length difference with transtibial prosthesis. Consider femoral lengthening to partially equalize knee heights. (2) If knee function is poor, knee fusion with foot ablation and fit with a knee disarticulation or transfemoral type prosthesis. (3) If ankle function is good, perform Van Nes rotationplasty.
	Unstable hip (complete or subtotal absence of the proximal femur)	Limb conversion: Knee fusion, with possible epiphysiodesis and foot ablation; fit with a knee disarticulation or transfemoral type prosthesis. If ankle function is good, consider a Van Nes rotationplasty.
Tibial		
	Total absence of the proximal tibia (with incomplete or no active knee extension)	Amputation: Knee disarticulation and fitting with a knee disarticulation or transfemoral type prosthesis. Possible distal femoral epiphysiodesis approximately 5 years before skeletal maturity to help equalize prosthetic knee height with unaffected side.
	Present proximal tibia (with full active knee extension), absent distal tibia, unstable ankle	Amputation and optimize lever arm of limb distal to knee: Foot ablation, consider concomitant or staged (when the tibia becomes ossified) distal fibular transfer to the proximal tibia if tibial length is very short. Consider proximal fibular head resection if proximal dislocation is symptomatic and fit with transtibial prosthesis.
	Distal tibia/fibula diastasis	Amputation: Foot ablation and fit with transtibial prosthesis.
Fibular		
	Stable ankle and foot with three or more rays	Equalize limb lengths: Lengthen short limb, shorten long limb, or a combination of both; shoe lift. Consider timed hemiepiphysiodesis to treat genu valgum.
	Unstable ankle and foot with two or fewer rays	Amputation: Foot ablation, consider timed hemiepiphysiodesis to treat genu valgum.

common mechanisms of injury are crush, lawn mower, power tool, other machinery, and motorized vehicle injuries. Pediatric injuries from firearms and explosives are less common in the United States but are very common in regions with land mines and conflicts. In general, multiple limb involvement is less common, and the level of amputation is closely tied to the degree of soft-tissue injury.

Lack-of-formation deficiencies are congenital, and the etiologies are poorly understood. In the recent past, it was believed that nearly all were sporadic events with no clear inheritable pattern. However, an increasing number of reports describe variable modes of inheritance of skeletal deficiencies, some with isolated phenotypes and others being part of a larger syndrome.[4] Examples include familial coxa vara,[5] longitudinal

fibular deficiencies,[6] longitudinal tibial deficiencies,[7,8] and split hand/split foot malformations.[9,10] This information is clinically important because parents often are very concerned about future offspring who may be affected. In addition, as young patients grow into adults they want to know if they are likely to pass along their traits to their own children.

Table 1 and **Table 2** list the common etiologies for congenital and acquired

Table 2 Acquired Limb Deficiencies

Etiology	Features	Treatment Guidelines and Options
Infection Purpura fulminans (purpuric rash, fever, hypotension, disseminated intravascular coagulopathy) associated with protein C deficiency, *Neisseria meningitides*, meningococcemia, Streptococcus, *Staphylococcus aureus*, or other pathogens	Often multiple limb and organ involvement that requires aggressive resuscitation. Skin necrosis can occur over healthy underlying soft tissues and does not predict amputation level. Soft-tissue necrosis commonly results in dry gangrene. Osteomyelitis is an uncommon feature but can occur. Growth plates can be affected, causing full or partial growth disturbance and subsequent angular deformity and/or limb-length discrepancy.	Early fasciotomies for compartment syndrome are generally not recommended because of a high postoperative infection rate. Surgical intervention for dry gangrene is commonly initiated after tissue necrosis is well demarcated. Limbs may require extensive skin grafting over healthy underlying tissue. Partial physeal arrest may require subsequent corrective osteotomies and/or completion of the physeal arrest to avoid recurrent deformities. Limb-length discrepancies should be monitored and treated according to the projected discrepancy.
Traumatic Lawn mower injuries Vehicle collisions Electrical or thermal burns Explosive devices	Compared with congenital deficiencies, multiple limb involvement is less common, and joint function proximal to the involved level is normal. Amputation through a long bone results in problems with overgrowth. Electrical burns commonly have deep soft-tissue involvement well proximal to the involved level of skin. Explosive devices often leave residual shrapnel that may be painful if near a nerve or subcutaneous bone.	Preserve knee function. Avoid residual limb overgrowth with amputations through joints or primary capping when possible. Late problems with overgrowth can be treated with a fibular head or an iliac crest osteochondral autograft. Consult plastic surgeons early in the planning phase of surgery because valuable skin grafts can sometimes be taken from the amputated limb.
Dysvascular Congenital band sequence Thrombotic event	Although congenital, residual limb overgrowth can occur because the level of amputation is often midshaft.	The ends of the residual limb may have inadequate soft-tissue coverage, which may require bone shortening, resection of a constriction band, or both.
Neurogenic Myelomeningocele Central or peripheral neuropathies	Charcot arthropathy or chronic recurrent infections occasionally result in amputation.	The level and type of amputation should focus on treating the underlying problem and creating a residual limb that will avoid pressure ulceration. Unlike in adults or individuals with diabetes, associated vascular disease does not occur, and wound-healing issues do not dictate the level of amputation.
Tumor resection Benign or malignant tumors Gigantism or focal limb hypertrophy syndromes (Klippel-Trenaunay syndrome)	Primary malignant bone tumors have a peak incidence in the first two decades of life and may undergo limb salvage or amputation. Large benign tumors, such as plexiform neurofibromas, or various types of focal limb hypertrophy can become so deforming that amputations provide better control of limb size than performing an epiphysiodesis.	The level of amputation is dictated by the stage of the tumor for malignancies and the size of the limb for overgrowth. Ray amputations can be done to decrease the width of hands or feet.

pediatric amputations along with the general clinical features and treatment options. These tables can serve as a quick reference for guidance but should not replace common sense when treating the individual.

Terminology

Many classifications for limb deficiencies exist, but none are perfect. The goal of a classification system should be to assist with accurate communication, provide divisions for clinical studies, and allow for prognostication. Few (if any) classifications are successful at achieving all three goals. Therefore, it is helpful to be familiar with multiple classifications and not be influenced by their inherent limitations.

Limb deficiencies can be described by their mode of acquisition (either lack of formation or acquired), specific etiology (for example, postmeningococcemia, thromboembolic event, posttumor resection), and anatomic or radiographic descriptions. Deficiencies are most broadly categorized as either congenital or acquired. It is important to note that these categories are not mutually exclusive. For example, a congenital band sequence is an acquired deficiency that occurs from external bands that constrict the developing limb in utero. This can result in a range of deficiencies, from a minor constriction band around the soft tissues that is purely a cosmetic issue to a complete transverse amputation in utero. Therefore, a congenital band sequence is both acquired and congenital. A vascular event in utero can result in either an acquired amputation if it occurs after the limb has formed or in aplasia or hypoplasia of limb tissue earlier during limb formation, resulting in a lack of formation. To some degree, the classification is semantic, but it also can be clinically useful. For example, a child with a congenital band sequence will share many characteristics with children who have other congenital deficiencies, particularly the multiplicity of limbs that can be affected. In addition, the social and psychological issues are similar to those of a child with an amputation since birth. However, congenital band sequences that result in an amputation through a long bone will also have problems associated with bony overgrowth. Understanding that the etiology is both congenital and acquired is helpful in predicting which issues may arise.

Many congenital deficiencies resulting from lack of formation have patterns of aplasia or hypoplasia. A widely used classification is the International Organization for Standardization (ISO) and International Society for Prosthetics and Orthotics (ISPO) classification that was developed first by the "Kay" Committee

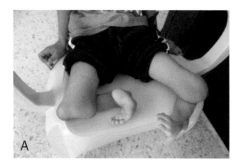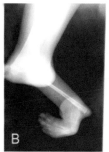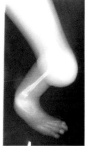

Figure 1 Clinical photograph (**A**) and AP radiograph (**B**) of a child with a congenital bilateral complete tibial longitudinal deficiency, with partial deletion of the midtarsals and full deletion of the medial first rays of the feet. This patient had no active knee extension. The recommended treatment was bilateral knee disarticulations with a transfemoral-type prostheses for ambulation.

in 1973; with some minor modifications, it became an international standard in 1989.[11] The classification satisfied a need for a logical, non-Greek- or non-Latin-based nomenclature that could be easily translated and would avoid ambiguity. The two major divisions within the classification are transverse deficiencies and longitudinal deficiencies. Transverse deficiencies have normal tissue development proximal to the level of the deficiency and are described by naming the bone segment at which the limb terminates followed by a description of the abnormal tissue distal to the level of termination, such as any additional finger buds. A longitudinal deficiency has a reduction of elements within the long axis of the limb and can involve multiple long bones. It is described in a proximal to distal fashion, naming only the affected bones. A partial deficiency is stated as such, with some approximation of the longitudinal fraction that is still present. The number of rays or digits present is described, starting from the preaxial (radial or tibial) side. **Figure 1** provides an example of how a longitudinal deficiency can be described with this classification.

Although the ISO/ISPO classification provides a major improvement in communication, it is important to be aware of its limitations. It is based on radiographic or bony anatomic features of the long bones; it does not attempt to describe soft-tissue defects and joint

motion. The joint muscle girdle, the stabilizing ligaments, and range of motion are crucial features that drive treatment options and should not be overlooked.

Surgical Planning
Goals
The three major goals of surgery are to (1) project and optimize function in adulthood, (2) optimize function during growth, and (3) minimize the number of major surgeries. The first two goals often are well aligned, and optimal management during growth yields optimal results in adulthood. However, circumstances exist when these goals are not well aligned, leading to the consideration of both situations separately. The priority is for optimal function in adulthood, but management during growth must be tolerable for both the patient and the family.

For example, consider a 3-year-old child with unilateral localized gigantism of a foot who will undergo a foot amputation. Without another procedure, the length of the residual limb just after surgery will be too long to accommodate a foot prosthesis. A short-term solution would be to perform a transtibial amputation. However, major problems with terminal residual limb overgrowth would occur, which would not be a good long-term result. A better option is to resect the distal tibia (including the growth plate) combined with a Boyd amputation. If the length of the tibia is already adequate for an adult transtibial residual limb, then a proximal tibial epiphysiodesis can be done at the same time. Immediately after surgery, the length of the residual limb will still be too long. However, several years later, the growth of the contralateral limb should provide a great enough difference to accommodate a standard transtibial prosthesis.

Projecting Limb-Length Discrepancies

The previous example also highlights the need to consider limb-length discrepancies at skeletal maturity. The first few clinic visits with a family who is facing elective treatment should be dedicated to developing a treatment plan that is acceptable to everyone. The current and projected limb-length discrepancies, both with and without treatment, will be a crucial component. Many publications are dedicated to the accurate projection of limb-length discrepancies, but details are beyond the scope of this chapter. However, some useful tools for rough estimates of limb lengths at maturity can be quickly used while performing the physical examination.

The first assumption is that infants with congenital deficiencies have limbs that will grow proportionally.[12] Therefore, if the long bone is 60% of the length of the opposite long bone at birth, it will be about 60% of the long-bone length at skeletal maturity. Another way to visualize this is to look at both limbs in full extension and see where the distal end of the limb is relative to the longer side. It will end at approximately the same place relative to the other limb when the child is an adult. With a little more information, the discrepancy in centimeters at maturity can be calculated. The average femoral/tibial length of normal individuals at skeletal maturity is 44/37 cm for males and 41/34 cm for females. If the affected limb is 60% of the length of the other side, multiply by 0.6 the average length of that bone at

maturity. This calculation will not provide a perfectly accurate number, but it will provide enough information to allow consideration of the major treatment options.

If trauma has caused complete growth arrest to the growth plate, the proportion rule cannot be used. Rather, the percentages of growth provided by that growth plate for the entire limb should be referenced, which are approximately as follows: proximal femur, 15%; distal femur, 35%; proximal tibia, 30%; and distal tibia, 20%. From this information, the average growth in millimeters per year from each femoral or tibial growth plate can be calculated, with the following two assumptions: (1) most growth ends in boys and girls at approximately 16 years and 14 years of age, respectively; and (2) the growth arrest is complete. Infections often cause a partial physeal arrest, so projecting the growth inhibition is not as straightforward because the rate of inhibition is unique to the level of involvement of the growth plate. In these circumstances, the growth inhibition method or Moseley's straight-line graph method can be used.

Surgical Timing

Ideally, surgical intervention occurs at a time that allows the child to reach normal motor milestones. To decrease the risks of anesthesia in infants, elective surgery is best delayed until the child is 9 to 12 months old. For example, in a child who will need an elective foot amputation for a fibular or tibial deficiency, surgery is delayed until the child is pulling to stand, which is typically between 10 and 14 months of age.

For limb deficiencies associated with hip dysplasia, the early remodeling potential of the hip should be considered and used to the patient's advantage. A femoral neck that is in varus may protect the hip to some degree from subluxation or dislocation if the acetabulum is dysplastic. However, severe coxa vara can

cause blunting of the lateral lip of the acetabulum with hip abduction and may even lever the head inferiorly out of the acetabulum. A valgus-producing proximal femoral osteotomy combined with femoral shortening to help relax the soft-tissue hip girdle should be performed when there is still remodeling potential for the acetabulum. A pelvic osteotomy also may be needed to ensure optimal hip development and prevent dislocation. Minimizing hip dysplasia in the future will benefit patients planning to undergo either a lower limb amputation or a lengthening procedure.

Psychological Considerations

For elective surgery, it is important that the family has accepted the need and is ready to have the child undergo the procedure. Parents often find it difficult to commit a child to an amputation because of the complex emotional issues. An amputation imparts a sense of finality. Drotar et al[13] described five stages of parental reactions following the discovery of a congenital anomaly: shock, denial, sadness and anger, adaptation, and reorganization. Many parents discover the anomaly at birth, although the frequency of antenatal diagnoses resulting from improvements in prenatal ultrasound is growing. Evidence shows that these parents experience the same stages of emotion, with many reaching the adaptation stage before birth.[14] It is reasonable to assume that parents will struggle with making any decisions before reaching the adaptation stage, so extensive counseling and multiple medical opinions are initially needed.

Parents often feel pressure to make a decision about an amputation as early as possible. Although it is reasonable to assume that amputations are psychologically easier for the child if done before long-term memory is developed, no evidence validates this assumption. Traditionally, this age was thought to be approximately 3 to 4 years. However, the model of how young children form memories has been recently challenged and suggests that even very early traumatic events can be recalled.[15] Finally, the well-being and self-esteem of the child is most closely tied to social support from classmates, parents, teachers, and friends.[16,17] Parental depression and anxiety and marital discord in families also have been associated with increased childhood depression and anxiety.[18] Therefore, parental well-being and comfort with the decisions they are making is paramount. A prosthesis or an orthosis can be fashioned to fit the extremity for functional purposes until the family is ready to make a decision about surgery. In these situations, patients and/or families often reach a point where they prefer a more cosmetic prosthesis or orthosis and will reconsider an amputation as a logical step toward that goal.

Surgical Principles of Pediatric Amputations
Principle 1: Amputate Through Joints When Possible

Children are at risk of terminal bony overgrowth after a transcortical amputation, with prevalence approaching 50%. The mechanism is thought to be from a periosteal reaction, with penciling of the terminal bone. Painful bursae can develop, or the soft tissues can telescope over the tip and externalize the bone. This phenomenon can occur in any skeletally immature patient; it often recurs despite multiple trimmings of the overgrowth, and recurrences sometimes continue into the third decade of life. It is a painful, recurrent problem and best avoided by ensuring that the bone end always has a native or grafted cartilage cap. Therefore, the first principle is to amputate through joints whenever possible and avoid transcortical amputations. Also, for traumatic amputations with a limited soft-tissue envelope that does not allow primary closure of the skin, long bones can be easily shortened by removing a segment

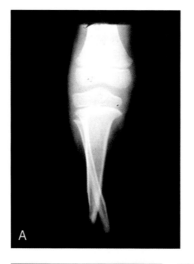
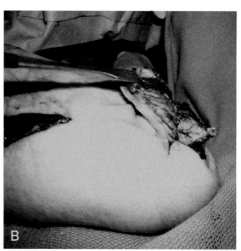
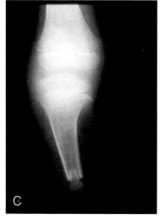
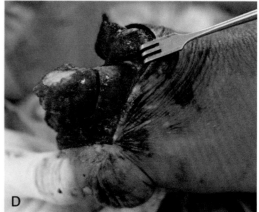

Figure 2   AP radiograph (**A**) and intraoperative photograph (**B**) of tibial residual limb overgrowth. AP radiograph (**C**) and intraoperative photograph (**D**) of osteochondral capping using an ipsilateral fibular head autograft (modified Marquardt technique as described by H. G. Watts). In the preoperative radiograph, the fibula appears longer, but the tibia is a subcutaneous bone and is often symptomatic first.

of the shaft that is fixed with a plate, allowing soft tissues to be advanced and closed over the articular cartilage.

For the unavoidable transcortical amputation, the first principle also includes primary capping with an osteochondral autograft, which can reduce the risk of overgrowth to approximately 10%. Capping was first described after Ernst Marquardt observed that overgrowth never occurred after amputations though joints[19,20] (**Figure 2**). Multiple biologic and synthetic grafts have been tried. Synthetic grafts have been problematic because of inflammatory foreign body reactions that may

require revisions.[21] Autografts from the iliac crest are successful, but patients may experience donor site pain. Fibular head autografts have been successfully used for tibial residual limb capping, and the procedure was well described in a recent series of 50 patients.[22] A metacarpal head and several centimeters of its shaft, if available from the amputated limb, also fits nicely into the canal of the tibia. The metatarsal shaft is pressed into the canal of the tibia, creating an interference fit that avoids the need for fixation. The periosteum of the recipient bed is sutured to the cartilage as reinforcement.

Principle 2: Preserve Joint Function, Especially at the Knee

Despite impressive advancements in computerized prosthetic devices, no substitute exists that can provide the functional range of motion and strength of a native joint controlled by the individual's own motor cortex. Energy costs are substantially increased for patients with transfemoral amputations compared with those with transtibial amputations; therefore, every effort should be made to salvage a functional knee. In comparison with unimpaired individuals, the mean oxygen consumption is 9% higher in individuals with a unilateral transtibial amputation and 49% higher in those with a unilateral transfemoral amputation.[23] Interestingly, when Jeans et al[24] compared gait in children with different lower limb amputation levels, children with knee disarticulations had similar rates of oxygen consumption and velocity compared with those who had transtibial amputations. However, the children in this study were evaluated when walking on level ground. On uneven terrain, the mechanical knee cannot quickly adapt, thus causing difficulty with gait. The second principle is to preserve joint function, especially at the knee.

Inadequate residual limb length below a joint can be a concern. Inadequate tibial residual limb length is a common reason for knee disarticulations or transfemoral amputations. However, if the child is still growing and the growth plate is preserved, the residual limb will naturally increase in length. Also, very short tibial residual limbs can be lengthened to improve prosthetic use. Similarly, very short femoral residual limbs can be lengthened to allow the individual to use a transfemoral prosthesis instead of a hip disarticulation prosthesis (**Figure 3**). The average length obtained with planar fixators is 8.7 cm in the femur and 6.9 cm in the tibia. After lengthening, most patients are able to wear a standard prosthesis

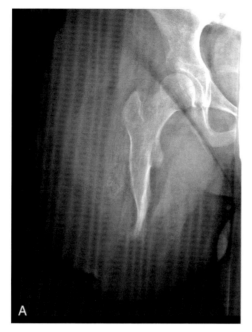 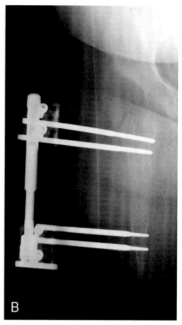

Figure 3 AP radiographs of a short femoral residual limb (**A**) that was associated with poor control of the prosthesis. The femur underwent an osteotomy and lengthening of 9 cm (**B**) with an external fixator. The amount of length achieved was limited by pain over the distal tip during the lengthening process, but this pain abated during the consolidation phase.

appropriate for their level of amputation.[25] It is important to perform the osteotomy for the lengthening distal to any tendon insertions, such as the iliopsoas or patellar tendon, to avoid contractures or dislocations. For very short segments, a step-cut or an oblique cut in the bone can be performed to avoid the tendon insertion site.

The lack of soft-tissue coverage also is a common reason for a higher-level amputation. However, in children, skin grafts can hypertrophy much more robustly compared with adults and should be given every opportunity to heal and adapt (**Figure 4**). Parry et al[26] showed in a retrospective study that functional outcomes and prosthetic use were excellent when skin grafts were used to preserve length in pediatric amputations.

Principle 3: Preserve Limb Length

In general, the longer the residual limb, the better the gait.[27] A longer limb provides a better lever arm for generating power and is crucial for a well-seated residual limb within a conventional prosthesis. Increased length of the distal segment also provides distribution of the contact forces between the limb and the prosthesis, thereby reducing pressure ulceration, which can be of particular concern for insensate skin grafts that do not have normal pliancy. The ideal length for an amputated long bone has not been studied. The minimum absolute value is based on the ability to keep the prosthesis in place, and this number changes with advancements in prosthetic liner types as well as transosseous integration methods. The maximum length is based on the desire for equal joint heights (such as the knee for a transfemoral amputation) and the bulk of the various prosthetic materials between the distal residual limb and the mechanical joint. Patients with variable knee heights have similar function when walking on level ground. In the experience of this chapter's author, minor problems have been reported with variable knee heights, such as difficulty fitting into stadium seating and pain under the longer thigh when sitting because of

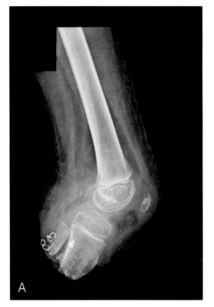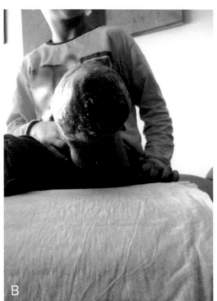

Figure 4   Lateral radiograph (**A**) and clinical photograph (**B**) of a 4-year-old boy who was injured by a bomb blast, resulting in a traumatic tibial amputation. The left tibial segment was extremely short with inadequate soft-tissue coverage, but the extensor mechanism remained intact. The full thickness tissue loss over the distal residual limb and the tibial periosteum was treated with skin graft. After the grafted tissue hypertrophies and matures, it will function well inside a standard transtibial prosthesis. With normal growth, the proximal tibia will increase by an additional 6 to 8 cm by skeletal maturity.

the short tibial segment and increased pressure from the chair on the posterior thigh.

When planning an amputation proximal to a growth plate, the future growth that will be lost should be considered. A common scenario is a midshaft femoral amputation in a small child where the residual femoral limb length is fashioned at the level that would be appropriate at skeletal maturity (approximately 5 to 10 cm above the opposite joint line). However, the distal femoral epiphysis contributes to 80% of the growth of the entire femur. Therefore, the residual limb will initially seem an appropriate length, but at skeletal maturity, it will be much too short.

Because it is important to preserve both limb length and growth plates, it should be remembered that a residual limb also can become too long. The space needed to accommodate a mechanical joint that is level with the contralateral side depends on the materials available. In general, the residual limb should be at least 5 cm shorter than the anticipated prosthetic joint line. An appropriately timed epiphysiodesis can be done if the child is still growing. An intercalary shortening with internal fixation of the shaft can be performed if the child is skeletally mature. A maximum of 5 cm can be removed in the femur and 3 cm in the tibia, with soft-tissue closure as the limiting factor.

Special Considerations
Upper Limb Deficiencies
Often, there is little need for surgical intervention of upper limb deficiencies, beyond the initial treatment of traumatic injuries. Individuals with congenital amputation often have nubbins on the terminal residual limb, which should not be removed unless they involve a specific issue, such as hygiene or repeat trauma. The nubbins can provide traction and sensation for the distal residual limb.

Patients with a unilateral upper limb deficiency often can compensate extremely well with a sound contralateral side, which has made the use of upper limb prostheses a controversial topic. A study by James et al[28] suggested no functional or quality-of-life difference for individuals with unilateral below-elbow disarticulations with and without prostheses. However, long-term follow-up studies showed that children with upper limb prostheses continued to use prostheses into adulthood. Interestingly, they also tended to choose the simplest device, even when exposed to a variety of prostheses.[29] Individuals with bilateral upper limb deficiencies often compensate surprisingly well by using the lower limbs and feet, especially if the deficiency was present since birth. It is important for the surgeon to carefully consider how foot function may substitute for hand function before considering any lower limb surgery in these patients. For bilateral hand amputations, the Krukenberg procedure should be considered.[30]

Syme Disarticulation Versus Boyd Amputation
Amputations about the ankle are achieved with either a Syme disarticulation or a Boyd amputation. Both procedures have been reported to achieve satisfactory results and have similar rates of complications, but each has advantages and disadvantages with regard to postoperative care and the types of complications encountered.

In a Syme ankle disarticulation, the medial malleoli often are resected in adults to decrease their prominence, but this is unnecessary in children because growth of the malleoli is typically diminished. The advantages of a Syme disarticulation are ease of the surgery, decreased acute postoperative wound complications, no need for a postoperative cast, and a shorter time to prosthesis fitting. The major disadvantages reported in the literature are an increased risk of posterior migration of the heel pad and a less reliable weight-bearing residual limb.[31,32] However, Birch et al[33] noted that posterior migration of the heel pad is typically asymptomatic and does not affect function within the prosthesis. If a Syme disarticulation is performed in a young child, Eilert and Jayakumar[31] advocated retaining the calcaneal apophysis and positioning the heel pad squarely beneath the distal tibia to avoid heel pad migration, which results in regeneration of the calcaneus so that the residual limb effectively becomes a Boyd-type amputation at maturity.

The Boyd amputation is a fusion of the calcaneus to the distal tibia, with resection of the talus. The advantages include a stable heel pad at the base of the residual limb that can reliably bear weight and improved prosthetic suspension. In adults with normal anatomy, this procedure results in a longer residual limb with a bulbous end compared with a Syme disarticulation, which is not always true for children because the residual limb is often hypoplastic. The total length of the residual limb will depend on any growth inhibition and the presence or the absence of the distal tibial growth plate. The distal tibia and its growth plate are often resected, which shortens the residual limb and allows for correct positioning of a subluxated calcaneus beneath the tibia while decreasing soft-tissue tension at wound closure. When performed in very young children, it can result in a residual limb that ends at the contralateral mid-calf level at skeletal maturity. Watts[34] previously reported that in such situations, any bulk from the calcaneus is nicely contoured as part of the calf within the prosthesis and provides a good cosmetic result as well as self-suspension within the prosthesis. The disadvantages of a Boyd amputation include the following: it is more technically demanding than a Syme disarticulation, postoperative wound complications are increased, nonunion may require a revision, a postoperative cast is required, and more

time is needed postoperatively before the limb can be fitted with a prosthesis. It also can result in a residual limb that is too long for a more sophisticated foot prosthesis and distal bulkiness can affect prosthetic cosmesis. The rate of complication is approximately 15%, most being soft-tissue healing that can be managed with local wound care.[35]

Congenital Tibial Pseudarthrosis

Special caution is needed in performing amputations in patients with congenital tibial pseudarthrosis in whom multiple attempts for a union have failed. It is tempting to amputate through the nonunion site; however, overgrowth may develop in the transtibial residual limb and nonunion may occur after a residual limb capping procedure. Amputation at the level of the ankle is recommended to improve the length of the residual limb as well as decrease symptoms from overgrowth. The nonunion may or may not persist after a Syme disarticulation or a Boyd amputation; however, the nonunion is rarely symptomatic within the prosthesis and may not require further treatment.[35-37]

Van Nes Procedures

A Van Nes rotationplasty substitutes a 180° rotated ankle for the knee in patients with a femoral deficiency. Borggreve[38] originally described the procedure in Germany for the treatment of tuberculosis of the knee, and Van Nes later modified the procedure to treat congenital femoral focal deficiency. The procedure also can be performed after primary tumor resection about the knee.[39,40] Long-term follow-up studies have shown excellent function and more energy-efficient gait parameters compared with similar patients who received a transfemoral amputation or conversion of a congenital deficiency to a transfemoral amputation. Cosmesis often is an initial concern; however, follow-up studies consistently report that a Van Nes rotationplasty is well accepted

by patients from a psychosocial and a cosmetic point of view.[41-43]

Various surgical techniques have been described for a Van Nes rotationplasty. Invariably, the knee joint is resected; typically one or both growth plates at the knee also are resected. The limb is rotated 180°, and then it is fused with an intramedullary rod and a temporary percutaneous cross pin, a plate, or an external fixator. A spica cast also can be used. Because ankle motion substitutes for the knee, the ankle must be stable with excellent function and range of motion before surgery. Mild fibular deficiency where the tip of the fibula ends at the mortise has shown good postoperative function in a case study (AV Cuomo, KC Perkins-Tiff, PR Scott-Wyard, et al, unpublished data presented at the Association of Children's Prosthetic-Orthotic Clinics Annual Meeting, Banff, Canada, 2012). Derotation of the limb can occur and sometimes requires a second procedure to rerotate the limb. Compensation of mild loss of rotation occurs through subtalar motion. The rotationplasty can be technically performed in Aitken types A, B, C, and D femoral deficiencies. Additional rotation can be achieved through the middle of the tibia as part of the primary procedure or to treat derotation (**Figure 5**). If there is a hip joint, treatment of any hip dysplasia or coxa vara should be considered to optimize hip function. Additional rotation can be achieved after the coxa vara is addressed. Patients with a stable hip generally do not require an ischial weight-bearing prosthesis.

Multiple Limb Deficiencies

The child with multiple limb deficiencies requires special consideration because the capability to perform tasks is dependent on how well other parts of the body can substitute for function. A holistic, team approach is particularly important for planning treatment. Surgery is rarely indicated for multiple

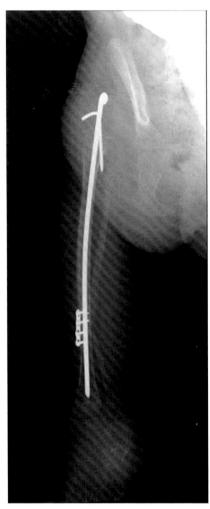

Figure 5 AP radiograph of a Van Nes rotationplasty performed in a child with a congenital femoral deficiency. The short distal tuft of the femur limited the extent of rotation through the knee fusion, and additional rotation was achieved with an osteotomy in the tibia. (Courtesy of Joseph Ivan Krajbich, MD, Portland, OR.)

congenital deficiencies. Amputation or surgical correction of the feet or remnants of the feet should not be done if they substitute for hands, even if surgery will provide better gait or improved prostheses use.

Summary

The etiology and management of pediatric and adult amputations differ substantially. By adhering to several surgical principles, an acceptable result can be achieved in pediatric patients undergoing amputation. These principles are based on the child's growth and its effects on residual limb length and the potential for terminal bony overgrowth. The treatment of children with congenital limb reductions and multiple-limb involvement often requires a multidisciplinary team approach. Surgical planning requires a thorough evaluation of the child, predictions of limb differences at maturity, and consideration of the family's needs and expectations.

References

1. Ziegler-Graham K, MacKenzie EJ, Ephraim PL, Travison TG, Brookmeyer R: Estimating the prevalence of limb loss in the United States: 2005 to 2050. *Arch Phys Med Rehabil* 2008;89(3):422-429.

2. Krebs DE, Fishman S: Characteristics of the child amputee population. *J Pediatr Orthop* 1984;4(1):89-95.

3. Conner KA, McKenzie LB, Xiang H, Smith GA: Pediatric traumatic amputations and hospital resource utilization in the United States, 2003. *J Trauma* 2010;68(1):131-137.

4. Ghanem I: Epidemiology, etiology, and genetic aspects of reduction deficiencies of the lower limb. *J Child Orthop* 2008;2(5):329-332.

5. Say B, Tunçbilek E, Pirnar T, Tokgözoglu N: Hereditary congenital coxa vara with dominant inheritance? *Humangenetik* 1971;11(3):266-268.

6. Brewster TG, Lachman RS, Kushner DC, Holmes LB, Isler RJ, Rimoin DL: Oto-palato-digital syndrome, type II: An X-linked skeletal dysplasia. *Am J Med Genet* 1985;20(2):249-254.

7. Czeizel AE, Vitéz M, Kodaj I, Lenz W: A family study on isolated congenital radial and tibial deficiencies in Hungary, 1975-1984. *Clin Genet* 1993;44(1):32-36.

8. Klopocki E, Kähler C, Foulds N, et al: Deletions in PITX1 cause a spectrum of lower-limb malformations including mirror-image polydactyly. *Eur J Hum Genet* 2012;20(6):705-708.

9. Babbs C, Heller R, Everman DB, et al: A new locus for split hand/foot malformation with long bone deficiency (SHFLD) at 2q14.2 identified from a chromosome translocation. *Hum Genet* 2007;122(2):191-199.

10. Gurrieri F, Everman DB: Clinical, genetic, and molecular aspects of split-hand/foot malformation: An update. *Am J Med Genet A* 2013;161A(11):2860-2872.

11. Day HJ: The ISO/ISPO classification of congenital limb deficiency. *Prosthet Orthot Int* 1991;15(2):67-69.

12. Amstutz HC: The morphology, natural history, and treatment of proximal femoral deficiencies, in Aitken GT, ed: *Proximal Femoral Focal Deficiency: A Congenital Anomaly.* Washington, DC, National Academy of Sciences, 1969, pp 50-57.

13. Drotar D, Baskiewicz A, Irvin N, Kennell J, Klaus M: The adaptation of parents to the birth of an infant with a congenital malformation: A hypothetical model. *Pediatrics* 1975;56(5):710-717.

14. Aite L, Zaccara A, Nahom A, Trucchi A, Iacobelli B, Bagolan P: Mothers' adaptation to antenatal diagnosis of surgically correctable anomalies. *Early Hum Dev* 2006;82(10):649-653.

15. Wang Q, Peterson C: Your earliest memory may be earlier than you think: Prospective studies of children's dating of earliest childhood memories. *Dev Psychol* 2014;50(6):1680-1686.

16. Varni JW, Rubenfeld LA, Talbot D, Setoguchi Y: Determinants of self-esteem in children with congenital/acquired limb deficiencies. *J Dev Behav Pediatr* 1989;10(1):13-16.

17. Varni JW, Setoguchi Y, Rappaport LR, Talbot D: Effects of stress, social support, and self-esteem on depression in children with limb

deficiencies. *Arch Phys Med Rehabil* 1991;72(13):1053-1058.

18. Varni JW, Setoguchi Y: Effects of parental adjustment on the adaptation of children with congenital or acquired limb deficiencies. *J Dev Behav Pediatr* 1993;14(1):13-20.

19. Marquardt E, Correll J: Amputations and prostheses for the lower limb. *Int Orthop* 1984;8(2):139-146.

20. Marquardt E: The multiple-limb-deficient child, in Bowker JH, Michael JW, eds: *Atlas of Limb Prosthetics: Surgical, Prosthetic, and Rehabilitation Principles*, ed 2. St Louis, MO, Mosby-Year Book, 1992, pp 839-884.

21. Tenholder M, Davids JR, Gruber HE, Blackhurst DW: Surgical management of juvenile amputation overgrowth with a synthetic cap. *J Pediatr Orthop* 2004;24(2):218-226.

22. Fedorak GT, Watts HG, Cuomo AV, et al: Osteocartilaginous transfer of the proximal part of the fibula for osseous overgrowth in children with congenital or acquired tibial amputation: Surgical technique and results. *J Bone Joint Surg Am* 2015;97(7):574-581.

23. Huang CT, Jackson JR, Moore NB, et al: Amputation: Energy cost of ambulation. *Arch Phys Med Rehabil* 1979;60(1):18-24.

24. Jeans KA, Browne RH, Karol LA: Effect of amputation level on energy expenditure during overground walking by children with an amputation. *J Bone Joint Surg Am* 2011;93(1):49-56.

25. Bowen RE, Struble SG, Setoguchi Y, Watts HG: Outcomes of lengthening short lower-extremity amputation stumps with planar fixators. *J Pediatr Orthop* 2005;25(4):543-547.

26. Parry IS, Mooney KN, Chau C, et al: Effects of skin grafting on successful prosthetic use in children with lower extremity amputation. *J Burn Care Res* 2008;29(6):949-954.

27. Waters RL, Perry J, Antonelli D, Hislop H: Energy cost of walking of amputees: The influence of level of amputation. *J Bone Joint Surg Am* 1976;58(1):42-46.

28. James MA, Bagley AM, Brasington K, Lutz C, McConnell S, Molitor F: Impact of prostheses on function and quality of life for children with unilateral congenital below-the-elbow deficiency. *J Bone Joint Surg Am* 2006;88(11):2356-2365.

29. Crandall RC, Tomhave W: Pediatric unilateral below-elbow amputees: Retrospective analysis of 34 patients given multiple prosthetic options. *J Pediatr Orthop* 2002;22(3):380-383.

30. Swanson AB: The Krukenberg procedure in the juvenile amputee. *J Bone Joint Surg Am* 1964;46:1540-1548.

31. Eilert RE, Jayakumar SS: Boyd and Syme ankle amputations in children. *J Bone Joint Surg Am* 1976;58(8):1138-1141.

32. Fulp T, Davids JR, Meyer LC, Blackhurst DW: Longitudinal deficiency of the fibula: Operative treatment. *J Bone Joint Surg Am* 1996;78(5):674-682.

33. Birch JG, Walsh SJ, Small JM, et al: Syme amputation for the treatment of fibular deficiency: An evaluation of long-term physical and psychological functional status. *J Bone Joint Surg Am* 1999;81(11):1511-1518.

34. Watts H: Surgical modifications of residual limbs, in Smith DG, Michael JW, Bowker JH, eds: *Atlas of Amputations and Limb Deficiencies: Surgical, Prosthetic, and Rehabilitation Principles*, ed 3. Rosemont, IL, American Academy of Orthopaedic Surgeons, 2004, pp 931-943.

35. Westberry DE, Davids JR, Pugh LI: The Boyd amputation in children: Indications and outcomes. *J Pediatr Orthop* 2014;34(1):86-91.

36. Guille JT, Kumar SJ, Shah A: Spontaneous union of a congenital pseudarthrosis of the tibia after Syme amputation. *Clin Orthop Relat Res* 1998;351:180-185.

37. Jacobsen ST, Crawford AH, Millar EA, Steel HH: The Syme amputation in patients with congenital pseudarthrosis of the tibia. *J Bone Joint Surg Am* 1983;65(4):533-537.

38. Borggreve J: Kniegelenkersatz durch das in der Beinlängsachse um 180° gedrehte Fussgelenk. *Arth F Orthop* 1930;28:175-178.

39. Kotz R, Salzer M: Rotation-plasty for childhood osteosarcoma of the distal part of the femur. *J Bone Joint Surg Am* 1982;64(7):959-969.

40. Krajbich JI, Carroll NC: Van Nes rotationplasty with segmental limb resection. *Clin Orthop Relat Res* 1990;256:7-13.

41. Alman BA, Krajbich JI, Hubbard S: Proximal femoral focal deficiency: Results of rotationplasty and Syme amputation. *J Bone Joint Surg Am* 1995;77(12):1876-1882.

42. Hanlon M, Krajbich JI: Rotationplasty in skeletally immature patients: Long-term followup results. *Clin Orthop Relat Res* 1999;358:75-82.

43. McClenaghan BA, Krajbich JI, Pirone AM, Koheil R, Longmuir P: Comparative assessment of gait after limb-salvage procedures. *J Bone Joint Surg Am* 1989;71(8):1178-1182.

Chapter 65

Prosthetic Considerations in the Pediatric Patient

Brian J. Giavedoni, MBA, CP, LP

Abstract

Pediatric prosthetics has become a well-established subspecialty within the field of prosthetics. The fitting of a limb-deficient child with a prosthesis is a complex process requiring a thorough knowledge of the child's underlying conditions and anatomic anomalies. Additional considerations in these children are the initial need for family-centered care and the long-term nature of care that will be required over the patient's lifetime.

Keywords: amputation; congenital limb difference; limb deficiency; pediatrics; prosthetics

Introduction

The prosthetic prescription for a child is very different than that for an adult with a similar level of limb loss. Congenital limb differences require an understanding of the anatomic anomaly and all of the associated developmental, physical, and physiologic implications. In the management of pediatric limb anomalies, the child is a continuously changing patient in whom body size, limitations, and physical potential mimic the age-appropriate developmental advances expected in able-bodied children. The support and participation of the patient's family, technologic advances, and the practitioner's skill and experience all contribute to the prosthetic fitting outcome.

Lifelong and family-centered care are two additional distinctions in the treatment of a child with a limb deficiency. Unlike their adult counterparts, children often have no input in initial surgical planning or prosthetic prescription. All decisions are made by parents in consultation with the treatment team, which often includes a physician, a prosthetist, a therapist, and a social worker.

Prosthetic issues unique to children with limb differences encompass anticipated physiologic growth, healing potential, and tissue metabolism.

The incidence of congenital limb deficiency is approximately 5 to 10 per 10,000 live births.[1] Children with upper limb deficiencies outnumber those with lower limb deficiencies by a ratio of 3:1, and they often have multiple limb anomalies and other comorbidities or syndromes (**Figure 1**). A comprehensive examination of a child with a congenital limb difference should include facial, spinal, and pelvic evaluations so that other conditions can be quickly identified. If a syndrome is involved, the limb difference may not be the most pressing medical issue.

Prosthetic Fitting Strategies
Lower Limb Fittings

The prosthetic socket is the foundation of a well-designed and functional prosthesis and must be intimate, anatomically correct, and comfortable. The socket represents the interface between the patient's body and technology. A poor socket fit will negate the advantages of

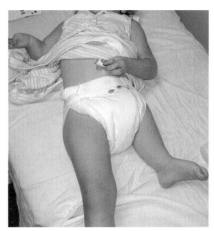

Figure 1   Photograph of an infant with multiple congenital limb anomalies, including left proximal focal femoral deficiency and right and left ulnar deficiencies.

good technology. Generally, a prosthesis for a child should be designed to last at least 12 months, although its useful duration is heavily dependent on the activity level and play habits of the child. A prosthesis that becomes unusable in less than 1 year may indicate that either the initial socket fit was too aggressive or it did not take into account both longitudinal and circumferential growth.[2] From a global perspective, the ability to "grow" a prosthesis to coincide with the child's physiologic growth is an important consideration for the prosthetist. Although manufacturers have provided an ever increasing number of prosthetic components, the most desirable options are those in which parts can be added to increase height or those made of materials that can be adjusted after fabrication.

Lower limb socket designs and components vary with the age, the activity level, and the functional requirements of the individual child. Most children

---

Mr. Giavedoni or an immediate family member serves as a board member, owner, officer, or committee member of the Association of Children's Prosthetic and Orthotic Clinics.

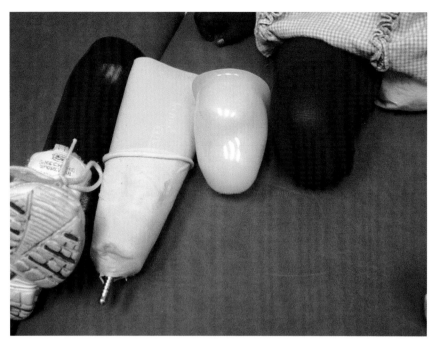

Figure 2   Photograph of the limb of a child with a very short transtibial amputation. A pin liner (center) can be used for suspension over a thin thermoplastic inner socket (right). The outer prosthesis is shown on the far left.

with a lower limb deficiency will want to walk, run, and play in the same manner as their able-bodied peers. Knowledge gained over the past 10 years has demonstrated that protecting a young child (6 years or younger) from falling by incorporating a locking knee into a transfemoral-level prosthesis is not only unnecessary but may prove counterproductive. Studies have suggested that early knee placement in a prosthesis can reduce the adaptation of clearance options during the development of ambulation.[3-5]

Although many component options are available for pediatric patients, the choice of whether to use a particular option must be based on sound clinical judgment. Manufacturers began producing pediatric component lines in the late 1980s and, over time, have substantially increased the variety of components available for most functional amputation levels.

Stance control knees, which are frequently selected for adult amputees, are often unnecessary for the child with

lower limb loss. For children, a step-over-step strategy for descending stairs is often impossible in a device with activated stance control. Step-over-step running is effortless if a child is exposed early to this activity, and it is hampered by a knee with prosthetic stance control. In the experience of this chapter's author, most children request deactivation of the stance control feature in their knees so that their activity level is not reduced. Similarly, although a locking knee may be appropriate for geriatric patients, it is rarely appropriate in the pediatric population. If increased knee stability is required, simple alignment modifications can be made to articulating knees to increase stability.

Although suction sockets provide an intimate, secure solution to both suspension and ease of donning for adults, these sockets are generally ill-suited to the growing child. Relatively small variances in volume can substantially affect both fit and the ability to maintain a vacuum seal. Similarly, although various types of gel liners provide comfort, these

liners increase the need for hygienic practices to avoid the commonplace occurrences of yeast and fungal infections. In addition, liners add weight and bulk to an already visually oversized prosthesis. However, if justified clinically, liners can afford both suspension and the ability to increase the lifespan of the prosthesis by allowing changes to the liner thickness to compensate for growth (**Figure 2**).

Experience has demonstrated that most healthy, active pediatric amputees easily achieve a K4 activity level through their developing years and into their 20s and 30s. Because of the high activity level of many children, pediatric lower limb components may be subjected to tremendous wear and tear. When catastrophic failure is not the reason for replacement of a prosthesis, physiologic growth is usually the inciting factor. Generally, a child will grow 12 inches (30.38 cm) per year, thus warranting the need to replace a prosthetic foot, and, in most cases, requiring a new socket or an entirely new prosthesis.

Upper Limb Fittings

In the child with an upper limb difference, early fitting with a passive prosthesis with a hand can assist in crawling and maintaining sitting balance by equalizing limb lengths. With the advent of small silicone sleeves for upper limb suspension, torso-shoulder harnessing is no longer necessary in early-stage fittings. Adequate suspension can be achieved by using a combination of a self-suspending socket design and a sleeve (**Figure 3**).

If the tools or benchmarks used to establish the success or failure of a pediatric upper limb prosthesis are flawed, then the expected outcomes will be unreliable. If an upper limb prosthesis is viewed as a tool that is specifically tailored to the needs of the individual child, then success should be measured based on the successful completion of tasks chosen by the child, not by the

© 2016 American Academy of Orthopaedic Surgeons

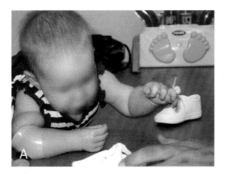 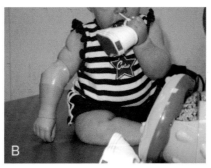

Figure 3 Photographs of a child with a transverse radial deficiency. **A,** A self-suspending three-quarter socket design provides equal arm lengths. **B,** The socket design allows for propping and balance.

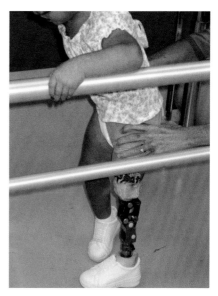

Figure 4 Photograph of a child with a lower limb prosthesis in which dynamic alignment has been achieved without the aid of alignment jigs or hardware because of space limitations.

clinician or tester. In a study by Crandall and Tomhave,[6] it was concluded that successful unilateral transradial amputees will choose a prosthesis on the basis of functions unique to their own specific needs, and that the most successful users have prostheses that provide multiple options. The study reported that 26 of 29 of the amputees (90%) reported using their upper limb prosthesis, with an mean daily use of 9.2 hours. Fourteen of the study participants reported using their prostheses on a fulltime basis throughout the year.

As technology advances, more prosthetic options are becoming available for patients with wrist disarticulations and partial hand amputations. Only a decade ago, individuals with partial hand amputation were considered ineligible for prosthetic fittings because of their very long residual limbs. Ten years later, based on the Client Centered Care System assessment, positive results were reported in preliminary research on 14 patients with congenital partial hand amputations who were fitted with the externally powered ProDigits (Touch Bionics) prosthesis.[7]

In both upper and lower limb prosthetic management, a common dilemma is whether to replace the entire prosthesis or only the failed or outgrown components. As a general rule, the entire device should be replaced if (1) the major components (hand, foot, or knee) have excessive wear and (2) the socket requires replacement because of growth or surgical revision. However, because the hands of children have a slower rate of growth than their feet, a prosthetic hand will continue to match the soundside hand for a longer period of time. An intact prosthetic hand may often be reused on a replacement prosthesis after the child has outgrown the prior device.

Growth Management in Children

Growth in children is a physiologic reality, and their open growth plates represent a major difference between children and adults. In adults undergoing amputation, adequate space can be allowed to accommodate both an optimal socket design and a good selection of prosthetic components. This is not the case in pediatric patients in whom transosseous amputations are rare. Rather, an elective amputation in a child with a congenital limb deficiency is usually performed through the most distal joint. Disarticulation preserves the distal growth plates, prevents residual bone overgrowth, and improves weight-bearing ability and the stability of the prosthetic socket on the residual limb. This approach, however, presents the prosthetist with the unique challenge of providing a prosthetic fitting for a very long upper or lower residual limb; optimal component selection is rarely a reality in this situation.

In the upper limb, the placement of myoelectric hardware within the forearm of a very long residual transradial limb is challenging. In the lower limb, prosthetic components that can be aligned are commonplace for adult amputees but are generally contraindicated in pediatric patients because of spatial limitations. The art of attaching a socket to a lamination plate directly with no built in alignment capability continues to be standard practice (**Figure 4**). When a knee disarticulation is performed, the lack of additional clearance for the knee results in a lower knee center than on the contralateral side. In some instances, the knee center can be better approximated by mounting the knee joint posterior to the distal aspect of the limb (**Figure 5**). Any level of knee bending allows for shortening of the overall length of the entire limb, which affords ground clearance for the swing-through phase of gait.

An underlying goal for all clinicians involved in the prosthetic care of children is to ensure that surgical management ultimately leads to the

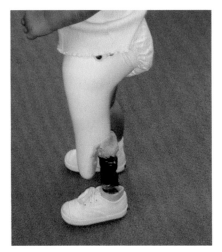

Figure 5 Photograph of a child with a proximal focal femoral deficiency fitted with a single axis knee. The knee center is better approximated by mounting the knee joint posterior to the distal aspect of the limb (on the heel).

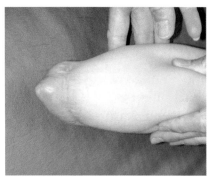

Figure 6 Clinical photograph shows terminal bony overgrowth that will require surgical intervention.

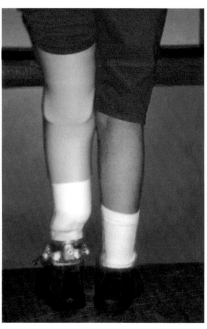

Figure 7 Photograph of a child with a prosthesis designed to provide proper alignment for angular issues. The patient had fracture nonunion and transtibial amputation.

best possible prosthetic outcomes in adulthood. When staged or timed appropriately, growth plate arrests can maintain the functional benefits of distal end bearing while creating increased clearance for prosthetic components over time. Growth plate arrest may be performed in patients treated with knee or ankle disarticulation. This practice of growth plate arrest varies depending on the medical center where the patient is treated, but it can provide the necessary space to allow for superior prosthetic components that would not otherwise be possible because of spatial limitations. The eventual creation of equal knee center heights is often more relevant to the mature amputee because of aesthetic concerns that usually manifest in young adulthood and functional concerns, such as a prosthetic knee that can accommodate the limited legroom on airplanes.

The use of socks to adjust or accommodate changes in limb volume is a common practice in both adult and pediatric patients. Initially, a parent will aid the child in donning and doffing the prosthesis. Proper alignment of the residual limb within the socket is critical for comfort and good function. Socks can range from 1 ply to 5 plies in thickness. Thermoplastic socket designs with frame support allow for increased flexibility and volume control by adjusting the socket with heat if necessary, or adding interface padding behind the inner socket to increase support areas.

In the upper limb, circumferential growth can be accommodated with the use of an onion skin transradial socket design that allows very thin layers of the inner socket to be peeled away. Based on the experience of this chapter's author, a growing infant tends to undergo longitudinal growth while baby fat is slimed or shed. This results in loss of socket suspension caused by the overall circumference reduction of the residual limb. The addition of a silicone upper limb sleeve can address this challenge.

Bony Overgrowth and Angular Deformities

Most elective amputations in children with congenital limb differences are planned to preserve bone growth by preserving the distal growth plates. In patients with traumatic or acquired amputations, a transdiaphysial amputation may be performed, resulting in eventual periosteal overgrowth[8] (**Figure 6**). In general, after bony overgrowth begins, prosthetic wearing tolerance quickly decreases and prosthesis nonuse is common. Very few prosthetic interventions are available to reduce the pain associated with such overgrowth. The presence of a small bursa, detected by palpation, is a classic sign of the onset of overgrowth. These bursae generally require surgical treatment. A number of surgical options are available, and some are more successful than others at preventing recurrences.

Angular deformities are very common in patients with congenital limb deficiencies. In a patient with longitudinal deficiency of the fibula, there is a high incidence of genu valgus, often resulting in angles greater than 35°. However, biomechanical principles dictate that the ground reaction force from a prosthetic foot pass near or through the center of the knee. With an angular deformity at the knee, the foot is outset to accommodate the limb. The resultant medial distal hump can be sizable, and it often poses a challenge in wearing pants. (**Figure 7**). Angular deformities can be treated with either guided growth surgery or osteotomy. Consultation between the

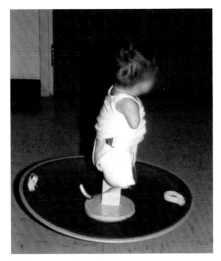

Figure 8 Photograph of a child with quadrilateral amputations using a prosthetic socket with a saucer setup for balance training and core trunk strengthening.

prosthetist and the pediatric orthopaedic surgeon is necessary to determine the need and timing of surgical interventions.

Bilateral Lower Limb Deficiencies

Prosthetic fitting for patients with bilateral lower limb loss requires clinical experience in recognizing the correct prosthetic pathways to optimize outcomes. In general, fitting of a bilateral transtibial or Syme ankle disarticulation prosthesis is initiated when the child reaches the pull-to-stand stage of development. Bilateral prosthetic fitting is similar to unilateral fitting except in alignment challenges. In a child with a bilateral longitudinal deficiency of the fibula, flexed knees are common and must be considered when aligning the prosthesis. Genu valgus may also be present and will require incorporation into the prosthetic alignment.

Patients with bilateral transfemoral amputations or knee disarticulations begin with short nonarticulated stubby prostheses (stubbies) or may start with knees incorporated into the devices. The decision of whether or not to initially add knees requires expertise and sound clinical judgment. The first prosthesis is usually best designed with stubby feet. This strategy provides the child the opportunity to develop balance and coordination with the prosthesis and frees the child's hands for other tasks. Historically, stubby feet were attached to a saucer. The rocker motion provided balance training and core strengthening. Although the saucer technique is now rarely used, it remains a sound viable practice for the quadrilateral amputee (**Figure 8**). After standing stability and good core strength are achieved, adding knees to subsequent prostheses has proven to be an effective transitional step as the child reaches developmental milestones.

Summary

The management of children with limb deficiencies is challenging and complex. Clinical practice guidelines for the pediatric patient are often anecdotal and based heavily on mentoring experiences. A child with bilateral congenital or acquired amputation warrants special consideration. Understanding the physical and physiological differences of a child with a limb deficiency is necessary to optimize prosthetic fittings and provide quality care over the lifetime of the patient.

References

1. Froster UG, Baird PA: Congenital defects of lower limbs and associated malformations: A population based study. *Am J Med Genet* 1993;45(1):60-64.

2. Morrissy RT, Giavedoni B, Coulter-O'Berry C: The limb-deficient child, in Wood W, Winter RB, Morrissy RT, Weinstein SL, eds: *Lovell and Winters Pediatric Orthopaedics.* Philadelphia, PA, Lippincott Williams & Wilkins, 2001, pp 1217-1272.

3. Geil M, Coulter C: Analysis of locomotor adaptations in young children with limb loss in an early prosthetic knee prescription protocol. *Prosthet Orthot Int* 2014;38(1):54-61.

4. Geil M, Coulter-O'Berry C: Temporal and spatial parameters of crawling in children with limb loss: Implications on prosthetic knee prescription. *J Prosthet Orthot* 2010;22(1):21-25.

5. Geil MD, Coulter-O'Berry C, Schmitz M, Heriza C: Crawling kinematics in an early knee protocol for pediatric prosthetic prescription. *J Prosthet Orthot* 2013;25(1):22-29.

6. Crandall RC, Tomhave W: Pediatric unilateral below-elbow amputees: Retrospective analysis of 34 patients given multiple prosthetic options. *J Pediatr Orthop* 2002;22(3):380-383.

7. Atkins D: A one year retrospective overview of partial hand patients using ProDigits. *Proceedings of the MEC'11 conference, UNB; 2011.* Available at: http://dukespace.lib.duke.edu/dspace/handle/10161/4760. Accessed October 9, 2015.

8. Aitken GT, Pellicore RJ: Introduction to the child amputee, in *American Academy of Orthopaedic Surgeons: Atlas of Limb Prosthetics: Surgical and Prosthetic Principles.* St. Louis, MO, Mosby-Year Book, 1981, pp 493-500.

Chapter 66

Occupational Therapy for the Child With an Upper Limb Deficiency

Wendy Hill, BScOT   Vivian J. Yip, OTD, OTR/L

Abstract

Comprehensive care of a child with an upper limb difference includes occupational therapy. To provide the best outcomes for this patient population, it is helpful to review prosthetic and nonprosthetic care and prosthetic and therapy options, as well as understand the role of the occupational therapist. The importance of family-centered care and involvement of a comprehensive team should be recognized. Considerations are needed to accommodate the uniqueness of each child, family, and situation.

Keywords: acquired amputation; congenital limb loss; limb difference; limb loss; occupational therapy; pediatric; prosthetics; training; upper limb deficiency

Introduction

Children are adaptable. A child born without an arm or a hand, with a limb difference, or who has an acquired upper limb amputation is capable of learning how to complete necessary tasks and participate in desired activities. If children are fitted with a prosthesis at an early age, encouraged to wear it, and taught how to use it, they will learn how to accomplish important activities using the prosthesis. If a child chooses not to wear a prosthesis, he or she will learn to do these activities in other ways, often using other parts of the body to compensate for the missing limb.

Unilateral congenital transradial limb deficiency is a common level of limb loss seen in pediatric prosthetic clinics throughout the world.[1-4] The treatment of upper limb deficiency differs slightly from clinic to clinic, but most clinics offer prosthetic fitting as a common treatment option for

children. Regardless of the decision to elect or decline a prosthetic fitting, the child should be regularly evaluated by the management team. The team of specialists in an upper limb clinic can assess the child as he or she develops and address concerns or issues that may arise. Experienced clinicians can be identified through the Association of Children's Prosthetic and Orthotic Clinics (ACPOC). This organization promotes multidisciplinary team development and collaboration and supports research and education for professionals involved in caring for children who need orthopaedic interventions.[5] Information on clinical teams who provide care for children with limb differences is available from ACPOC and can serve as an additional resource.

The prosthetic options for children with upper limb loss include passive or cosmetic prostheses, body-powered or cable-activated prostheses, and

externally powered prostheses. When children become involved in extracurricular activities and sports, more than one type of prosthesis may be required. Children who are fitted with a prosthesis often have an active-grasping prosthesis for daily use and may also have a passive prosthesis with activity-specific recreational attachments or a passive cosmetic option.

It is important to be aware of the psychological effect experienced by a family or a child with a limb deficiency. The desire to have a prosthesis may be rooted in the child's or the family's desire to appear "normal" to the outside world, possibly to avoid stares and questions from strangers or to assuage the guilt parents may feel regarding the cause of the limb deficiency. A prosthesis may help the child and/or the family come to terms with the child's condition, and a cosmetic prosthesis may promote comfort in social situations.

As children age, they will decide if they need a prosthesis and what type of prosthesis they prefer. Being fit with prostheses during childhood allows the exploration of various options and provides experience on which to base prosthetic decisions later in life.

The Team and First Assessment

The members of the clinical team will vary depending on the clinic but may consist of a physician (pediatrician or physical medicine specialist), an orthopaedic surgeon, a prosthetist, an occupational therapist (OT), a physical therapist, a social worker, a case

Neither of the following authors nor any immediate family member has received anything of value from or has stock or stock options held in a commercial company or institution related directly or indirectly to the subject of this chapter: Ms. Hill and Dr. Yip.

manager, a child-life therapist, a nutritionist, a psychologist, and a psychiatrist. The first encounter with the clinical team can be intimidating for families, so it is important not to overwhelm them by introducing too many care providers at the initial meeting. One of the main goals of the first meeting is to build rapport with the family and child because the clinic may be providing care for many years. Some clinics treat children until they are 18 years of age, whereas others follow the patient into adulthood. If the family is having difficulty accepting or coping with the limb loss, further psychosocial counselling should be recommended.

Pediatric care involves the entire family unit. The activities or interests that are important to the family will form the basis of the child's treatment by the team. If the family wants the child to be fit with a prosthesis, information and appropriate prosthetic options should be presented by the prosthetist and/or the OT. When funding is secured, the prosthetist will begin building an appropriate prosthesis. The OT typically has a role in evaluating the child as he or she works with a temporary prosthesis and may provide feedback to assist the prosthetist so that the device can be fabricated in the most ideal functional position. The child and the family will then attend prosthetic training sessions with the OT to learn how to use the prosthesis and incorporate it into daily activities.

The role of an OT is to maximize independence in occupations (meaningful and purposeful everyday life activities).[6] These include the activities of daily living (ADLs) and the instrumental activities of daily living (IADLs). ADLs are activities oriented toward taking care of one's own body. For a child, this may include bathing, grooming, hygiene, toileting, dressing, and feeding. IADLs may include play participation, exploration, school activities, and social participation with peers and the community.[6] As

Table 1 Items That May Be Included in the Team Assessment
Birth history
Medical history
Previous therapy interventions
Health history of parents, siblings, and other extended family members who may have a limb difference
Developmental status
Cognitive function
School-grade level and performance
Socioeconomic status of parents and/or guardians
Family and child's daily routine
History of the patient's use of a prosthesis if one was previously used
Activities of daily living assessment and instrumental activities of daily living assessment—how they are completed (with assistance, using equipment, age appropriateness)
Identification of individuals who provide the most care for the patient
Patient and parent social skills, thoughts about limb difference, coping skills and techniques
Inspection of the residual and sound limbs related to skin integrity, residual limb length, pain, edema, bony prominences, range of motion, and strength
Discussion of interests, goals, and the things the family wants the child to accomplish (with or without a prosthesis) (aesthetics versus function)
Information about prostheses and other adaptive equipment and strategies, as appropriate

children develop, these activities will change and may include participation in hobbies, sports, and work activities. The OT provides skilled services in collaboration with the family and the team to facilitate full engagement in the child's everyday life activities. For a child with upper limb loss, the OT assists the family in solving problems in accomplishing ADLs and/or IADLs with or without a prosthesis. The OT evaluates the development, behavior, and performance skills of the child to establish family-centered goals and interventions and provides information and resources to educate the family so that the child can work toward optimal participation in ADLs and IADLs.

The involvement of other team members can help the family to accept and cope with the limb difference. The OT will follow the child's development, help the parents focus on the child's strengths and abilities, and address concerns about the child's ability to participate in future activities.[7] Many aspects of the child's life, health,[8] and relationships may be included in the team assessment (**Table 1**).

Unilateral Transradial Deficiency

Prosthetic Considerations

When a family decides to pursue prosthetic fitting for their child, the options for appropriate types of prostheses should be presented at the first consultation appointment and at subsequent appointments over the years as new technologies or components become available. The options for a prosthesis are dependent on the age of the child, the level of amputation, and the availability of funding. Practice guidelines vary regarding the age when the first prosthesis is prescribed. A 2006 review of the literature determined that the age of the first fitting varied worldwide, with the age ranging from 2 months to 25 months.[9] The aim of the study was to determine if fitting a prosthesis before 2 years of age was related to lower rates of rejection and better functional outcomes at an older age. The authors concluded that the currently used guidelines for prosthetic prescription procedures are based on experience, not on evidence.

Shaperman[10] conducted a survey of fitting practices for children with transradial limb loss in pediatric prosthetic clinics throughout North America. She concluded that most children with unilateral transradial limb absence have their first fitting when they can sit (approximately at age 6 months) and are later fit with an active-grasping prosthesis when the child demonstrates awareness of cause and effect and attempts to hold objects (between ages 10 and 18 months). Because there is limited evidence-based research on the best age for fitting the first prosthesis, it is important to collaborate with the child's parents to determine what is in the best interest of their child and family.

There are various reasons why children with congenital upper limb differences may be fitted with a prosthesis at different ages or stages of development. The home situation may be overwhelming for some families, and they may be unable to comply with the requirements of prosthetic care when the child is a toddler. A family may want to wait until the child is able to verbalize his or her wants and needs or may not have access to care when the child is young. Regardless of the reason, prosthetic fitting in an older child has its own considerations. The child will likely be able to express his or her opinions, and his or her level of motivation will need to be considered. It is likely that an older child will have adapted to efficiently completing ADLs with compensatory techniques and will not find a prosthesis useful for these tasks. If fitted, the child may only consider a cosmetic option for special occasions or an activity-specific

prosthesis to participate in sports or recreational pursuits of particular interest. If the child decides to incorporate an active prosthetic option into ADLs and IADLs, he or she must be prepared to allot time for training with the prosthesis to achieve proficient use.

The First Passive Prosthesis

The goals of fitting the first passive upper limb prosthesis at an early age are twofold. First and foremost, it allows the family to establish a consistent wearing pattern and become accustomed to incorporating the prosthesis into the family's lifestyle. When a child age 2 or 3 years is fit with a prosthesis for the first time, parents often must struggle to keep the prosthesis on the child. This may be because the child is accustomed to using his or her residual limb in daily activities and the added weight and heat of the prosthesis forces the child to do tasks in an unfamiliar manner. Second, a prosthesis that is fitted around the time the child is mastering sitting can be incorporated into the acquisition of gross motor skills. It provides length extension and support on the missing side to aid with sitting balance, reaching forward while sitting, prone play, crawling, and pulling to a standing position (**Figure 1**).

When a child wears a prosthesis as a regular part of the daily routine, he or she learns to manipulate toys in the true midline of the body, instead of a skewed midline closer to the missing limb when a prosthesis in not worn. The prosthesis helps establish a more upright posture from a young age and encourages body symmetry. The neuronal group selection theory of brain development described by Meurs et al[9] implies that if a child wears a prosthesis during the early phases of development, a representation of the limb with a prosthesis will be established in the brain. If the prosthesis is used as the child develops motor skills, the child will have motor functioning abilities with and without

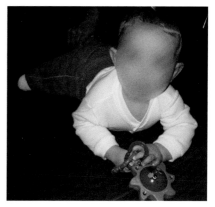

Figure 1 Photograph of a child with a passive upper limb prosthesis that provides support in prone play.

the prosthesis.[9] The clinical experiences of the authors of this chapter reinforce this theory because children who establish an early prosthesis wearing pattern tend to incorporate the use of the device into their daily routines and use it to accomplish daily tasks.

The prosthetist and OT provide the parents with a home program when the passive prosthesis is fitted. This program should include instructions for initial wearing time and how to progress to full-time wear. At the Atlantic Clinic for Upper Limb Prosthetics, New Brunswick, Canada, full-time wear is considered all waking hours, with removal of the prosthesis for napping and bathing. The parents should monitor the child for signs (such as localized areas of redness around the brim of the socket or on the distal end of the residual limb) that the prosthesis is becoming too small and in need of adjustment.

The home program should also provide instruction for hygiene and cleaning of the residual limb and the prosthesis. The inner socket should be cleaned daily with a soft, moist cloth (with a mix of soap and water or alcohol and water) or a baby wipe. The outside of the prosthesis should be cleaned as often as the child's hand is cleaned, such as when there is obvious dirt or food on it. Certain types of prosthetic gloves are more prone to staining than others. If there is a polyvinyl chloride glove covering the hand, it will be easily stained by food dyes, ink, clothing dyes, and other agents. Stains should be cleaned promptly with alcohol or they will be very difficult to remove. Many of the newer prosthetic hands and gloves for children are made of silicone and do not stain easily.

As part of a home program, it is helpful to include a list of toys or activities that will encourage use of the prosthetic arm in bimanual play. If the child does not pay attention to the side with the prosthesis, interesting toys can be attached over the hand with straps or handles. Toys that can be placed in the mouth or that make noise may be highly interesting to very young children. A fun game can be made by placing toys with large handles on the prosthetic hand and encouraging the child to remove them. The child can be encouraged to hold down a toy with the prosthesis while playing with or manipulating the toy with the other hand. Deep pots or buckets filled with blocks or smaller toys to dump or pick up are fun for some children. Playing with large balls or large stuffed animals encourages bimanual arm use, as does playing pat-a-cake or other rhyming songs with arm gestures.

Regular follow-up with the family is essential to monitor progress with the wearing schedule, comfort, and fit of the prosthesis as well as the child's achievement of developmental milestones. These will be factors in deciding when to fit the next prosthesis. If the prosthesis is too snug before the child is considered developmentally ready, the prosthesis can be lengthened or the socket can be adjusted to allow more time for the development of gross motor skills and improved cognitive readiness.

It is important that the fitting process does not have unnecessary delays that would leave the child without a prosthesis after a wearing schedule has been established. If possible, the fitting for a new prosthesis should be started before the previous device has been completely outgrown. This will ensure any progress made in wearing and using the prosthesis is not lost.

The First Active Prosthesis

The appropriate time to fit a child with the first active prostheses varies among practitioners and in different parts of the world. Some centers follow a developmental approach to fitting a child with a myoelectric hand, meaning that the child is considered ready if he or she is cognitively ready and is walking and no longer requires arm extension for balance. Other centers fit a body-powered prosthesis when the child meets their readiness criteria; an externally powered prosthesis would be considered if the child proves to be a good user of the body-powered device. In Germany, the family is given the choice of either a myoelectric or body-powered prosthesis when the child is between the ages of 2 and 4 years.[11] In the United Kingdom, prosthetic centers follow guidelines established by the British Society for Rehabilitation Medicine. These guidelines recommend fitting children for a first passive prosthesis between the ages of 4 to 15 months, and then fitting the first active prosthesis, either a body-powered device or a myoelectric device, between the ages of 15 months and 3 years.[12]

When a child has outgrown the passive prosthesis and is considered ready for a prosthesis with active prehension, the team, including the family, must determine what type of prosthesis will best meet the child's needs. To ensure the child's success with an active prehension prosthesis, the family must be committed to attending the training appointments and complying with the requirements of the home program.

Body-Powered Prostheses for Young Children

When the child has outgrown the first passive prosthesis and/or has demonstrated a readiness to use a terminal device for grasping, an active-grasping prosthesis should be considered. The criteria to determine readiness are as follows: (1) the child can follow simple one- or two-step directions; (2) he or she has an attention span of at least 5-10 minutes; (3) the child attempts to put objects in his or her hand or the terminal device; and (4) the child tolerates being handled by the OT.[13,14]

During general development, the child may be ready for formal training between 20 and 26 months of age.[13,14] The child's behavior, ability to attend to simple instructions, and motor development will influence the progress during prosthetic training. A home program for the family will guide parents in how to assist the child in learning the control motions of opening and closing the terminal device and promote follow-through with using the prosthesis.

Toddlers with a transradial deficiency are typically fit with the elbow preflexed in the socket. This allows the terminal device to be in a midline position without the child exerting much effort, and the prosthesis will be prepositioned adequately for two-handed activities. When the prosthesis is positioned with the elbow in extension, which is more appropriate for adults or older children, toddlers tend to ignore the prosthesis, and more effort is needed for appropriate midline use of the prosthesis.[13,14] A well-balanced harness that is slightly snug and does not have a center ring will help the very young child easily learn the control motion.

Initial prosthetic training should begin at a height-appropriate table for the child to learn the basic control motion. The OT should sit behind the child and use both hands, one hand on the shoulder joint for stabilization and one hand on the forearm of the prosthesis to assist with humeral flexion for opening the terminal device[13,14] (**Figure 2**). The therapist should call attention to the open terminal device with verbal cues. The child is encouraged to use the sound hand to place an object in the open terminal device while the OT guides the prosthesis from humeral flexion to humeral extension to close the terminal device securely on the object. It is important to use repetitive bimanual tasks to teach the control motion, including activities such as stringing beads, opening nesting barrels, and opening markers. The child should be encouraged to use the prosthesis for gross motor activities and all daily tasks.

As the child progresses and understands the basic control motion, he or she needs to learn various prosthetic skills and refinements. These include prepositioning the terminal device, accurate placement of objects inside the terminal device, opening the terminal device close to the body, keeping the terminal device closed when reaching forward, and refining the basic control motion to include shoulder abduction. All of these skills are learned by the child through practice and performing age-appropriate bimanual activities on a daily basis and during prosthetic training with the OT. Training activities and functional tasks described in the following section on externally powered prostheses also can be used in body-powered prosthesis training.

Externally Powered Prostheses for Young Children

Externally powered prostheses generally refer to those devices operated using myoelectric control. However, activation also can be accomplished with switches, touchpads, or linear transducers. Children with longitudinal deficiencies who have digits at the distal end of the residual limb may prefer to use the movement they have in the distal end to push against or activate a switch or touchpad to control a prosthetic hand.

Egermann et al[11] described the following keys to success in a pediatric upper limb prosthetic rehabilitation program. A myoelectric prosthesis should be fitted at a specialized center,

and the child should be managed by a specialized multidisciplinary team. The child should train with an OT and be regularly monitored to assess use of the prosthesis and for changing prosthetic needs. The center should provide timely support for maintenance and repair of the prosthesis.

Myoelectrode Site Selection
When fitting a young child with the first myoelectric prosthesis, a simple one-muscle system is often used to operate the hand. When the muscle is contracted, the hand opens. When the muscle is not contracting, the hand closes and remains closed. This is often referred to as the "cookie crusher" control strategy. Initially, the electrode sensitivity will be set quite high so that any activity of the muscle will cause the hand to open. This is intentional because it draws attention to the hand and reinforces the cause-effect concept.

When fitting a toddler or very young child with a myoelectric prosthesis, finding appropriate muscle sites to place an electrode is generally not challenging. The muscles can be palpated during the assessment; however, the electrode is generally placed on the forearm extensors close to the lateral epicondyle. The size of the standard electrode will usually encompass much of the extensor muscle belly, producing a strong signal when the muscle is contracted.

During the appointment to select the myoelectrode site, it is a good idea to place an electrode on the forearm in the approximate location on the extensor muscle and secure it with a cuff or strap if the child allows. A single-function toy modified to operate with a standard electrode can be used to establish the cause-effect concept at this early stage. A toy that lights up, makes sounds, or moves is highly reinforcing for young children (**Figure 3**). When the child is asked to wiggle his or her "little arm," the child sees that something happens as a result. This will encourage the child

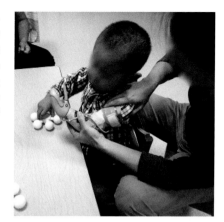

Figure 2 Clinical photograph of a therapist positioning a transradial prosthesis to assist with terminal device operation.

to continue to activate the muscle to see the resulting action of the toy. This technique works well when the child is sitting quietly, either with the parents or with the OT, and is able to attend to the toy. A small room with a limited number of people is recommended for this training. The OT may want to gently hold the child's forearm when he or she is being asked to wiggle it so the child does not wiggle the whole arm instead of the muscles in the forearm. A child's prosthetic hand also can be used in place of the toy for the purpose of site selection and cause-effect training. Some children respond well to a prosthetic hand as opposed to a toy; however, because the hand is not attached to the child's forearm, operating a hand this way is still an abstract concept and may not generalize into the ability to control the prosthetic hand after the prosthesis is fabricated.

When the child is old enough to have a sustained attention span of at least 10 minutes and the ability to follow simple instructions, the myoelectrode site selection process and socket fitting can take place with the aid of computer software. Several manufacturers have software for evaluating and visualizing muscle signals, but the MyoBoy tester (Ottobock) is most often used for pediatric patients because it is the only software with a

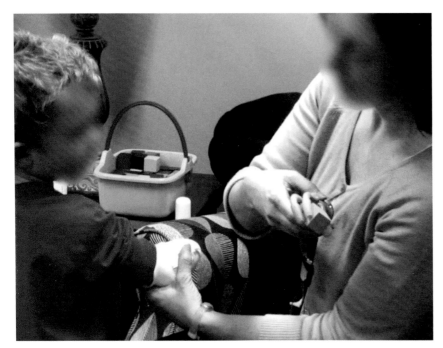

Figure 3 Clinical photograph of a therapist using a test socket with a prosthetic hand during myoelectrode site selection.

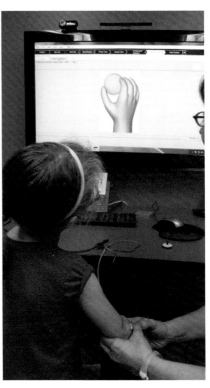

Figure 4 Clinical photograph of a therapist working with a child to determine myoelectrode site selection using computer software. The child can see a virtual hand moving in real time as the electrode is activated.

virtual child's prosthetic hand.[15] The MyoBoy tester allows muscle signals to be viewed in real time, and the child can see a virtual hand moving in real time as he or she activates the electrode (**Figure 4**). If the child can isolate the muscle on command, the electrode sensitivity can be adjusted to an appropriate level, eliminating guesswork. For young children, the computer software may not be motivating, so attention will be quickly lost. If this happens, it is more important to know that the child understands the concept of contracting the muscle to cause something to happen than to sit for extended periods of time practicing this control. It may be necessary to distract the child with other toys or games to ensure that he or she keeps the socket on long enough to ensure a good fit and intimate contact with the electrode.

Control Training
When a toddler is fit with the first active-grasping prosthesis, it will likely be used in a passive manner initially. It is important to manage the expectations of the parents so they do not assume that the child will immediately be able to pick up objects with the prosthesis and manipulate them voluntarily. This will occur gradually over time and will require regular prompting and intervention by the parents and/or the OT.

When the prosthesis is completed and the prosthetist is satisfied with the fit and suspension, training can begin. Training should occur in a small but comfortable room with the parents, child, and OT; the number of distracting toys or people should be limited. Toys or objects brought in for training should be kept out of sight until needed by the OT. If the child is shy or anxious, he or she can be seated on a parent's lap. If comfortable with the OT, the child can be seated on the floor facing the OT or at a small child-size table. The OT may at times want to be behind the child to hold the prosthesis or to demonstrate actions.

The child is asked to wiggle the "little arm" within the socket. If the parents use different terminology to refer to the residual limb, the OT should use the familiar term so the child understands the instructions. Sometimes, using a sticker on the outside of the socket close to the distal end of the residual limb on the side where the electrode is located can help the child understand the motion required. The child can be asked to try to "touch" the sticker or move toward it with the little arm. When he or she sees that the hand moves, it will reinforce the muscle movement. The OT should draw attention to the movement of the hand when the child activates the muscle. Repetition is important at this early stage. The OT should continue to ask the child to wiggle or move toward the sticker, and the child should be praised for opening the hand. The child's attention span will dictate how long this training will last.

If the child opens the hand consistently, small toys, such as blocks, play animals, plastic rings, and colorful paper, can be placed in the opened hand to maintain interest. Often the child will want to remove the object from the hand. By extending the arm to pull a toy away, the extensor muscles will contract causing the hand to open. This also reinforces the control of the hand. If the child enjoys the repetitiveness of dropping toys on the floor, the game of putting objects in the hand and having the child drop them can be a fun training activity.

At the first myoelectric prosthesis fittings, it is helpful to have a parental access switch incorporated into the prosthesis in a discreet location on the forearm. This switch bypasses the electrode and will allow the parents or OT to open the hand to place objects inside or help release an object if the child becomes frustrated. This is especially helpful if the child is attempting to grasp an object and cannot maintain the contraction long enough to place it in his or her hand or if the hand is stuck on an object or the child's clothing.

When the child wants to move around the room, toys with handles, such as ride-on toys (a rocking horse or tricycle) or push-toys (grocery carts, strollers, or toy lawnmowers), should be introduced. These toys encourage bimanual play. It is safer and easier to hold on with both hands while on a ride-on toy. If the child allows, the OT or parent should help position the prosthetic hand on the handle of the toy. It is important to let the child explore using the hand in his or her own way for periods of time and watch closely for opportunities to intervene. When the OT helps to position the hand on objects or handles, it demonstrates to the child how the hand can be useful. This is important even if the child is not at a stage when he or she can consistently open the hand when asked. By pointing out these opportunities to parents during training sessions, the OT can reinforce how the parent can continue training in the home environment.

With very young children, it is important to give frequent breaks during training or to have multiple short training sessions. The OT must recognize signs of resistance and judge when to push the child to attempt to use the hand and when to pull back and allow the child to play independently. If the OT is too demanding, the child may pull the arm away or hide it behind his or her back and use only the sound arm for play. Training progress can be lost if the child resists wearing the arm or bringing it into play because people are paying too much attention to the activation of the hand.

If the child is resistant to training strategies to open the hand, it is best to let the child explore through play and use the prosthesis passively as he or she has done in the past. This will allow the child to become comfortable with the weight and size of the prosthetic arm and the sounds that occur when the hand is opened. If cognitive awareness is present and the OT is confident that the child has made the connection between contracting the muscle and activating the hand, success has been achieved. This may be the only expectation at the first training session. Some children make the connection within the first 10 minutes of training, whereas others may need several sessions to fully understand how to activate the hand.

Over the course of weeks or months through a detailed home program and the support of the OT, the child is expected to progress from using the hand passively to using it actively. The process of learning to use a myoelectric hand can be categorized into the following stages that require specific skills.[16,17] (1) The awareness that moving the muscle causes the prosthetic hand to open and close. (2) The ability to open the hand on command, although the child tends to use it passively for support. (3) The child attempts to place objects in the hand or position the hand but requires assistance or support because of

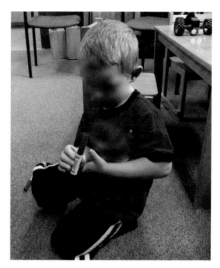

Figure 5 Clinical photograph of a boy using body support for the initial control of a terminal device.

the weight of the prosthesis. Support may be provided by the side of the body (**Figure 5**), a tabletop, the parent, the OT, or someone else. (4) The ability to successfully grasp objects spontaneously, without needing support for the weight of the prosthesis. (5) The ability to hold and carry objects while keeping muscles quiet and releasing objects when desired (**Figure 6**). (6) The ability to grasp objects in various positions around the body and at different heights. (7) The ability to coordinate use of both hands smoothly and spontaneously. (8) The ability to adjust the opening width of the prosthetic hand based on the size and softness of the object being grasped (grasping delicate objects without crushing them). (9) The ability to grasp and/or release objects while the arm is moving or the object is moving (**Figure 7**). (10) The ability to grasp, hold, or release objects when not looking at the hand.

Children progress at different rates, and their individual personalities and age of maturation are factors in how they use their prostheses. Some children learn to activate the hand and will do this when commanded or reminded; however, they tend to use the prosthesis in a passive manner most

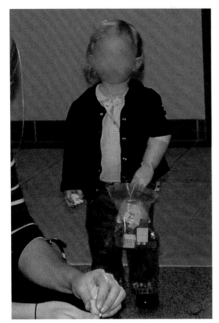

Figure 6 Photograph of a child carrying an object with her prosthetic hand. The muscle must be kept quiet to prevent release of the object.

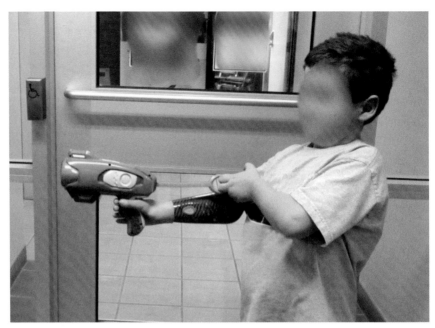

Figure 7 Photograph of a child controlling a terminal device while his arm is in motion.

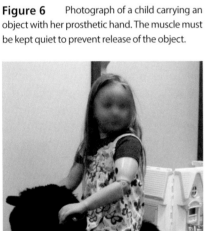

Figure 8 Clinical photograph of a child using a rocking horse, a toy that encourages bimanual play.

Table 2 Suggested Activities to Encourage Bimanual Play

Holding onto a rolling pin to roll out dough

Pinch dough to make marks

Hold handles on push toys, such as a stroller, a grocery cart, or a lawnmower

Hold onto riding toys, such as bouncers, tricycles, or a play car with a steering wheel

Hold containers, such as a bag of chips, a box of raisins, a bottle of bubbles, a bag of toys, a small pail for sand and water

Hold a pot to stir

Hold a bag or purse to put items in or to empty

Play with two-handed musical instruments, such as a toy drum, maracas, and cymbals

of the time. Others require very little prompting to use the hand for grasping and will routinely use it to complete bimanual tasks, although they still will require assistance to position the wrist appropriately.

Much of the training and progression of skills occurs at home. The home program should reinforce what has been discussed during training sessions, such as expectations for wearing and using the prosthesis, care and maintenance information, and the implementation of suggested activities that encourage use of the prosthesis. Some activities to encourage bimanual play (**Figure 8**) are described in **Table 2**.

When activities are chosen for training, it is important to note the opening width of the prosthetic hand. All items should easily fit into the prosthetic hand for bimanual play, including handles on toys. The smallest size prosthetic hands have a limited opening width. Parents should be made aware that the smallest size prosthetic hands have a limited opening width and should take this into account when purchasing toys for the home.

Subsequent Prostheses and Changing Control Strategies

As the child develops and ages, the ability to follow instructions improves and the possibilities for controlling a prosthesis also increase. When the first myoelectric prosthesis is outgrown, a decision must be made about when to introduce a two-muscle control system. Children are usually ready to switch to a two-site control system at 4 years of age or older. At this point, they have better control over movement of the distal end of the residual limb and have generally outgrown the behavioral challenges characteristic of many 2- and 3-year-old children. Their attention spans are longer and they follow instructions well. The age for introducing a two-muscle control system is variable because it depends on how well the child has learned to control the one-muscle system and how well the prosthesis has been integrated into daily use at home. If the child continues to require prompting to use the hand for grasping and struggles with consistent control, it is not appropriate to switch to a more difficult control strategy.

When introducing a two-muscle control system, the forearm extensors and flexors are used if possible. The child must learn to activate and relax each muscle separately for independent control of the opening and closing functions of the hand. Initially, the OT should explain to the child how to move the residual limb to activate the muscles by flexing and extending the wrist on the intact arm. For some children, asking them to close their eyes and move both sides in the same manner will help them to achieve this technique. For some children, holding the residual limb and asking them to make a muscle on one side of the arm and then the other will be effective. For others who have soft tissue or nubbins at the end of the residual limb, it is helpful to draw a face on the end of the arm and have them move the tissue in different ways to make changes to the face. This may reinforce the desired muscle action.

When the muscle bellies can be palpated and the child understands the action required to contract both muscles, visual feedback can be very helpful to practice the motions. Computer software can be used to show signals or a virtual hand in real time.[15] Initially, it is useful to show the signals and have the child concentrate on making contractions with one muscle and then the

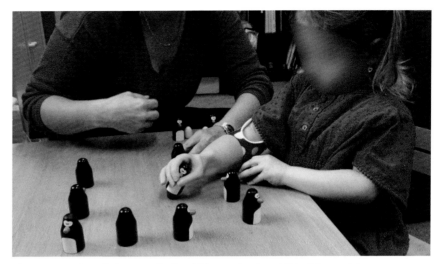

Figure 9 Clinical photograph of a child engaging in a skill-building activity to encourage repetitive use of her prosthetic hand.

other. There are training games within the software that reinforce sustaining signal strength while relaxing the opposing muscle. Frequent breaks may be required during training because of muscle fatigue. If the computer software is confusing or too abstract for the child, a prosthetic hand can be used at this stage of training.

In some children with congenital limb loss, the anatomy of the musculature in the residual limb is not the same as the intact limb and sometimes there are co-contractions of the extensor and flexor muscles. This may delay the change to a two-site control strategy or it may make it impossible to make the change. In these cases, alternative control strategies can be considered, depending on the prosthetic components being used. For example, in a rate-sensitive control system, a big or fast contraction of a muscle opens the hand and a small or slow contraction of the same muscle closes the hand. The Vario (Ottobock) one-muscle control system operates much like a "cookie crusher" system but provides proportional control over the speed of opening the hand by contracting the muscle and proportional control over closing the hand by the rate of muscle relaxation. When the child is able to use

these alternative control methods, he or she will have finer control of opening and closing the hand. This allows more confidence when using the hand for everyday activities.

Progression of Training

When the basic operation of the hand has been mastered, the use of the hand can be refined. Activities presented in therapy should initially require repetition to ensure that the hand is working properly and that the child is consistently able to open and close the hand. Some ideas for initial skill-building activities include moving or stacking blocks or cones, playing tic-tac-toe with wooden blocks, playing board games that require the movement of objects (**Figure 9**), and removing caps from markers for coloring. During these initial skill-building activities, the arm may require support from the OT or the child to remove the weight factor when activating the hand. These activities encourage the child to use the hand in a dominant manner and provide opportunities to operate the hand. If the activities are motivating and fun, most children will willingly participate. When the fit of the prosthesis and function of the hand are deemed to be satisfactory, training can continue using functional activities to

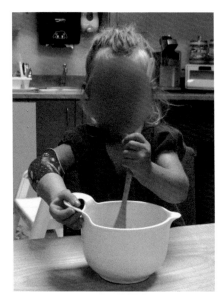

Figure 10 Photograph of a child stirring a pot. This task provides bimanual functional activity training.

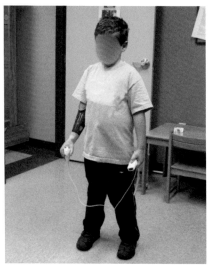

Figure 11 Clinical photograph of a child demonstrates that active video games requiring movement in three dimensions can be used to provide function training that encourages movement of both arms.

reinforce more natural use of the hand in the home environment.

Functional Activity Training

Training activities should be fun and relevant to the child's age and developmental level. For preschool-age children, imaginative play and gross motor activities are popular. Tabletop and gross motor activities should vary to keep the child's interest and attention. Children at this age enjoy many activities, such as drawing; coloring; building with construction blocks; blowing bubbles; playing simple card games; pretend play in a kitchen, workshop, or grocery store; dressing in costumes or adult clothing; parachute games; playing with dolls or stuffed animals; making objects with dough; and participating in outdoor playground activities. Self-care skills, such as fastening buttons, zippers, or laces, can be practiced by dressing up in oversized clothes or dressing and undressing dolls or stuffed animals. This is easier for the children initially, and they can progress to practicing these skills on themselves.

As children approach school age, attention should be given to skills required in the school setting such as cutting with scissors, tying shoelaces independently, starting zippers on coats, and stabilizing and opening bags with zippers and individually wrapped snack items. Outdoor play and learning to skip rope are important as well.

Children near school age or slightly older may enjoy time spent baking or helping to prepare snacks or food. Younger children may be able to hold a bowl and stir to make pudding (**Figure 10**) or roll out dough to make cookies. Many bimanual tasks can be practiced in the kitchen, such as opening packages, measuring, pouring, cutting food, washing hands and dishes, spreading out a tablecloth, putting on an apron, and wrapping and putting away food.

One of the factors to consider in training is whether the prosthesis will stay on the child and function appropriately when the child is active and sweating. Games or sports involving running and full-body movement can be used to evaluate this concern. Racquet

sports such as badminton and tennis or catching and throwing games are a good choice because they require the use of both hands. Swinging, playing on a teeter-totter, and climbing up ladders or rope walls are also good choices. When space is limited or the child prefers video games, active games that require movement in three dimensions can be effective in encouraging children to use both hands to hold remotes while moving in a limited space (**Figure 11**).

Unilateral Transhumeral and Shoulder Disarticulation-Level Deficiencies

First Passive Prosthesis: Fitting and Training

The choice of whether or not to fit a child with a unilateral transhumeral or shoulder disarticulation congenital deficiency with a prosthesis is the same as for children with a unilateral transradial deficiency. If the family is motivated to pursue prosthetic fitting, committed to attending follow-up appointments for therapy, and amenable to participating in a home program for the child, a passive fitting can be considered at the same developmental timeframe as that previously described for a child with a transradial deficiency. The goal of the first prosthesis is to establish a wearing pattern, accustom the child to the weight of the prosthesis, and include it during play.

A passive prosthesis at this deficiency level consists of an intimately fitted socket, a humeral segment, a passive friction elbow, a forearm segment, a wrist, and a terminal device. The terminal device options include a passive hand, a mitt, or a voluntary-opening terminal device (for example, a passive hook or Child Amputee Prosthetics Project terminal device [CAPP TD#1] with an adult to assist with passive grasping ability).

A passive arm with a friction elbow and wrist can provide support and help with balance as a child learns to sit and, eventually, to walk. It should be worn throughout the child's waking hours as long as it does not interfere with gross motor skills. Most children with a limb loss at this level will not crawl on all four limbs. They usually learn to scoot on their bottoms and use other methods to transition to a prone posture or standing. A physical therapist may be consulted if there is a delay in the child achieving gross motor milestones. The parent will need to position the forearm of the prosthesis for various activities. For example, the elbow should be in an extended position to help with balance in sitting or when reaching forward to play. When the child begins walking, the elbow should be positioned in extension to help with balance. When the child is comfortable walking, he or she can be encouraged to bring the terminal device forward to push or carry large items.

The First Active Prosthesis
The readiness criteria used for determining when to transition to an active prosthesis for the child with a transhumeral limb loss is the same as for the transradial level. The prosthesis is intended to be used as an assisting or "helper" hand. This is especially true when referring to higher-level upper limb loss. As the function of more joints needs to be replaced, it becomes more complicated and time consuming to control these motions. For children with a deficiency at the transhumeral level, elbow flexion and extension, wrist rotation, and hand grasp and release need to be considered. When fitting a child, especially with the first active-grasping prosthesis, the hand or terminal device will be the focus of control, with the other joints remaining as passive friction joints that are manually positioned.

Body-Powered Prosthesis: Transhumeral Level
The first transhumeral prosthesis for a young child will operate with a single control cable. It is initially easier for a young child to focus only on operating the terminal device and then learn how to operate the elbow lock at a later stage. The same control motions (shoulder flexion and extension) are used for transradial and transhumeral prostheses. After the child has learned how to consistently open and close the terminal device on objects, prepositioning of the wrist and elbow or forearm are introduced. The length of the residual limb will affect the type of prosthetic elbow used. There are two types of elbow units available for children–an internal elbow with a turntable and an elbow with outside joints. The elbow joint with a turntable is used if an older child is able to tolerate the extra weight and if the residual arm length is short enough to accommodate the size of the component. The overall length of the prosthesis should not compromise the child's comfort and functional position at a table when performing two-handed activities. A young child is usually fit with outside elbow joints with a pull tab to lock and unlock the elbow when the child is not developmentally ready and does not have adequate shoulder depression and extension to activate the elbow lock from the control strap on the harness. The child or an adult caring for the child can activate the pull tab to preposition the elbow for activities.

An older child who is able to use his or her sound hand on the pull tab to activate the elbow lock can use his or her ipsilateral leg or a table to assist with prepositioning the forearm. If an older child has adequate shoulder depression and extension, the elbow lock control strap may be attached to the harness. The child may initially need hands-on assistance to learn the control motions of shoulder depression and extension. The terminal device at the wrist will be prepositioned in the same way as for a transradial prosthesis. For example, the terminal device with be rotated upward (supinating the terminal device instead of upward and downward movement) for holding cards or rotating it downward (pronating the terminal device) for holding onto a rolling pin or a bike handle.

The developmental readiness criteria that should be met before adding a dual-control cable system are usually accomplished at age 4 to 5 years and include (1) mastering operation of the terminal device; (2) ability to tolerate one full rubber band on the hook; (3) understanding the control motion for elbow lifting and locking; and (4) attaining adequate strength and range of motion to operate the dual-control cable system.

The child should be taught the control motions of humeral flexion and scapular abduction. The combination of these two motions helps maintain the forearm in a certain position after lifting. When the elbow is locked, humeral flexion will allow the terminal device to open. When the elbow is unlocked, humeral flexion lifts the forearm and scapular abduction keeps the forearm in position before locking the elbow. The elbow-lock cable is separate from the dual-control cable system. The child may need a more hands-on approach to learn shoulder extension and scapular depression to control the elbow lock. The OT can stand in front or in back of the child and guide the prosthesis through the control motion. Learning this motion takes time and practice. It is important to provide a variety of bimanual activities in standing and sitting positions that require the child to preposition the forearm, such as buttoning a shirt, tying shoelaces, or pushing a cart.

Externally Powered Prostheses: Transhumeral Level
The options for controlling a prosthesis at the transhumeral level depend on the anatomic presentation of the residual limb. If the child has a longitudinal deficiency and there are residual

digits present, the considerations will be different. The digits should then be used to activate control of the terminal device within the socket using either force-sensing resistors or switches. If the child has a transverse deficiency, the triceps muscle is usually chosen for myoelectric control of the opening function of the prosthetic hand. Physiologically, this is the muscle most closely associated with opening the hand. Extending the elbow and opening the hand is more natural than flexing the elbow to open the hand. Also, when the triceps is used in a one-site control system, it is easier to learn to quiet this muscle than the biceps to allow the hand to maintain a grasp while carrying objects. When children lift large objects, it often triggers activation of the bicep muscle. Therefore, in the first myoelectric prosthesis, the triceps is the muscle of choice, and when the child is ready to switch to a two-muscle control system, the biceps is a logical choice for activating the closing function of the hand.

When teaching the child to activate the appropriate muscle, the terminology used must be consistent with the terms that the parents use at home to refer to the residual limb or any nubbins that might be present. As with a transradial-level deficiency, the child must learn to move the tissue at the distal end of the residual limb to activate the muscle. If there are nubbins present, it is much easier for the child to understand the instruction of "move your nubbins up like you are trying to hold something" or "move your nubbins down like you are stretching them out." Touching or tickling the area to be activated may help. It may also be helpful to hold the residual limb so the child does not misunderstand and activate shoulder muscles.

When the child seems to understand the action required, an electrode can be placed on the desired muscle belly and held in place with a cuff or strap. It can then be used to activate either a modified toy or prosthetic hand to reinforce the concept of moving the muscle to cause some action and, eventually, to open the hand.

The fitting process for this deficiency level is the same as described in the transradial section. A cast is taken encapsulating the shoulder, a trial socket is fabricated, and the final prosthesis is then fabricated to match as closely as possible the length of the intact arm for the humeral and forearm segments. A chest strap is used to secure the prosthesis and aid with suspension.

The strategies for training with an externally powered transhumeral prosthesis are the same as those used with a transradial prosthesis. The focus is on learning to control the hand. Initially the OT or parents will need to position the elbow and wrist in an optimal position for using the hand. Eventually, the child will be able to preposition the hand to function independently (**Figure 12**).

Elbow and wrist units for children will remain as passive or manually locking joints, unless there is a reason to switch to a powered elbow. Powered components such as elbows and wrists add a substantial amount of weight to the prosthesis and are often unnecessary for children who have an intact contralateral hand to use for positioning the prosthetic hand. If an externally powered elbow is considered, control of the elbow should be separate from control of the hand. A simple method is to incorporate a pull switch into the chest strap harness attached to the humeral segment so that when the child abducts the arm, the elbow moves.

Body-Powered Prostheses: Shoulder Disarticulation Level

The readiness criteria used for a young child with a transradial deficiency is similar to activating/fitting a child with a shoulder disarticulation–type prosthesis. As with transradial and transhumeral prostheses, the initial focus is on control of the terminal device.

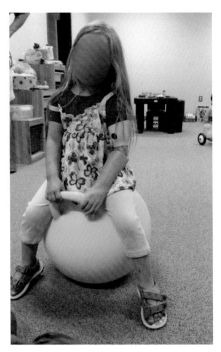

Figure 12 Clinical photograph of a child with a transhumeral prosthesis demonstrates the importance of positioning the prosthetic forearm so that the child can focus on functional use of the terminal device.

However, in adolescents with a shoulder-level deficiency, positioning of the prosthetic shoulder in flexion/extension and abduction/adduction need to be considered, as well as control of the elbow, wrist, and terminal device. The shoulder may initially be placed in a fixed position of slight flexion and abduction to aid with function and simplify positioning. The young child needs to be able to tolerate some frustration and have a good power source to control the terminal device. A single-control cable with a contralateral thigh strap is recommended for initial active operation of the terminal device. The terminal device will operate with shoulder girdle elevation and trunk rotation, which is a difficult motion for a young child to perform. When teaching the control motion, it is necessary to stabilize the lower trunk and have the child use trunk flexion to open the terminal device. Because the shoulder disarticulation prosthesis has limited function, it will take much effort by the family to encourage the child to wear and use this type of prosthesis. The OT will use the same techniques and provide the child with bimanual activities to encourage use and skill development.

The readiness to learn how to operate the forearm lift and elbow lock operation is the same for a transhumeral prosthesis. The prosthesis will need a dual-control cable rather than a single-control cable, and the elbow lock can be connected to a chin nudge control. The child will use shoulder girdle elevation and trunk rotation on the prosthetic side, while stabilizing the lower trunk to lift the forearm. The elbow lock will be locked and unlocked when the nudge button is pushed by the child's chin. The child should learn the motion as a combined motion of forearm lifting and elbow locking from the beginning. A flexion stop, which limits the full range of motion of the forearm, may initially be used for safety. When the child has established good control of the forearm motion, the flexion stop may be removed.

Externally Powered Prostheses: Shoulder Disarticulation Level

When the shoulder joint is absent, the muscles chosen to operate the terminal device for myoelectric control must be proximal to the shoulder. The orientation of the electrode on the muscle fibers of the chosen muscle will be important to consider. Myoelectric control at this level becomes more complex because the muscles required to operate the functions of the prosthetic hand are not physiologically associated with the intended function and are sometimes confusing for a child to learn.

Other options for control at this level are use of push switches or force-sensing resistors; the latter provide proportional control based on proportional pressure on the surface of the touchpad. Push switches can be used when the child can elevate, depress, protract, and retract his

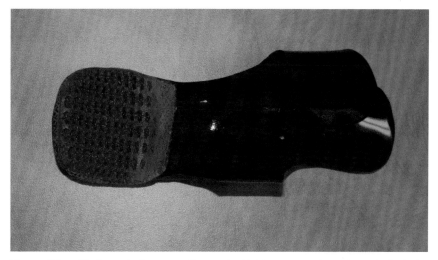

Figure 13   Photograph of an opposition post, which is a commonly used prosthetic device for a child with a partial hand deficiency. The device attaches to the limb with a distal and proximal bracelet and provides a flat, hard surface and a post for opposition.

or her shoulder to activate control over various prosthetic components. A single switch can be used with a simple "cookie crusher" control circuit to operate a prosthetic hand. Dual-action switches can be used to operate elbow motion, where a small shoulder motion activates elbow flexion and a larger shoulder motion activates elbow extension.[18] When fitting a child at this level, it is best to begin simply with control of the terminal device as the only powered component.

Transcarpal and Partial Hand Deficiencies

Amputation levels distal to the wrist have many functional advantages over those above the wrist. If the length of the forearm is equal to the contralateral limb and the wrists are equal in length, body posture will be symmetric. The limb can be very useful as a support for holding objects while manipulating objects with the dominant hand. If there are any nubbins present on the residual limb, they may also be used to manipulate objects.

Many children with a deficiency at this level prefer to use their residual limb and do not tolerate full-time wear of a prosthesis. The advantages of kinesthetic feedback and proprioception will usually outweigh the grasping function

of a prosthesis. It is important, however, to offer prosthetic options to these children because their needs and desires will change as they age.

The most common choice for an assistive device for these children is an opposition post (**Figure 13**), which is sometimes referred to as a paddle or opposition splint. This is a simple device that attaches to the limb with a distal and proximal bracelet and provides a flat, hard surface to oppose the distal residual limb. The pad of the post can be covered with a friction surface to assist with more adequate grip. The opposition post allows the child to hold objects using the remaining part of the palm by flexing at the wrist. Using utensils, markers, toothbrushes, and toys with handles becomes much easier with the ability to hold with both "hands." The opposition post typically needs to be customized for thin, medium, or thick objects. A child may be fit with multiple posts for different activities. An opposition post for thin objects, such as paper or playing cards, will not be able to hold large objects, such as a baseball bat or bike handle (**Figure 14**). A push-button multipositional post may be used so that the child can be fit with one post for various activities.

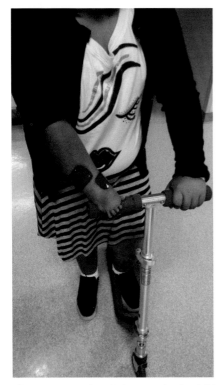

Figure 14 Clinical photograph of a child using a larger-sized opposition post that fits the handle of a scooter.

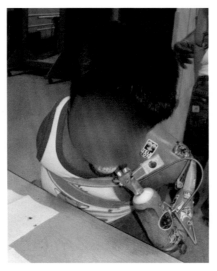

Figure 15 Clinical photograph of a child with a bilateral upper limb deficiency using a shoulder disarticulation prosthesis with a hook for self-feeding.

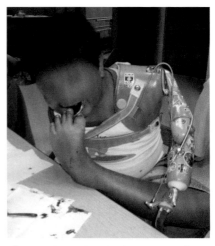

Figure 16 Clinical photograph of the child in Figure 15 using his foot for self-feeding.

Some parents or children will want to pursue prosthetic fitting despite the fact that the prosthesis will likely be longer than the contralateral limb. Before proceeding with a fitting, it may be helpful to demonstrate the expected overall length to parents using a drawing of the limb with the additional space required for wrist units and a terminal device. The parents can then make an informed choice to continue with the fitting or to explore other options and adaptations.

If a myoelectric prosthesis is chosen, site selection and training will follow the same process as described in the transradial section of this chapter.

Bilateral Upper Limb Deficiency

The team approach is crucial in the care of a child with bilateral or multiple limb loss. The therapist, prosthetist, and team can provide assistance with home activities, instructions, adaptive equipment, and psychosocial support. A child with high-level congenital limb loss may not reach developmental milestones within the typical time frames. He or she may need additional time to acquire gross and fine motor skills and will perform tasks in an adapted manner. The child should be encouraged to move and use all available limbs during play. Parents should be reminded not to overdress the child because there is less skin surface area for heat dissipation. Excessive clothing also restricts the child's movements, making it difficult to achieve motor skills. Ample range of motion and flexibility in the trunk and remaining lower limbs will be helpful to complete tasks and activities.

For a child with high-level bilateral upper limb loss, prostheses may assist with eating, writing, and limited dressing and hygiene; however, prostheses cannot provide complete independence. The child will need to rely on modified body movements, adaptive equipment, mouth use, and foot use for many self-care tasks. The development of foot skills will occur naturally if the child is given the opportunity to use his or her feet. Providing age-appropriate fine motor activities will enhance the dexterity and use of the child's toes. The feet provide sensory feedback and precision that prostheses do not provide. Most children prefer to use foot skills over using their prosthesis/prostheses (**Figures 15 and 16**).

For a child missing both arms with residual arm lengths that can touch each other, the child will likely become accustomed to using a bimanual pattern to perform daily tasks. The child is able to feel the objects in his or her residual arms and can manipulate the objects to incorporate them into activities, including self-feeding with a fork or spoon, teeth brushing, grooming, hygiene, and writing (**Figure 17**). If the child chooses not to use prostheses, he or she will use compensatory techniques and may require adaptive equipment to complete some tasks.

Prosthetic Considerations

If a family decides to pursue fitting for their child with one or two prostheses, early fitting is preferable to establish a consistent wearing pattern. Often, early fitting is not possible because of the child's delays in attaining motor skills and family concerns. For children with bilateral upper limb loss, there is not a formula or standard method of fitting because each case is different and often complex. In some instances, it is beneficial to fit the child with one

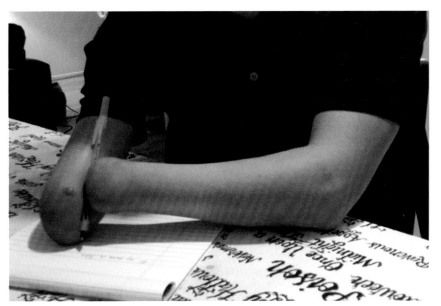

Figure 17 Clinical photograph of a child demonstrates bimanual use of residual limbs.

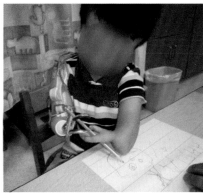

Figure 18 Clinical photograph of a child with bilateral limb deficiencies using his dominant limb to position an object in the terminal device of his prosthesis.

prosthesis initially to evaluate how he or she adapts before considering fitting both arms. It may be beneficial to fit the nondominant side if there is some functional use of the dominant side (**Figure 18**). Alternatively, it may be beneficial to fit the side with more length and range of motion to better incorporate the prosthesis into specific tasks or activities. Many factors must be taken into consideration by the team during the prosthetic prescription phase. It is extremely important that the prosthesis or prostheses do not interfere with the child's development. The prostheses should be made as lightweight as possible by using endoskeletal prosthetic components. Terminal devices should be carefully chosen because the prosthesis will be used for dominant-hand tasks. It is important to establish a consistent wearing pattern; however, it should be expected that the prosthesis will not be worn full time.

Passive Prosthetic Fitting

For a child with bilateral transradial limb deficiencies, he or she can be fit with a prosthesis when good sitting balance has been achieved. The team and family can decide if one or two prostheses are

beneficial for the child because the child will likely use the prostheses to support body weight and perform simple tasks. For a child with bilateral transhumeral loss or amelia, the child is more likely to be fit when he or she is safely walking. Children with bilateral amelia or those with very short transhumeral limb deficiencies may need to wear a helmet for protection when learning to walk because of the inability to protect themselves from falls.

The child with amelia at the shoulder level can be fit with one prosthesis initially. Typically, the single prosthesis will be fit on the side opposite of the child's dominant foot so that the dominant foot may assist with positioning of the prosthesis. This prosthesis will not be used to support body weight for activities such as crawling.

Bilateral Transradial Body-Powered Prostheses

The criteria for readiness for fitting with an activated prosthesis is the same as the readiness criteria for a unilateral fitting.

Initial control training for bilateral transradial cable-activated prostheses begins with the OT assisting as one prosthesis is moved into humeral flexion

to demonstrate how the terminal device opens and then placing an object into the terminal device. This training continues until the child initiates the control motion and the OT assists the child in closing the terminal device. When the child is at a table, he or she can learn to push objects with the opposite limb or with the second prosthesis (if both sides are fit) into the open terminal device. The child needs to learn to time the closure of the terminal device with the grasping of the object. The child will continue to practice until the control motion is refined. He or she is then taught the second control motion, biscapular abduction to open the terminal device near the midline of the body. More advanced skills include learning how to preposition the terminal devices adequately, eliminating cross-control, refining the size of the opening and closing of the terminal device, and repositioning an object in the terminal device by using one hook to position the other hook (**Figure 19**).

Bilateral Transhumeral Body-Powered Prostheses

The length of the residual transhumeral limb, shoulder range of motion, and strength all must be adequate for the child to successfully operate transhumeral prostheses. A child with short residual limb length and weakness

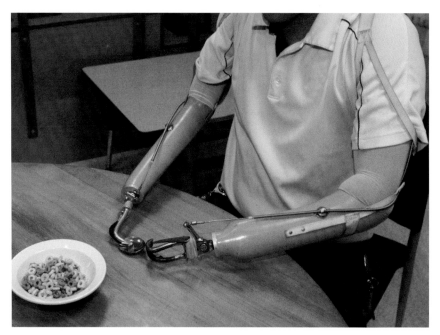

Figure 19 Clinical photograph of a bilateral upper limb amputee using one hook to position a utensil in the second hook.

typically has difficulty lifting the weight of the prostheses to place the terminal device in the best position for function and gains little from the prostheses.

Initial prosthetic control training should begin with a single-control cable system and a pull tab to operate the elbow. The single-control cable system requires less force to open the terminal device when the forearm is at 90° of flexion. Children between the ages of 2 and 3 years typically do not have the range of motion, strength, or understanding to operate a dual-control cable system. The training on how to open and close the terminal device is the same as that given for a transradial prosthesis. An adult assists with prepositioning the forearm with the pull tab to operate the elbow.

When the child has mastered opening and closing the terminal device, he or she will next be taught how to preposition the terminal devices, preposition the turntable on a positive locking elbow (if one is used), eliminate cross-control (if possible), transfer an object from one terminal device to the other, and refine the size of the opening of the terminal device.

Bilateral Amelia at the Shoulder Level

If a child with bilateral amelia at the shoulder level is fitted, the child will likely only be fitted on one side. The child may progress to bilateral fitting; however, this is not recommended because of the excessive weight, discomfort, decreased mobility, and lack of functional use of the prostheses. The child is more likely to be fitted with bilateral cosmetic prostheses rather than bilateral functional prostheses.

The child with bilateral amelia is more likely to be fitted with electric components for an active prosthesis. The push-button switch control will be placed at the top part of the shoulder disarticulation socket. The child will use shoulder elevation to activate the button to open the terminal device. When the child relaxes the shoulder away from the button, the terminal device will close.

The OT assists the child in learning the control motion and places objects in the terminal device. The OT or other adults may need to assist the child to preposition the shoulder, elbow, and wrist. The child may incorporate the

prosthesis into play, learning how to grasp and release objects from a table, carry lightweight objects, scribble, color with markers, or eat with a swivel spoon secured inside the terminal device.

A shoulder disarticulation prosthesis for children is typically limited to use in tabletop activities. The goals of functional prosthetic training should include eating, printing, writing, typing, and carrying objects. These children may need adaptations to the environment and may use adaptive equipment, foot skills, and compensatory techniques to complete most activities of daily living.[14]

Acquired Upper Limb Deficiency

In children with an acquired amputation, the OT interventions and strategies used will vary based on the child's age and the amputation level. Considerations for acquired amputations will be very similar to amputations in adults. After surgery, areas to address include wound management, edema control, desensitization, range-of-motion exercises, and maximizing independence in ADLs. Depending on when the OT becomes involved in the care of the child, some of these areas may have been addressed. The child will likely be seen by therapists in an acute care setting before being referred to a prosthetic center.

When the child is first seen in the prosthetic clinic, the acute care instructions should be reviewed. The OT should review desensitization techniques and procedures for mobilization of scar tissue, address phantom sensation or phantom pain, and review range-of-motion exercises for all of the joints of the upper limb (not just the closest joint to the amputation). For example, in a child with a transradial amputation, shoulder range of motion is as important as elbow range of motion. The limb should be wrapped with a self-adhering elastic bandage until edema is controlled. If the bandage is not being applied evenly or consistently at home, a silicone liner can be used instead. The silicone liner also can be helpful in keeping scar tissue supple and for shaping the limb in preparation for prosthetic fitting.

When the wound has healed and edema is resolved, a prosthesis can be considered. The prosthetic options for a child with an acquired amputation are the same as previously discussed for congenital limb deficiencies. If the child is older, he or she may prefer to have an active-grasping prosthesis as the first primary device because all of the child's experience before the amputation was accomplished with two-handed performance of tasks. Replacing the grasp on the amputated side will be viewed as necessary to continue to do things in the accustomed manner. If the child is younger, the grasping patterns may not have been as well established and the perception of need for a prosthesis may not be the same.

For a child with a very short residual limb or with sensitive areas on the residual limb, an active-grasping prosthesis may not be immediately tolerated. The weight of an externally powered prosthesis may cause too much stress on the short residual limb. Also, the forces transferred to the residual limb when using a body-powered or externally powered prosthesis to lift or carry objects may not be tolerated. For these children, a passive or cosmetic prosthesis may be a better initial option, or they may prefer not to wear a prosthesis.

Time should be allocated to address concerns about performing ADLs. For the older child who was previously independent in self-care activities, adaptations should be considered to allow the child to regain independence, even before a prosthesis has been fabricated. This may mean adding zipper pulls to coats to allow the child to use the residual limb to pull up a zipper, using elastic shoelaces or teaching one-handed methods to tie a shoe, and addressing grooming concerns. For the child who has lost the dominant hand, strategies for changing hand dominance for writing, eating, and other daily tasks should be addressed.

OT Intervention When a Prosthesis Is Not Worn

There are many reasons why an individual will choose to wear or not to wear a prosthesis, and there are studies demonstrating that children will function well whether they wear a prosthesis or not.[4,19-24] However, it is important to continue to discuss prosthetic options and new technologies and components as they become available so that families can make informed decisions for the best care of their children.

For children who decline prosthesis wear, regular monitoring by the team remains necessary because the needs of the child and family may change over time. The factors that affect the decision of whether to try a prosthesis may change. In some instances, family issues or other medical concerns make prosthetic fitting a lesser priority, or the functional benefits are not perceived by parents to be sufficient to warrant fitting at an early age. The personality of the child may be a factor. In a rambunctious toddler who is already having problems with general behavioral management, the parents may find prosthesis fitting and training an unrealistic expectation.

Although the child may function well in performing daily tasks without a prosthesis, the OT should determine how tasks are accomplished so that bad habits, such as poor posture and overusing other body parts (especially teeth for opening packages), can be addressed early to prevent long-term problems. Modifications may be beneficial to allow the child to be independent in dressing. For example, pulling up pants may be easier to accomplish if a loop is sewn into the pants on the side of the short arm. Zippers on jackets may be easier to fasten with a zipper pull that fits the residual limb. The child can be taught to tie shoelaces with one hand, or shoes

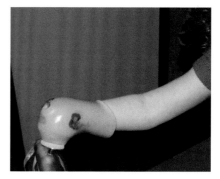

Figure 20   Photograph showing an example of adaptive equipment. A special socket is mounted on the handlebar of a bicycle so that the residual limb can fit into the socket to provide better steering control.

can be adapted with elastic laces or fabric hook-and-loop closures.

The OT can help anticipate functional issues and find solutions for performing daily activities. Often, learning to ride a bicycle is a concern because the child must be able to securely grip the handlebars. In this case, a special socket can be made to mount on the bicycle so that the residual limb can fit into the socket to provide better steering control (**Figure 20**).

Starting school may be another concern for parents, especially concerns about using playground equipment and meeting requirements for music or gym classes. It is important for the OT to maintain open communication with the parents and to be available as a resource to the parents and school and/or daycare as functional issues arise. For example, swinging on monkey bars is very difficult when using a prosthesis because maintaining suspension of the prosthesis is usually a concern when it is supporting the child's body weight. A modified strap or metal hook can be attached to the residual limb for use on monkey bars; however, this solution is often unsuccessful (**Figure 21**). If the child wants to play a musical instrument, a strap may be devised to aid in supporting the instrument. Holding a skipping rope may require the rope to be tied around the residual limb, or the

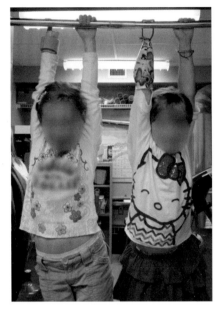

Figure 21 Clinical photograph of two children with unilateral prostheses with custom adaptations for use on playground equipment.

handle of the rope can be modified with a fabric hook-and-loop fastener or elastic strap. In some instances, children need to attempt a desired task before they realize it is not practical or realistic.

Summary

The care of children with upper limb differences has a variety of considerations. The OT and prosthetist provide the family with the education and knowledge to make appropriate prosthetic fitting decisions for their child. There is no single plan of care for every child with an upper limb difference, and there may be trials and errors before the ideal plan is realized. The plan of care is dynamic and should adapt as the child progresses through different stages of development. There may be stages of wearing and not wearing of a prosthesis throughout childhood. The OT should be available to assist with changes in the child's functional ability. The OT will assist with learning to use a prosthesis and incorporating it into ADLs if that is the choice of the child and family. The OT also helps to ensure that the child is able to independently complete ADLs

and IADLs that are important to the family, whether or not the child wears a prosthesis.

Because each child is unique, the care for children with upper limb differences is best provided by a unified team of specialists in an upper limb clinic where the needs and goals of the child and the family are the central part of the treatment plan.

References

1. Burger H, Marincek C: Upper limb prosthetic use in Slovenia. *Prosthet Orthot Int* 1994;18(1):25-33.

2. Curran B, Hambrey R: The prosthetic treatment of upper limb deficiency. *Prosthet Orthot Int* 1991;15(2):82-87.

3. Davids JR, Wagner LV, Meyer LC, Blackhurst DW: Prosthetic management of children with unilateral congenital below-elbow deficiency. *J Bone Joint Surg Am* 2006;88(6):1294-1300.

4. Kuyper M-A, Breedijk M, Mulders AH, Post MW, Prevo AJ: Prosthetic management of children in The Netherlands with upper limb deficiencies. *Prosthet Orthot Int* 2001;25(3):228-234.

5. The Association of Children's Prosthetic-Orthotic Clinics. Mission-Vision-Objectives. Available at: http://www.acpoc.org/mission.asp. Accessed August 25, 2015.

6. American Occupational Therapy Association (AOTA): Occupational therapy practice framework: Domain and process (3rd edition). *Am J Occup Ther* 2014;68(suppl 1):S1-S48.

7. Hubbard S: Powered upper limb prosthetic practice in paediatrics, in Mazumdar A, ed: *Powered Upper Limb Prostheses: Control, Implementation, and Clinical Application.* Heidelberg, Germany, Springer-Verlag, 2004, pp 85-115.

8. Canavese F, Krajbich JI, LaFleur BJ: Orthopaedic sequelae of childhood meningococcemia: Management

considerations and outcome. *J Bone Joint Surg Am* 2010;92(12):2196-2203.

9. Meurs M, Maathuis CG, Lucas C, Hadders-Algra M, van der Sluis CK: Prescription of the first prosthesis and later use in children with congenital unilateral upper limb deficiency: A systematic review. *Prosthet Orthot Int* 2006;30(2):165-173.

10. Shaperman JL: Early upper limb prosthesis fitting: When and what do we fit. *J Prosthet Orthot* 2003;15(1):11-17.

11. Egermann M, Kasten P, Thomsen M: Myoelectric hand prostheses in very young children. *Int Orthop* 2009;33(4):1101-1105.

12. Ibbotson V: Abstract: Congenital upper limb deficient children: Fitting philosophies in the UK. *Instructional Course Abstract: ISPO World Congress, Vancouver, Canada, 2007.* Brussels, Belgium, International Society for Prosthetics and Orthotics, 2007, p 27.

13. Patton J: Occupational therapy, in Smith DG, Michael JW, Bowker JW, eds: *Atlas of Amputations and Limb Deficiencies: Surgical, Prosthetics, and Rehabilitation Principles,* ed 3. Rosemont, IL, American Academy of Orthopedic Surgeons, 2004, pp 813-829.

14. Shaperman J: *Child Amputee Prosthetics Project Manual: Regents of the University of Los Angeles.* Los Angeles, CA, Shriners Hospital for Children-Los Angeles Unit, 1997.

15. Ottobock website. MyoBoy: Measure–Train–Simulate–Document. Available at: http://professionals. ottobock.ca/cps/rde/xchg/ob_us_en/hs.xsl/6961.html?id=teaser2#teaser2. Accessed September 23, 2015.

16. Hermansson LM: Structured training of children fitted with myoelectric prostheses. *Prosthet Orthot Int* 1991;15(2):88-92.

17. Hermansson LL: *Assessment of Capacity for Myoelectric Control*

Manual. Orebro University Hospital. Orebro, Sweden, Liselotte Hermansson, 2011.

18. Hubbard S: Myoelectric prostheses for the limb-deficient child, in Jaffe K, ed: *Physical Medicine and Rehabilitation Clinics of North America.* Philadelphia, PA, WB Saunders, 1991, pp 847-866.

19. Biddiss EA, Chau TT: Upper limb prosthesis use and abandonment: A survey of the last 25 years. *Prosthet Orthot Int* 2007;31(3):236-257.

20. de Jong IG, Reinders-Messelink HA, Janssen WG, Poelma MJ, van Wijk I, van der Sluis CK: Mixed feelings of children and adolescents with unilateral congenital below elbow deficiency: An online focus group study. *PLoS One* 2012;7(6):e37099.

21. Deans S, Burns D, McGarry A, Murray K, Mutrie N: Motivations and barriers to prosthesis users participation in physical activity, exercise and sport: A review of the literature. *Prosthet Orthot Int* 2012;36(3):260-269.

22. James MA, Bagley AM, Brasington K, Lutz C, McConnell S, Molitor F: Impact of prostheses on function and quality of life for children with unilateral congenital below-the-elbow deficiency. *J Bone Joint Surg Am* 2006;88(11):2356-2365.

23. Routhier F, Vincent C, Morissette MJ, Desaulniers L: Clinical results of an investigation of paediatric upper limb myoelectric prosthesis fitting at the Quebec Rehabilitation Institute. *Prosthet Orthot Int* 2001;25(2):119-131.

24. Vasluian E, de Jong IG, Janssen WG, et al: Opinions of youngsters with congenital below-elbow deficiency, and those of their parents and professionals concerning prosthetic use and rehabilitation treatment. *PLoS One* 2013;8(6):e67101.

Chapter 67

Pediatric Physical Therapy

Colleen P. Coulter, PT, DPT, PhD, PCS

Abstract

Children with congenital and acquired limb deficiencies receive the best care when a multidisciplinary team specializing in pediatrics evaluates the child, provides appropriate interventions, and recognizes the challenges in working with this patient population. Using knowledge of growth, motor development, and orthopaedics, pediatric physical therapists play an integral role in the team treating children with limb loss. The physical therapist often serves as a liaison between the family and other team members and promotes family-centered care that focuses on the child's function and participation in the home and the community.

Keywords: amputation; exercise; pediatric; physical therapy; limb salvage; rehabilitation; rotationplasty

Introduction

The World Health Organization recognizes that children experience rapid growth and substantial changes in physical, social, and psychological development during their first 2 decades of life and that a child's development depends on and is influenced by factors in the child's environment as well as the wishes, beliefs, and actions of parents and caregivers.[1] In addition, children experience the intensity and effects of disability and health-related conditions differently from adults.[1] The Children and Youth Version of the World Health Organization's International Classification of Functioning, Disability and Health (ICF-CY) uses terminology that classifies these challenges and problems in the following areas: body structures and function, activity limitations, and participation. Healthcare providers use the ICF-CY framework and terminology to document and measure health-related issues and design interventions for their young patients that include both the child and his or her family.

Within this construct, surgeons, orthotists, prosthetists, and therapists are very aware of and comfortable with identifying, measuring, and treating impairments of body structure and function, such as limb differences, the physiologic effects of trauma and disease, limitations to joint range of motion, vital signs, and pain. Although such limitations of body structures and function need to be addressed, these are best accomplished with goals that consider and optimize a child's function and engage the child within his or her family, school, and community environments. The ultimate goal of pediatric rehabilitation is for children to participate in activities with their families and within their schools and communities.

During the past 10 years, children with limb deficiency or loss have reaped the benefits associated with the increased societal awareness of adults with limb loss and the subsequent technological advances of prosthetic components. An unfortunate benefit of war has been the increased number of wounded soldiers who are seeking rehabilitation and prostheses that enable them to resume function beyond what was previously imagined. Similarly, children with amputations and limb differences continue to challenge their capabilities by participating in camps, events, and activities designed specifically to meet their needs.

Manufacturers have assisted in meeting these demands by developing various pediatric prosthetic components, such as running feet for children[2,3] and adaptive feet for rock wall climbing and cycling.[4] In addition, developments in pediatric suspension systems now allow children to wear prostheses without the need for suspension belts. However, a persistent major gap remains in the development of pediatric prosthetic knee technology that will keep up with the ever-growing demands and wear and tear placed on prosthetic components during a child's everyday activities and play.

By providing surgical options besides amputation, advances in surgical reconstruction and limb salvage techniques continue to influence the decisions of families of children in whom bone tumors are diagnosed.[5] Even children diagnosed with congenital longitudinal deficiencies of the femur, tibia, and fibula are benefiting from these surgical innovations. Physical therapists and prosthetists should be aware of these advances to fully understand the options available to each family as they make difficult decisions for their patients.

In pediatric patients with acquired limb loss, the physical therapist's role is well defined. The primary goal is to restore both children and adolescents

Dr. Coulter or an immediate family member serves as a board member, owner, officer, or committee member of the Association of Children's Prosthetic and Orthotic Clinics.

to the function they possessed before the trauma or surgery that precipitated the amputation. This restoration is initially done through wound care, edema control, shaping of the residual limb, preserving range of motion, and strengthening and functional exercises.

For children with congenital limb loss, the physical therapy goals and management strategies are different. These children naturally develop abilities to perform age-appropriate activities by incorporating the impaired limbs into their movement stratgies.[6] Because children with congenital limb loss do not know any differently, learning to move with a deficient limb is "normal" for them as they automatically integrate their affected limbs into their motor, sensory, and cognitive development. Regardless of the type of deficiency, the size, shape, strength, and flexibility of the deficient limb provides both sensory and motor input that guides the child's motor development. Even infants and toddlers with moderate to severe lower limb deformities will attempt to pull to stand and cruise if they have intact neurologic development. Accordingly, the physical therapist needs to be knowledgeable in all areas of gross motor, fine motor, and cognitive development and be able to anticipate the limitations that may be caused by a limb deficiency.[7] The physical therapist also should be aware of current pediatric prosthetic technologies and surgical options available for the different classifications of limb deficiencies.

In children with congenital limb deficiencies, the physical therapist often acts as an advocate, teacher, and mentor to the child and his or her family, anticipating immediate and future functional challenges. In centers specializing in pediatric limb deficiencies, the physical therapist frequently acts as a liaison between the family and other team members, empowering the parents to be the primary providers of care and promoting family-centered care.

Home programs are generally necessary for optimal surgical and/or prosthetic outcomes and to enable the parents and family to assist in the care of a child who is limb deficient. Many factors determine the education provided to parents and the frequency of physical therapy visits, including the degree of the child's limb deficiency as well as the child's age, flexibility, strength, associated medical and/or neurologic impairments, and developmental achievements. The distance the family lives from the center and their ability to actively participate in a home program will further influence the amount of clinical interaction. Videotaping therapy sessions is an excellent teaching tool for both parents and any community-based physical therapists involved in the treatment of a child. Digital photography makes it easier to personalize therapy sessions, communicate with the community-based therapist, and document progress. Commercially available exercise manuals adapted for infants and children with limb deficiencies can provide excellent resources for home therapy programs.[8,9]

Postoperative Considerations

Postoperative swelling is common in children with both acquired and elective amputations. Edema control begins with postoperative dressings and continues with elastic bandage wraps and shrinkers after the wound is adequately healed. Properly applied dressings may control postoperative edema and facilitate prosthetic fitting.[6,7] The type of postoperative dressing is determined by the surgeon based on the age and activity level of the child, parent preference, and the distance of the child's residence from the treatment center.

Soft postoperative dressings may work well for young children, but for infants and toddlers undergoing amputations, many centers prefer to use a rigid dressing, which provides a greater degree of protection. The goals for rigid dressings are to (1) protect the residual limb from additional trauma because infants and toddlers resume activity very quickly after surgery, (2) maintain bony alignment after revision procedures, (3) reduce edema, (4) shape the residual limb, and (5) keep the dressing intact during the postoperative period as swelling decreases.[6,7] The cast is usually changed within 2 weeks and may be followed by another cast or soft dressing with an elastic bandage wrapping.

Soft dressings can be used in older children but need to be reinforced and reapplied frequently as the child's activity level increases. Elastic wrapping over a soft dressing may assist in early edema management.

After the wound is healed, edema control remains important. The principles for elastic wrapping in infants and children with an amputation are approximately the same as those for adults with an amputation.[10] Differences include the size of the elastic bandages, the use of tape strips to secure the shape of the elastic bandage as it is being wrapped, and extending the wrap around proximal structures to provide greater stabilization for security because of the child's increased activity during the postoperative period (**Figure 1**). Because most children are too small for commercially available over-the-counter prosthetic shrinkers, custom-sewn shrinker socks may be made from soft elastic tubular stocking of various sizes. Applying a commercially available one-ply prosthetic sock over the wrap as an additional barrier also is beneficial to prevent a child from unwrapping the bandages or scratching at the incision site. Infants and young children placed in soft dressings after surgery may tolerate leggings and spandex bicycle-style shorts that are modified to be worn over the residual limb. These products provide additional control of the wrap and protection for the residual limb. Detailed written instructions on the techniques

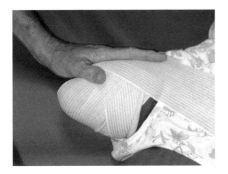

Figure 1 Clinical photograph of elastic wrapping of the residual limb of an 8-year-old child with a short transfemoral amputation after revision for femoral overgrowth. The elastic bandage is wrapped around the waist for stabilization and high on the adductor area to control edema proximally.

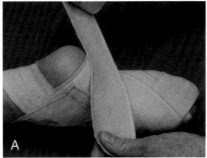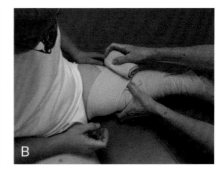

Figure 2 Clinical photographs of elastic bandage wrapping techniques for a 12-year-old boy after rotationplasty. **A,** The foot and ankle are wrapped, including the toes. **B,** The elastic bandage extends up the limb in a figure-of-8 pattern and includes the proximal thigh. An additional elastic bandage is necessary to continue around the waist for stabilization of the wrap and for edema control proximally.

of applying elastic wrappings should be provided to both parents and caregivers.

Children undergoing rotationplasty as treatment of trauma, tumors, or congenital anomalies require a unique wrapping technique to control edema and shape the limb proximally (**Figure 2**). Typically, substantial swelling occurs in the foot, ankle, and calf areas as well as above and below the surgical incision. The foot is wrapped, incorporating the toes and ankle separately as is done for an acute ankle sprain.[11] The wrapping continues up the limb in a figure-of-8 configuration, extending beyond the surgical site proximally and, if possible, around the waist to secure the wrapping. Control of proximal swelling that typically occurs after a rotationplasty is managed by using custom-sewn tights from elastic tubular stockings, compression shorts, and, even, support stockings. The amount of compression should allow an adequate degree of wound healing and should take into consideration the child's tolerance to pressure.

Physical Therapy Treatments

Range-of-motion, strengthening, gait training, and functional activities depend on a child's age, medical and neurologic condition, motivation, and interests as well as the family's ability to assist in the child's care. The following factors should be considered when developing therapy goals and home programs: (1) Every child is unique and develops at his or her own rate; (2) a child with multiple limb loss has special needs, and treatment interventions must be prioritized; (3) the environment needs to be adapted to the child for maximal function; (4) the child with a limb deficiency may have associated medical, neurologic, or orthopaedic impairments that will influence function and intervention; and (5) surgical amputations and revisions may take place at different developmental ages, so treatment should be centered on age-appropriate functions.[5,7,12] General expectations and limitations associated with common congenital lower limb deficiencies are listed in **Table 1**.

Early intervention is recommended to provide optimal outcomes and prevent the development of secondary disabilities. Family-centered services provide for maximal intervention.[9] Exercise programs should be created with the parents' input and consistent with their ability to perform the recommended interventions. Goals should be age appropriate, functionally based, and within the limits of the degree of the limb deficiency. With positive parental input, the child is likely to become a successful prosthesis wearer.[6,13]

Infants (Birth to <12 Months)

When a child is born with a limb deficiency, where available, a referral should be made to a limb deficiency center that specializes in the management of congenital limb differences.[12-15] At the center, the family meets with the physician and other team members to identify the infant's strengths and briefly outline possible future surgical, prosthetic, and therapeutic strategies that address the infant's physical impairments. Intervention should focus on assisting the infant to achieve motor and cognitive milestones in the context of his or her physical limitations.[7]

Families often come to their first clinic visit with a multitude of questions and fears about their child's deficiency. This information is often gathered from many sources, including well-meaning family and friends plus the Internet and social media. It is common to encounter parents and extended family members who have engaged in conversations on the Internet with other families, each having varying opinions about their infant's care. The physical therapist can help and, if needed, correct the family's understanding of their child's condition by using dolls with differing levels of amputations, samples of prostheses (similar to the child's first prosthesis), videos, and photographs of children wearing prostheses. All are useful teaching tools for parents and can ease

Table 1 Lower Limb Functional Outcomes and Special Considerations in Children With Lower Limb Deficiencies[a]

Deficiency	Outcomes and Considerations
Unilateral Syme disarticulation	No limitations are expected in daily activities.
	Able to participate in age-appropriate activities and sports, such as bicycling, skiing, dancing, and gymnastics.
	Assistive devices are not required.
	No limitations are expected in daily activities.
Unilateral transtibial level	No limitations are expected in age-appropriate daily activities.
	Able to participate in age-appropriate sports and activities, such as bicycling, skiing, dancing, and gymnastics.
	Assistive devices are not required.
Bilateral transtibial level	Slight limitations are expected on uneven surfaces, curbs, and stairs.
	Participates in age-appropriate sports with limitations.
	May require adaptive physical education or wheelchair for sports.
	Rides a bicycle with adaptations.
	Assistive devices are not required for ambulation.
	Uses a wheelchair as backup.
Unilateral knee disarticulation or transfemoral amputation level	May have limitations in age-appropriate daily activities.
	Requires adaptation to ride a bicycle; may ride without prosthesis.
	Able to participate in sports; adaptations may be required.
	Assistive devices are not required; uses crutches as backup.
Bilateral knee disarticulation or transfemoral level	Some limitations expected on uneven surfaces, curbs, and stairs or with kneeling.
	Encounters difficulty riding a bicycle; needs adaptations.
	Adaptive physical education is required.
	Uses a wheelchair for sports and as backup.
	Has limitations in sports and age-appropriate activities.
	May require assistive devices, although most do not.
Unilateral hip disarticulation	Limitations are expected on uneven surfaces, curbs, and steps. (Children with congenital deficiencies are quite functional; children with acquired loss have more difficulties.)
	Bicycling is difficult with prosthesis; may ride without prosthesis.
	Has limitations in running and sports; requires adaptations in sports.
	Uses a wheelchair for sports and as backup.
	May use crutches or cane for moderate to longer distances.
	May use crutches and no prosthesis.
Bilateral hip disarticulation	Wheelchair is used for primary mobility; power mobility may be necessary if associated upper limb involvement.
	Prosthesis use is for standing, exercise, and short-distance mobility.
	Requires assistive devices.
	Uses a wheelchair for sports.

[a]Multiple limb loss, medical conditions, trauma, and neurologic impairments may influence the functional outcomes.

Adapted with permission from Coulter O'Berry C: Physical therapy management in children with lower extremity limb deficiencies, in Herring JA, Birch JG, eds: *The Child With a Limb Deficiency*. Rosemont, IL, American Academy of Orthopaedic Surgeons, 1998, pp 319-330.

their anxiety and fears concerning the surgical, prosthetic, and therapeutic management of their child. The bond between the physical therapist and the family begins at this point.

Introducing the family to other families with children who have similar impairments is one of the most powerful interventions.[6,7,13] The effects of family networking are lasting and help ease parental fears and concerns for their child's future. However, the therapist needs to monitor the amount of information given to parents because not every parent is ready for all the available information at the first visit. Too much initial information increases parental anxiety and fosters fears for the child's future because it focuses on disabilities rather than abilities.

An infant with a congenital limb deficiency will benefit greatly from early intervention. According to the American Physical Therapy Association, early intervention is based on six important principles: (1) The rapid growth and development in the first years of life provide the foundation for later development; (2) infants can actively interact, form attachments, and are capable of learning; (3) parents are the main providers of care and early learning experiences; (4) parents of children with special needs may require assistance or instruction in caring for their children; (5) the interaction between the biologic insult and environmental factors influences the developmental outcome; and (6) structured programming may improve the abilities of infants and young children.[16]

Intervention should begin by evaluating the infant's gross and fine motor development to establish baseline records range of motion, strength, neurologic function, and movement patterns. In addition, the infant's ongoing motor development should be monitored regularly as he or she grows and learns to roll, sit, pull to stand, and walk.[12,17] These assessments should include any changes to range of motion, functional strength, weight bearing, and symmetry of both posture and movement.

Among infants with congenital limb deficiencies, asymmetry of movement is common. When asymmetry is present, parents and caregivers can be taught exercises for positioning, handling, and play so that they foster symmetric movements as the infant develops. Parents are encouraged to move their infants to both sides and not be afraid of further deformity or injury to the involved limb. They are taught to help the infant roll and transition into and out of sitting, kneeling, and standing equally to both sides. Symmetry and balance of movements during early motor activities are precursors to weight shifting in standing, cruising, and walking.[6,7,12,17]

In infants with congenital limb deficiencies or acquired limb amputations, range-of-motion exercises are designed to minimize the development of contractures and prepare the limb for future prosthetic fitting and function. With certain levels of limb deficiency, characteristic contractures and deformities are present. For example, longitudinal deficiencies of the tibia and the fibula are commonly associated with anomalies of the foot and the ankle. These deficiencies affect prosthetic and orthotic management and hinder gross motor development. Foot contractures, for example, may rule out the future option of a rotationplasty in an infant with a proximal femoral focal deficiency (PFFD), also known as a longitudinal deficiency of the femur, partial,[18] or affect the results of future limb lengthening in those with longitudinal deficiency of the fibula.

Similarly, hip flexion, abduction, and external rotation contractures are anticipated in infants with PFFD and those with short transfemoral limb loss.[6,12,13] Instruction should be provided regarding both positioning and range-of-motion exercises. Early prosthetic fittings should be considered if the loss is unilateral. Parents and caregivers can be taught how to maintain mobility at the hips, knees, and ankles during simple caregiving activities such as diapering, picking up the infant, dressing, feeding, and play.[6,7,13,19]

Parents should be instructed in range-of-motion and positioning exercises.[6,7,12,17] Hip and knee flexion contractures are common in infants who are born with short residual limb segments of the femur and the tibia, respectively, resulting from constrictive amniotic bands or from sustaining a traumatic amputation.[6,7,12,17] Prosthetic fittings have been used to manage knee flexion tightness in an infant as young as 6 months who was born with a very short unilateral transtibial amputation.[6,7]

Prosthetic fitting is recommended after the infant begins to pull to stand, typically at approximately age 8 to 12 months.[13,14,19,20] During this period, infants with longitudinal tibial and fibular deficiencies often have undergone elective amputations and are ready for the initiation of prosthetic fittings. Postoperative wound care, edema control, limb protection, and range-of-motion exercises constitute the important physical therapy considerations at this stage. The benefits of early fittings are threefold: (1) Flexion contractures are minimized; (2) symmetric weight bearing may be achieved for early, age-appropriate crawling, kneeling, and standing activities; and (3) the infant receives early sensory and proprioceptive feedback that truly prepares him or her for more functional prosthetic fittings at later developmental stages. An added benefit is that parents are involved early in the management of their child's care.[6,7] To maximize the benefits of a more anatomic prosthesis as the infant grows, it is recommended that the infant who would benefit from early prosthetic fitting have regular physical therapy to work on transitions and activities that are preparatory for crawling, standing, and walking.

Matching an infant's function with available prosthetic components allows the infant to parallel normal development. Infants with knee disarticulation and transfemoral amputation levels have demonstrated the ability to control a prosthetic knee and incorporate knee functions in early developmental activities, such as creeping and crawling, pulling to stand, half kneeling, and tall kneeling play[21-25] (**Figure 3**). Even infants with PFFD have demonstrated the ability to control prosthetic knee function in an unconventional prosthetic fitting with a short prosthetic tibial section using a hinged knee or an internal knee, depending on the length of the limb segments[21-23] (**Figure 4**). Prosthetic alignment should consider the developmental activities of the infant and may need to be modified frequently as the infant

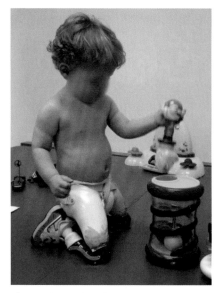

Figure 3 Clinical photograph of a 16-month-old child with congenital bilateral longitudinal deficiencies playing in a kneeling position. Knee disarticulations were performed at age 9 months, with prosthetic fitting at age 11 months. This child crawls, pulls to stand, cruises, and pushes a walker. The prostheses are not finished cosmetically because of the need for frequent alignment changes as the child develops.

develops and motor skills mature. The physical therapist and the prosthetist should work closely together to address alignment issues for the infant.

Infants born with multiple limb deficiencies with or without neurologic and medical involvement will require frequent therapeutic interventions and may take longer to acquire motor skills. Intervention should begin as soon as possible, focusing on all developmental parameters. Where available, referral to early intervention services is highly recommended as well as monthly monitoring by the limb deficiency team to update home programs and record changes in development, range of motion, and strength.[6,7,13,16]

Toddlers (12 to <36 Months)

By the first year, the toddler should be pulling to stand and, if appropriate, wearing a definitive prosthesis. Surgical intervention may be necessary at this

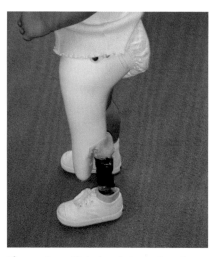

Figure 4 Clinical photograph of an 18-month-old child with a proximal femoral focal deficiency (PFFD) fitted in a traditional high proximal socket for containment of the hip because of the PFFD. A knee unit is placed distally. Although there is a short tibial segment, the knee is used appropriately in gait and all functional developmental activities.

age to correct deformities or perform a primary elective amputation. When surgeries are performed, postoperative management remains imperative for optimal prosthetic fit and function. When the toddler is ready for prosthetic fitting, instructions are given for donning and doffing, skin care, and wearing of the prosthesis. It is common for infants and young children with knee disarticulations and transtibial amputations to reject their prostheses. Initially, the prosthesis interferes with mobility and hinders overall movements, such that toddlers are more mobile in crawling and creeping activities without it. It is not until the toddler spends more time in standing and cruising activities that the prosthesis is readily accepted. The use of articulating knees in infants and toddlers has decreased some of these frustrations, allowing more normal gross motor functions by providing freedom and symmetry in patterns of movement through the actions offered by the prosthetic knee.[26] Gait studies in which toddlers are observed in developmental play situations document

prosthetic knee function during climbing up and sliding down a small slide, squatting in play, transitioning up to stand, and playing on the floor[21-25] (**Figure 5**).

A therapy program for a toddler at the prewalking and early walking stages should stress symmetry of posture and movement as well as control of weight shifting over the prosthesis.[12-17] Developmental screening and assessment tools make excellent treatment guidelines and assist in forming home programs.[7-9,27-30] Exercises should be fun and incorporated into a toddler's everyday play. Push toys and walkers are adjuncts to treatment. Most toddlers with single limb deficiencies do not require special assistive devices, but adaptations may be necessary to assist in ambulation for those with multiple limb loss.

Preschool and Young Childhood Years (36 Months to <6 Years)

As the child begins walking with the prosthesis, treatment again focuses on age-appropriate activities. Activities such as marching to music, climbing on small gym equipment, and riding a tricycle are excellent gross motor activities. Home exercise programs still include range of motion to prevent the progression of contractures.

The frequency of therapy visits at this stage will depend on the child's mastery of walking, the child's age-appropriate function, and the family's ability to follow through with home exercise programs. The physical therapist should monitor the child's development during clinic or prosthetic visits approximately every 4 to 6 months and make recommendations for changes of prosthetic components that parallel the child's motor development.[7,19] The prosthesis should be closely monitored for appropriate fit and function as the child grows. Feet with dynamic-response keels as well as feet that enable considerable adaptability to uneven terrain in all planes continue to become available

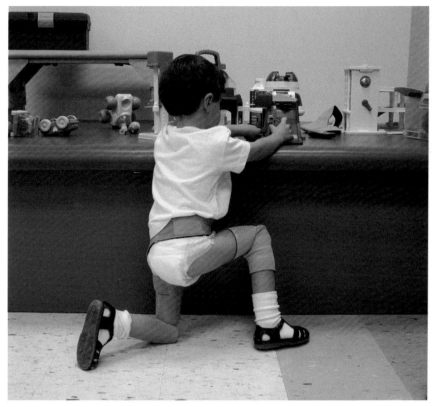

Figure 5 Clinical photograph of a 2-year-old child with congenital bilateral tibial deficiencies playing in a half-kneeling position. Note the knee disarticulation level on the left side and the Syme ankle disarticulation level on the right side. This child was fitted with an articulating knee unit at age 11 months. He was walking independently by age 15 months.

If possible, gait training should begin with the aid of parallel bars, teaching the child how the prosthetic components work, such as bending and straightening the prosthetic knee and learning how to sit, stand, and squat. Multidirectional weight shifts and stepping patterns progressing to walking on level surfaces with or without assistive devices should be instructed.

At approximately 7 years of age, the child's gait parallels that of an adult.[5,12,17] The child is able to participate actively in an exercise program and is less dependent on his or her parents. After the child is walking and the prosthesis is fitting well, outpatient physical therapy for this age group is best performed in a community or sports orthopaedic setting, using a developmental approach that motivates and challenges the child appropriately; avoid a setting that is equipped for infants and younger children. If possible, school visits by a therapist from a limb deficiency center are a helpful way of acquainting the child's teacher, school therapists, and classmates with his or her new prosthesis. Again, instruction and exercises should focus on age-appropriate activities, sports, and recreation.

in smaller and smaller sizes and may be indicated at this stage.[31]

Physical therapy can take place at the child's preschool or home and is an effective means of educating the child's teachers, classmates, and other family members. Preschool staff will be less apprehensive about having a child with special needs if they are well informed and taught strategies on managing the prosthesis and adapting the environment as needed. Toilet training is a major obstacle at this age for children with transfemoral or knee disarticulation prostheses. Typically, belts are required for suspension, making it difficult to pull pants up and down. Therapy can address this issue as well as dressing at home and in school.

In addition, certain surgical interventions, such as a Van Nes rotationplasty for the child with PFFD, can be introduced at this age. After each surgical intervention, wound healing, edema control, pressure wrapping, and range-of-motion and functional strengthening exercises are implemented. The child may require additional physical therapy postoperatively until independent function is restored.

Elementary Years (6 to 12 Years)

Initial amputations secondary to trauma or bone tumors commonly occur from 6 to 12 months of age.[5,6,19,20,32] In addition, children with congenital limb deficiencies may undergo surgical revisions for overgrowth or to correct developing deformities. At this stage, if available, children with legacy limb amputations should receive technologically advanced prosthetic components that may require additional gait training and balance exercises.[7,24,25]

Rotationplasty

Rehabilitation of the child with a rotationplasty is both challenging and rewarding. Children who have a rotationplasty from trauma or bone tumors with no associated hip pathology have gait patterns similar to those with transtibial function.[33] Children receiving rotationplasty for the treatment of PFFD have issues relating to hip and knee instability, including physiologic derotation that may be addressed either surgically or with prosthetic fitting.[18,34] These issues influence the gait pattern of the child. Regardless of the underlying etiology, range-of-motion and strengthening exercises of the hip, ankle, foot, and toes are imperative. Immediate postoperative management typically includes 6 to 8 weeks of no weight bearing, with instruction in isometric, active, and active-assisted hip, ankle, and foot range-of-motion exercises. Because the child attends frequent physical therapy for postoperative care, the physical therapist may be asked to monitor and assist the surgeon and family with wound care.[7]

As with the treatment of amputations and other reconstructive surgeries, after the bone has advanced into the healing stage and the surgeon gives clearance, then edema control; limb shaping; range-of-motion exercises of the hip, foot, ankle, and toes; and isometric strengthening of the hip and ankle are initiated. The child's orthopaedic surgeon should guide the progression of active and active-assisted exercises, weight bearing, and overall activity, which requires ongoing communication between the physical therapist and the surgeon. Open and closed chain hip strengthening and weight-bearing exercises can be initiated after the osteotomy site is healed. Healing is different in every child, with delays in wound healing commonly observed in children receiving chemotherapy for the treatment of bone cancer. Although both flexibility and strength are imperative for optimal prosthetic knee function, flexibility of the ankle, foot, and toes should precede strengthening. Ankle range of motion that restricts prosthetic knee function will interfere with proper gait and, in some children, cause pressure marks, skin breakdown, pain, and foot and midfoot breakdown. In extreme situations, tearing of the Achilles tendon has occurred. Similarly, tightness of the plantar fascia will influence toe and foot function. Toes are excellent initiators of prosthetic knee motion and act to stabilize the foot inside the socket. If the centers of the anatomic ankle-foot complex and the prosthetic knee are not equal, tightness is created inside the foot because of the inability to flex the prosthetic knee.[12]

Ankle dorsiflexion of 0° to 30° is adequate for prosthetic knee function. Optimal plantar flexion beyond 50° to 60° is desired.[6,7,12,17,33] The greater the available plantar flexion, the more streamlined is the relationship of the foot with the proximal segment, creating a larger excursion of prosthetic knee motion. Strength of the hip, ankle, foot, and toes leads to optimal prosthetic knee power after adequate range of motion is achieved. Exercises are necessary to facilitate ankle movements at speeds, excursions, and strengths common to knee function, using the foot's anatomy in an opposite orientation (**Figure 6**).

Limb Lengthening

Surgical management to address limb-length discrepancies of the femur, the tibia, or the fibula is typically initiated during the elementary years if the deficient limb is appropriate for lengthening. Limb equalization procedures include lengthening the short limb, shortening the sound limb through epiphysiodesis, surgically guided growth, bony resection, or a combination of these methods. Such limb lengthening procedures can be staged across several years, requiring extensive physical therapy and guidance for the child and the family. Common goals for therapy include maintaining range of motion in the joints above and below the external fixator, strengthening the limb, encouraging weight bearing, increasing endurance and overall conditioning, and restoring function and activity level during application of the external fixator.[6,35-39] These children should be kept as active as possible, attending school and participating in recreational activities as permitted.

Adolescence (13 to 17 Years)

Malignant bone tumors are most common in the first and second decades of life.[5,6] Children and their families are faced with surgical options for limb salvage, amputation, or rotationplasty depending on the size, location, and

characteristics of the tumor as well as the activity and functional levels of the child, taking into account cultural, psychological, and family issues.[7] Because physical therapists may play a role in educating the child and the family about the functional outcomes of each surgical procedure and the early and late effects of chemotherapy, therapists should be knowledgeable about these challenges.

The child who undergoes a limb salvage procedure encounters numerous physical challenges. Physical therapy goals include regaining mobility and strength, progressive weight bearing, improving cardiovascular endurance, pain management, scar mobility, and independence in transfers.[40] Age-appropriate activities, which include activities of daily living, are incorporated in the exercise program. The therapist must always remember, however, that the primary goal for a child with a bone tumor is to survive the malignancy. The aggressive nature of these tumors and the morbidity associated with their treatment can substantially limit the goals of physical therapy. Each limb salvage procedure is unique, and therapy must be performed under the close direction of the orthopaedic surgeon.[40]

For a child who elects or requires an amputation for local control of a tumor, an immediate postoperative prosthesis may be used if appropriate. Postoperative physical therapy treatment includes edema control; wound healing; and range-of-motion, strengthening, and balance exercises necessary to prepare the child for prosthetic fit and function.

At this age range, preadolescents and adolescents with congenital limb deficiencies may undergo surgical reconstructions and revisions to correct deformities and overgrowth in limbs that are less functional. This is often the child's choice, based on potential improvements with regard to function and cosmesis. When necessary, the ongoing management of longitudinal

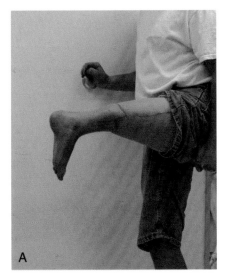
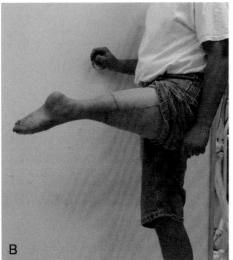
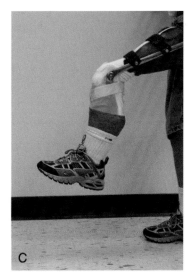

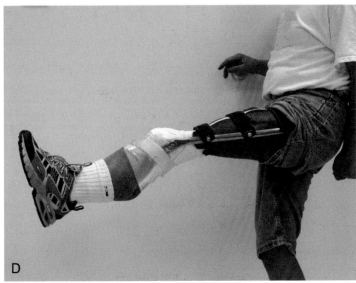

Figure 6 Clinical photographs of a 15-year-old boy who underwent a rotationplasty because of osteosarcoma using his foot and ankle to power a prosthetic knee 12 weeks after surgery. **A,** The foot in plantar flexion. **B,** The foot in dorsiflexion. **C** and **D,** The same foot and ankle positions with the boy wearing the prosthesis. The prosthesis is not cosmetically finished because of the need for frequent alignment changes to accommodate gains in plantar flexion and range of motion.

deficiencies of the femur, the tibia, and the fibula may require a continuation of the limb-lengthening processes described earlier.

Phantom limb sensation is common in adolescents with acquired amputations resulting from trauma and tumors[7,12,17,41] but is less frequent in those with congenital limb deficiencies after reconstructions or elective ablations. Phantom limb sensations typically do not interfere with function. The treatment guidelines for phantom sensations in children are similar to those for adults. Appropriate prosthetic fitting

and weight bearing may help decrease phantom limb sensations.[41]

Learning to drive a car is a very age-appropriate activity for adolescents. The physical therapist should know of local resources to assess the adolescent's abilities and the need for adaptations and modifications to the car. Accessibility issues are more apparent as the adolescent prepares for college and independent living away from his or her family. Universities and colleges typically have a department dedicated to students with special needs and accessibility issues.[42,43]

Sports and Recreation

Children and adolescents of all ages with amputations or limb deficiencies should be encouraged to participate in sports and recreational activities with their peers. The psychological effects of sports participation should be recognized.[44] Improving self-esteem and confidence; gaining independence; learning to compete, win, and lose; developing decision-making and problem-solving skills; and participating as a team member are a few of the benefits that individuals carry throughout their lives as they participate in recreational and

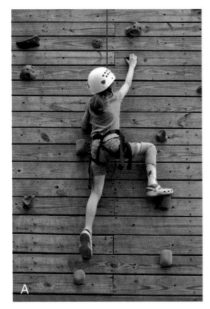 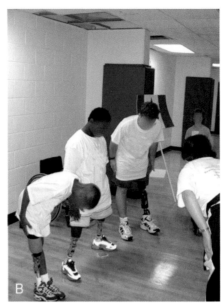

Figure 7   **A,** Photograph of an adaptive climbing program for children with physical challenges. **B,** Photograph of a karate class for children with limb deficiencies.

competitive sport programs. Improvement in physical fitness; the development of balance, strength, coordination, and motor skills; increased endurance; and weight control also are benefits of physical activity.[6] Adaptive sports and recreational programs have developed throughout the United States for individuals with all types of physical impairments.

In the United States, laws have been enacted that require children and adolescents to be educated in the least restrictive environment. The Individuals with Disabilities Education Act, provides free and appropriate education for children with disabilities.[6,12,17] Physical therapy and adaptive physical education in schools are included in this legislation. In addition, special adaptations and sports prostheses are available, depending on the degree and level of impairment. Advances in prosthetic technology are assisting people with amputations to compete in major sporting events on national and international levels.[45-48] The Challenged Athletes Foundation is an excellent resource for geographically located programs.[49] The Orthotic and Prosthetic Activities

Foundation provides financial and technologic assistance to individuals with physical disabilities who require orthotic and prosthetic services.[50] Exposing children and adolescents to these opportunities and referring them to local sports and recreational programs is one of the most important roles of a therapist (**Figure 7**).

Multiple Limb Loss With and Without Neurologic Impairments

Infants, children, and adolescents with congenital or acquired multiple limb loss have special needs. They require more intensive and regular therapeutic interventions.[7,17,41,51] Typically, delays in development occur, the severity of which often depends on the degree of limb loss and other associated medical or neurologic impairments. Special mobility aids, wheelchairs, and adaptations to the environment may be necessary. Prioritization of surgical, prosthetic, and therapeutic interventions is required to meet the goals of both the child and the family. It is important not to overburden the child with multiple new prosthetic devices at the same time.[6,7]

In infants, children, or adolescents with both neurologic involvement and amputation, the neurologic impairment has a greater influence on functional limitations than the amputation, whether acquired or congenital. Examples of acquired limb loss with neurologic pathology include a traumatic head injury with traumatic amputation, prematurity with intravenous infiltrate causing ischemia leading to amputation, meningococcemia causing brain and musculoskeletal insults, and myelomeningocele (spina bifida) with amputation. Treatment should focus on neurologic function as well as balance and stability associated with the prosthesis. Typically, the prosthetic limb is the more sound and stable limb. Strong communication and collaboration are necessary between the family, the school, the community, and the limb deficiency team for optimal outcomes.

Summary

Each infant, child, and adolescent is different and has expectations and goals unique to his or her needs. Many factors influence the goals when treating these patients. Age-appropriate functional activities that meet patient and family goals should guide physical therapy interventions. Treatments should be fun, meaningful, and coordinated with the child's family, schoolteachers, and community physical and occupational therapists. Physical therapists who work with infants, children, and adolescents are teachers, coaches, mentors, and advocates for the child and the family.

References

1. World Health Organization: ICY-CY International Classification of Functioning, Disability and Health: Children and Youth. Available at: http://apps.who.int/iris/bitstream/10665/43737/1/9789241547321_eng.pdf. Accessed October 14, 2015.

2. Össur: Feet. Available at: http://www.ossur.com/prosthetic-solutions/products/feet. Accessed October 14, 2015.

3. Cheetah Junior. Available at: https://www.ossur.com/prosthetic-solutions/products/feet/feet/cheetah-junior. Accessed November 4, 2015.

4. Catalyst Sports Adapted Climbing Clinics. Available at: http://www.go-catalystsports.org. Accessed October 14, 2015.

5. Dormans JP: Limb-salvage surgery versus amputation for children with extremity sarcomas, in Herring JA, Birch JG, eds: *The Child With a Limb Deficiency.* Rosemont, IL, American Academy of Orthopaedic Surgeons, 1998, pp 289-302.

6. Morrissy R, Giavedoni B, Coulter-O'Berry C: The child with a limb deficiency, in Morrissy R, Weinstein SL, eds: *Lovell and Winter's Pediatric Orthopaedics,* ed 6. Philadelphia, PA, Lippincott Williams & Wilkins, 2006, pp 1329-1382.

7. Coulter-O'Berry C: Physical therapy, in Smith DG, Michael JW, Bowker JH, eds: *Atlas of Amputations and Limb Deficiencies: Surgical, Prosthetic, and Rehabilitation Principles,* ed 3. Rosemont, IL, American Academy of Orthopedic Surgeons, 2004, pp 831-840.

8. Jaeger L, Ascher G, Atlee J, eds: *Home Program Instruction Sheets for Infants and Young Children,* ed 3. Tucson, AZ, Therapy Skill Builders, 1987.

9. Diamant RB, ed: *Positioning for Play: Home Activities for Parents of Young Children.* Tucson, AZ, Therapy Skill Builders, 1992.

10. VA/DoD Clinical Practice Guideline for Rehabilitation of Lower Limb Amputation. VA access to full guideline: http://www.oqp.med.va.gov/cpg/cpg.htm; DoD access to full guideline: http://www.qmo.amedd.army.mil/pguide.htm. Accessed October 15, 2015.

11. Taping, bandaging, orthotics, in Hunter-Griffin LY, ed: *Athletic Training and Sports Medicine,* ed 2. Rosemont, IL, American Academy of Orthopaedic Surgeons, 1991, pp 647-704.

12. Stanger M, Coulter-O'Berry C, Giavedoni B: Limb deficiencies and amputations, in Campbell S, Vander Linden D, Palisano R, eds: *Physical Therapy for Children.* St. Louis, MO, Saunders/Elsevier, 2006, pp 385-414.

13. Gillespie R: Principles of amputation surgery in children with longitudinal deficiencies of the femur. *Clin Orthop Relat Res* 1990;256:29-38.

14. Fisk JR, Smith DG: The limb deficient child, in Smith DG, Michael JW, Bowker JH, eds: *Atlas of Amputations and Limb Deficiencies: Surgical, Prosthetic and Rehabilitation Principles,* ed 3. Rosemont, IL, American Academy of Orthopaedic Surgeons, 2004, pp 773-777.

15. Krebs DE, Fishman S: Characteristics of the child amputee population. *J Pediatr Orthop* 1984;4(1):89-95.

16. Effgen SK, Bjornson K, Chiarello L, Sinzer L, Phillips W: Competencies for physical therapists in early intervention. *Pediatr Phys Ther* 1991;3(2):77-80.

17. Stanger M: Orthopedic management, in Tecklin JS, ed: *Pediatric Physical Therapy,* ed 3. Philadelphia, PA, Lippincott Williams & Wilkins, 1999, pp 378-428.

18. Guidera KJ, Novick CD, Marshall JG: Femoral deficiencies, in Smith DG, Michael JW, Bowker JH, eds: *Atlas of Amputations and Limb Deficiencies: Surgical, Prosthetic, and Rehabilitation Principles,* ed 3. Rosemont, IL, American Academy of Orthopaedic Surgeons, 2004, pp 905-915.

19. Tooms RE: The amputee, in Lovell WW, Winter RB, eds: *Pediatric Physical Therapy,* ed 3. Philadelphia, PA, Lippincott Williams & Wilkins, 1999, pp 378-428.

20. Kalamchi A, ed: *Congenital Lower Limb Deficiencies.* New York, NY, Springer-Verlag, 1989.

21. Geil M, Coulter C: Analysis of locomotor adaptations in young children with limb loss in an early prosthetic knee prescription protocol. *Prosthet Orthot Int* 2014;38(1):54-61.

22. Geil MD, Coulter-O'Berry C, Schmitz M, Heriza C: Crawling kinematics in an early knee protocol for pediatric prosthetic prescription. *J Prosthet Orthot* 2013;25(1):22-29.

23. Geil MD, O'Berry C: Temporal and spatial parameters of crawling in children with limb loss: Implications on prosthetic knee prescription. *J Prosthet Orthot* 2010;22(1):21-25.

24. Giavedoni BJ, Coulter-O'Berry C, Geil M: Movement masters. *Adv Dire Rehabil* 2002;11:43-44.

25. Giavedoni BJ: *The Use of Prosthetic Knees in Infants and Toddlers: Alignment.* Winnipeg, Canada, Canadian Association for Prosthetics and Orthotics, 2000, pp 25-26.

26. Wilk B, Karol L, Halliday S, et al: Transition to an articulating knee prosthesis in pediatric amputees. *J Prosthet Orthot* 1999;11:69-74.

27. Bayley N, ed: *Bayley Scales of Infant Development.* New York, NY, Psychological Corporation, 1969.

28. Folio MR, Fewell RR, eds: *Peabody Developmental Motor Scales.* Nashville, TN, George Peabody College for Teachers, 1974.

29. Frankenburg WK, Dodds JB, Fandal AW, eds: *Denver Developmental Screening Test: Manual.* Denver, CO, University of Colorado Medical Center, 1970, revised.

30. Furuno S, O'Reilly K, Hoska C, et al: *Hawaii Early Learning Profile (HELP): Activity Guide.* Palo Alto, CA, VORT Corporation, 1979.

31. College Park Industries: Truper Foot. Available at: http://www.college-park.

com/prosthetics/truper. Accessed October 10, 2015.

32. Krebs DE, Edelstein JE, Thornby MA: Prosthetic management of children with limb deficiencies. *Phys Ther* 1991;71(12):920-934.

33. Gupta SK, Alassaf N, Harrop AR, Kiefer GN: Principles of rotationplasty. *J Am Acad Orthop Surg* 2012;20(10):657-667.

34. Ackman J, Altiok H, Flanagan A, et al: Long-term follow-up of Van Nes rotationplasty in patients with congenital proximal focal femoral deficiency. *Bone Joint J* 2013;95-B(2):192-198.

35. Catagni MA, Guerreschi F: Management of fibular hemimelia using the Ilizarov method, in Herring JA, Birch JG, eds: *The Child With a Limb Deficiency*. Rosemont, IL, American Academy of Orthopaedic Surgeons, 1998, pp 179-193.

36. Paley D: Lengthening reconstruction surgery for congenital femoral deficiency, in Herring JA, Birch JG, eds: *The Child With a Limb Deficiency*. Rosemont, IL, American Academy of Orthopaedic Surgeons, 1998, pp 113-132.

37. Simard S, Marchant M, Mencio G: The Ilizarov procedure: Limb lengthening and its implications. *Phys Ther* 1992;72(1):25-34.

38. American Physical Therapy Association: Guide to physical therapist practice: Part 1. A description of patient/client management. Part 2: Preferred practice patterns. *Phys Ther* 1997;77(11):1160-1656.

39. Coglianese DB, Herzenberg JE, Goulet JA: Physical therapy management of patients undergoing limb lengthening by distraction osteogenesis. *J Orthop Sports Phys Ther* 1993;17(3):124-132

40. Shehadeh A, El Dahleh M, Salem A, et al: Standardization of rehabilitation after limb salvage surgery for sarcomas improves patients' outcome. *Hematol Oncol Stem Cell Ther* 2013;6(3-4):105-111.

41. Seymour R, ed: Clinical use of dressings and bandages, in *Prosthetics and Orthotics: Lower Limb and Spinal*. Philadelphia, PA, Lippincott Williams & Wilkins, 2002, pp 123-142.

42. Best US Colleges and Universities for Wheelchair Accessibility. Available at: http://www.oocities.org/ketchum4/bestcollegesanduniversitiespg2.htm. Accessed October 14, 2015.

43. CHASA: Children's Hemiplegia and Stroke Association website. Available at: http://chasa.org/. Accessed October 14, 2015.

44. Fergason JR, Boone DA: Prostheses for sports and recreation, in Smith DG, Michael JW, Bowker JH, eds: *Atlas of Amputations and Limb Deficiencies: Surgical, Prosthetic, and Rehabilitation Principles*, ed 3. Rosemont, IL, American Academy of Orthopedic Surgeons, 2004, pp 633-640.

45. Radocy R: Prosthetic adaptations in competitive sports and recreation, in Smith DG, Michael JW, Bowker JH, eds: *Atlas of Amputations and Limb Deficiencies: Surgical, Prosthetic, and Rehabilitation Principles*, ed 3. Rosemont, IL, American Academy of Orthopedic Surgeons, 2004, pp 327-338.

46. Michael JW, Gailey RS, Bowker JH: New developments in recreational prostheses and adaptive devices for the amputee. *Clin Orthop Relat Res* 1990;256:64-75.

47. Anderson TF: Aspects of sports and recreation for the child with a limb deficiency, in Herring JA, Birch JG, eds: *The Child With a Limb Deficiency*. Rosemont, IL, American Academy of Orthopaedic Surgeons, 1998, pp 345-352.

48. Miller K: Sports implications for the individual with a lower extremity prosthesis, in Seymour R, ed: *Prosthetics and Orthotics: Lower Limb and Spinal*. Philadelphia, PA, Lippincott Williams & Wilkins, 2002, pp 281-310.

49. Challenged Athlete's Foundation: Available at: http://www.challengedathletes.org. Accessed March 4, 2015.

50. Orthotic & Prosthetic Activities Foundation: Available at: http://www.opafonline.org. Accessed March 4, 2015.

51. Watts H: Multiple limb deficiencies, in Smith DG, Michael JW, Bowker JH, eds: *Atlas of Amputations and Limb Deficiencies: Surgical, Prosthetic, and Rehabilitation Principles*, ed 3. Rosemont, IL, American Academy of Orthopedic Surgeons, 2004, pp 923-929.

Chapter 68

Congenital Transverse and Intersegmental Deficiencies of the Upper Limb

Ee Ming Chew, MBBS   Michelle A. James, MD

Abstract

Congenital transverse and intersegmental deficiencies of the upper limb are considered malformations based on the Oberg, Manske, and Tonkin classification. Although these deficiencies are morphologically easy to recognize, they may represent proximal continuums of symbrachydactyly and longitudinal deficiencies. Unilateral upper limb deficiencies are generally not associated with other anomalies and do not require further evaluation. Because bilateral upper limb deficiencies may be part of a known syndrome, a genetic consultation and a systemic workup for other congenital problems are warranted.

In carefully selected patients, hand function may be augmented with reconstructive surgery, including web space deepening, arthrodesis, nonvascularized toe phalanx transfers, distraction lengthening, and free vascularized toe transfers. Revision amputation, such as removal of residual hypoplastic fingers (nubbins), is rarely indicated. In the past, some surgeons believed that the appearance of a traumatic amputation was preferable to the appearance of a malformation and recommended revising a malformation so that it appeared to be a traumatic amputation. Currently, this belief is not widely accepted by surgeons, parents, or individuals with upper limb differences. The limited benefits of these procedures must be weighed against their risks, including donor defects. Prostheses may help with social acceptance and may be useful as tools for specialized activities.

Keywords: intersegmental deficiency; prosthesis; reconstruction surgery; transverse deficiency

Introduction

Congenital transverse and intersegmental deficiencies are classified as malformations under the extended version of the Oberg, Manske, and Tonkin (OMT) classification scheme[1,2] (**Figure 1**). These terms describe failure of upper limb formation in the proximal-distal axis. Transverse deficiencies are easily categorized according to the last remaining bone segment. Proximal forearm (below-elbow) deficiencies are the most common type, followed by transcarpal, distal forearm, and transhumeral deficiencies.[3,4] Intersegmental deficiency, also known as phocomelia, is categorized according to the segment (total, proximal, or distal) that failed to form.[5]

Clinical Features

The diagnosis of transverse deficiency is readily apparent, although proximal forearm deficiencies exhibit variability in the length of the residual forearm. The elbow generally has full flexion and extension. Forearm rotation is frequently restricted by proximal radioulnar abnormalities. The residual limb is usually well cushioned, with rudimentary nubbins or dimpling often found at the distal end (**Figure 2**). This condition is almost always unilateral, occurs sporadically, and is rarely associated with other anomalies.[3] Children with a proximal forearm deficiency generally have normal cognition and developmental milestones, except that a child with a very short arm may not crawl.

Kallemeier et al[6] suggested that a transverse deficiency through the forearm represents a proximal continuum of symbrachydactyly. In their review of 291 patients with an upper limb transverse forearm deficiency, most of the limbs had one or more features of symbrachydactyly, including soft-tissue nubbins, skin invaginations, and hypoplasia of the proximal radius and ulna.

Transverse deficiency may be confused with constriction band syndrome (**Figure 3**). In the latter condition, children will have other manifestations, including multiple bands involving other limbs, acrosyndactyly, clubfoot, scoliosis, body wall defects, and cleft lip or cleft palate.[7]

Intersegmental deficiency or phocomelia is characterized by a hand that is attached directly to the thorax or humerus or with the forearm and hand attached directly to the thorax (**Figure 4**). Other than the epidemic of congenital malformations related to prenatal exposure to thalidomide during the 1950s and occasional association with thrombocytopenia-absent radius (TAR) syndrome, phocomelia remains exceedingly rare.

Dr. James or an immediate family member serves as a board member, owner, officer, or committee member of the American Board of Orthopaedic Surgery. Neither Mr. Chew nor any immediate family member has received anything of value from or has stock or stock options held in a commercial company or institution related directly or indirectly to the subject of this chapter.

I. MALFORMATIONS
    A. Abnormal axis formation/differentiation—entire upper limb
        1. Proximal-distal axis
            i.   Brachymelia with brachydactyly
            ii. Symbrachydactyly
                 a) Poland syndrome
                 b) Whole limb excluding Poland syndrome
            iii. Transverse deficiency
                 a) Amelia
                 b) Clavicular/scapular
                 c) Humeral (above elbow)
                 d) Forearm (below elbow)
                 e) Wrist (carpals absent/at level of proximal carpals/at level of distal carpals) (with forearm/arm involvement)
                 f) Metacarpal (with forearm/arm involvement)
                 g) Phalangeal (proximal/middle/distal) (with forearm/arm involvement)
            iv. Intersegmental deficiency
                 a) Proximal (humeral – rhizomelic)
                 b) Distal (forearm – mesomelic)
                 c) Total (Phocomelia)
            v.   Whole limb duplication/triplication

        2. Radial-ulnar (anterior-posterior) axis
            i.   Radial longitudinal deficiency - Thumb hypoplasia (with proximal limb involvement)
            ii. Ulnar longitudinal deficiency
            iii. Ulnar dimelia
            iv. Radioulnar synostosis
            v.   Congenital dislocation of the radial head
            vi. Humeroradial synostosis - Elbow ankyloses
            vii. Madelung deformity

        3. Dorsal-ventral axis
            i.   Ventral dimelia
                 a) Furhmann/Al-Awadi/Raas-Rothschild syndromes
                 b) Nail Patella syndrome
            ii. Absent/hypoplastic extensor/flexor muscles

        4. Unspecified axis
            i.   Shoulder
                 a) Undescended (Sprengel)
                 b) Abnormal shoulder muscles
                 c) Not otherwise specified
            ii. Arthrogryposis

    B. Abnormal axis formation/differentiation — hand plate
        1. Proximal-distal axis
            i.   Brachydactyly (no forearm/arm involvement)
            ii. Symbrachydactyly (no forearm/arm involvement)
            iii. Transverse deficiency (no forearm/arm involvement)
                 a) Wrist (carpals absent/at level of proximal carpals/at level of distal carpals)
                 b) Metacarpal
                 c) Phalangeal (proximal/middle/distal)

        2. Radial-ulnar (anterior-posterior) axis
            i.   Radial deficiency (thumb - no forearm/arm involvement)
            ii. Ulnar deficiency (no forearm/arm involvement)
            iii. Radial polydactyly
            iv. Triphalangeal thumb
            v.   Ulnar dimelia (mirror hand – no forearm/arm involvement)
            vi. Ulnar polydactyly

        3. Dorsal-ventral axis
            i.   Dorsal dimelia (palmar nail)
            ii. Ventral (palmar) dimelia (including hypoplastic/aplastic nail)

        4. Unspecified axis
            i.   Soft tissue
                 a) Syndactyly
                 b) Camptodactyly
                 c) Thumb in palm deformity
                 d) Distal arthrogryposis
            ii. Skeletal deficiency
                 a) Clinodactyly
                 b) Kirner's deformity
                 c) Synostosis/symphalangism (carpal/metacarpal/phalangeal)
            iii. Complex
                 a) Complex syndactyly
                 b) Synpolydactyly— central
                 c) Cleft hand
                 d) Apert hand
                 e) Not otherwise specified

II. DEFORMATIONS
    A. Constriction ring sequence
    B. Trigger digits
    C. Not otherwise specified

III. DYSPLASIAS
    A. Hypertrophy
        1. Whole limb
            i.   Hemihypertrophy
            ii. Aberrant flexor/extensor/intrinsic muscle

        2. Partial limb
            i.   Macrodactyly
            ii. Aberrant intrinsic muscles of hand

OMT Classification – Updated 28th January 2015

Figure 1   Listing showing the Oberg, Manske, and Tonkin (OMT) classification of congenital hand and upper limb anomalies. This classification was updated in January 2015. (Reproduced with permission from the Oberg, Manske, Tonkin (OMT) classification, 2015. International Federation of Societies of Surgery of the Hand. Accessed Oct. 14, 2015. Available at http://www.ifssh.info/2015_OMT_Classifiction_Congenital_Report.pdf.)

B. **Tumorous conditions**
  1. **Vascular**
     i. Hemangioma
     ii. Malformation
     iii. Others

  2. **Neurological**
     i. Neurofibromatosis
     ii. Others

  3. **Connective tissue**
     i. Juvenile aponeurotic fibroma
     ii. Infantile digital fibroma
     iii. Others

  4. **Skeletal**
     i. Osteochondromatosis
     ii. Enchondromatosis
     iii. Fibrous dysplasia
     iv. Epiphyseal abnormalities
     v. Others

IV. **SYNDROMES***
  A. **Specified**
     1. Acrofacial Dysostosis 1 (Nager type)
     2. Apert
     3. **Al**-Awadi/Raas-Rothschild/Schinzel phocomelia
     4. Baller-Gerold
     5. Bardet-Biedl Carpenter
     6. Beales
     7. Catel-Manzke
     8. Constriction band (Amniotic Band Sequence)
     9. Cornelia de Lange (types 1-5)
     10. Crouzon
     11. Down
     12. Ectrodactyly-Ectodermal Dysplasia-Clefting
     13. Fanconi Pancytopenia
     14. Fuhrmann
     15. Goltz
     16. Gorlin
     17. Greig Cephalopolysyndactyly
     18. Hajdu-Cheney
     19. Hemifacial Microsomia (Goldenhar syndrome)
     20. Holt-Oram
     21. Lacrimoauriculodentodigital (Levy-Hollister)
     22. Larsen
     23. Leri-Weill Dyschondrosteosis
     24. Moebius sequence
     25. Multiple Synostoses
     26. Nail-Patella
     27. Noonan
     28. Oculodentodigital dysplasia
     29. Orofacialdigital
     30. Otopalataldigital
     31. Pallister-Hall
     32. Pfeiffer
     33. Pierre Robin
     34. Poland
     35. Proteus
     36. Roberts-SC Phocomelia
     37. Rothmund-Thomson
     38. Rubinstein-Taybi
     39. Saethre-Chotzen
     40. Thrombocytopenia Absent Radius
     41. Townes-Brock
     42. Trichorhinophalangeal (types 1-3)
     43. Ulnar-Mammary
     44. VACTERL association

  B. **Others**

*The specified syndromes are those considered most relevant; however, many other syndromes have a limb component categorized under "B. Others".

OMT Classification – Updated 28th January 2015

Figure 1 (continued) Listing showing the Oberg, Manske, and Tonkin (OMT) classification of congenital hand and upper limb anomalies. This classification was updated in January 2015. (Reproduced with permission from the Oberg, Manske, Tonkin (OMT) classification, 2015. International Federation of Societies of Surgery of the Hand. Accessed Oct. 14, 2015. Available at http://www.ifssh.info/2015_OMT_Classifiction_Congenital_Report.pdf.)

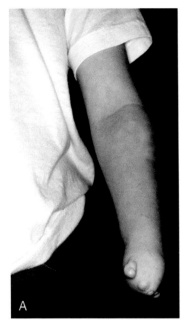
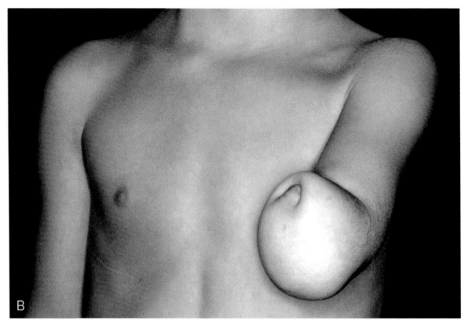

Figure 2   Photographs of patients with transverse deficiency of the upper limb. **A,** A deficiency at the metacarpal level, with residual nubbins. **B,** Dimpling is seen at the proximal forearm level.

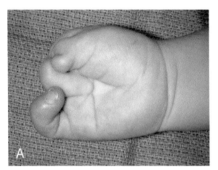
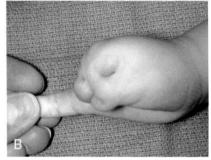
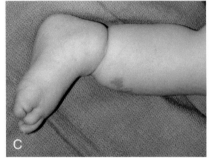

Figure 3   Photographs of the limbs of a child with constriction band syndrome, which may be confused with a transverse deficiency. This child has congenital amputation and acrosyndactyly of the radial four digits of the right hand (**A** and **B**) and banding of the left leg (**C**).

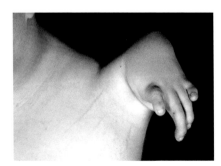

Figure 4   Photograph of the upper limb of a child with phocomelia. The forearm and hand are attached directly to the thorax.

It is difficult to account for a true intersegmental deficiency from the perspective of developmental biology.

Goldfarb et al[8] suggested that intersegmental deficiencies may represent forms of radial and ulnar longitudinal deficiencies. The authors retrospectively reviewed 41 patients (60 upper limbs) with a previous diagnosis of phocomelia. They concluded that all the deficiencies could be categorized into the following three main groups: proximal radial longitudinal deficiency (group 1), proximal ulnar longitudinal deficiency (group 2), and severe combined dysplasia with either absence of the forearm (group 3A) or absence of the forearm and upper arm (group 3B). Systemic and additional musculoskeletal anomalies

were present in the study's patients, suggesting that a complete workup is warranted.

Management
General Workup
Because unilateral transverse deficiency is usually not associated with other abnormalities, further specific workup of the patient is usually unnecessary.[9] However, bilateral deficiencies may be part of an identified condition such as TAR syndrome or VACTERL (V = vertebral, A = anal, C = cardiac, T = tracheal, E = esophageal, R = renal, L = limb) association. It is important to diagnose TAR syndrome

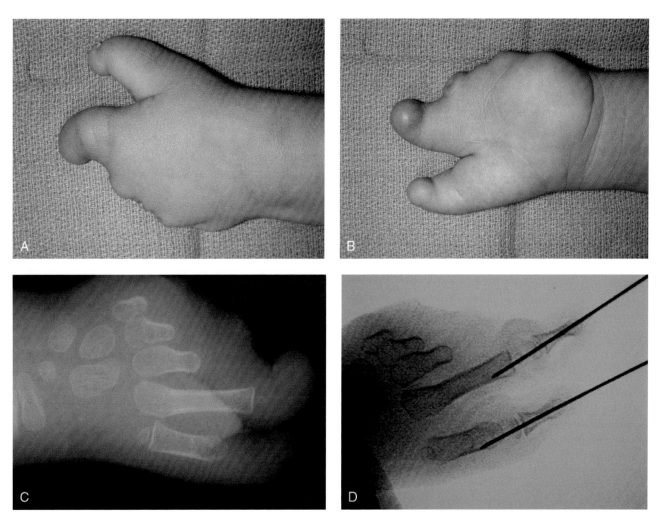

Figure 5   Dorsal (**A**) and palmar (**B**) photographic views of the hand of a child with a transverse deficiency of the left hand at the metacarpal level. The child was treated with a nonvascularized free toe phalanx transfer for digital reconstruction. **C,** Preoperative AP radiograph of the affected hand. **D,** Postoperative AP radiograph of the hand with toe phalanges held in place with Kirschner wires.

preoperatively because thrombocytopenia may persist and platelet transfusions may be necessary prior to surgery, even in later childhood. Consultation with a geneticist and a systemic workup is indicated to exclude other congenital problems. A special effort should be made to detect renal problems because the limbs and kidneys share the same developmental stage from the fourth to the eighth weeks of gestation, and both have a mesodermal origin.[10]

Surgical Options
Early Decisions
Parents occasionally request removal of the infant's nubbins. Nubbins on the

ridge of the terminal residual limb are easily injured. Small nails are difficult to trim, may grow abnormally, and can become irritated or infected. In addition, nubbins may be objects of curiosity to other children and may cause the child discomfort in social situations. Nubbin excision also may smooth the contour of the residual limb. However, older children rarely request removal of their nubbins. The nubbins provide sensory feedback and may be used to manipulate small, light objects. Nubbins that can provide volitional control and those that are large enough for later augmentation with bone and soft tissue should not be removed.

Later Decisions
Digital reconstruction may be considered in children who have some structures distal to the carpus. Nubbins that lack bony support and are large enough to accept bone graft can be augmented with nonvascularized free toe phalanx transfers[11] (**Figure 5**). This technique offers a limited means of increasing the length of digits, stabilizing soft-tissue nubbins, and improving function.[12] However, graft resorption, donor-site morbidity, functional problems with footwear, and a high rate of emotional problems with foot appearance must be balanced against the limited gains.[13,14]

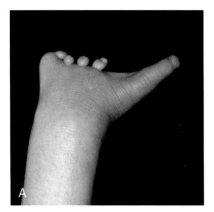 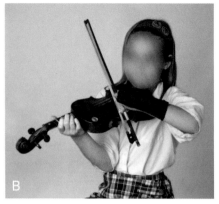

Figure 6 Photographs of a child with a transverse deficiency of the ulnar four fingers (**A**) using an adaptive prosthesis for playing a violin (**B**).

There is a very limited role for distraction lengthening in the management of digital insufficiency.[15] The desire for improved appearance must be weighed against the high morbidity of this procedure and the risk of functional loss. Lengthened digits that are thinner, stiffer, and scarred do not provide better function. Lengthening against atrophic distal soft tissue results in ulceration, which requires additional soft-tissue coverage or shortening back to a comfortable level. There have been isolated reports of forearm lengthening for transverse short transradial deficiencies; however, this procedure has a high complication rate and has not proved beneficial for functional improvement or prosthetic fitting.[16,17]

In appropriately selected children with transverse deficiency at the metacarpal level, free vascularized toe-to-hand transfers may be beneficial. The goal of this procedure is to provide a basic hand with two opposable digits or a chuck pinch. Although this complex procedure is accompanied by many potential difficulties, good functional results have been reported.[18,19] It must be recognized that transferred toes will still have the appearance of toes, not fingers.

The Krukenberg procedure is rarely indicated. In this procedure, the radius and ulna are separated and the muscles are reattached so that the radius pinches against the ulna. This procedure

is purported to be most useful in blind individuals with bilateral distal forearm congenital deficiency or traumatic loss because it provides unilateral prehension with sensory feedback. Occasionally, it may be indicated for a sighted child with a transradial deficiency and a long forearm.[20] Although opinions differ, one of the authors of this chapter (MAJ) believes that the Krukenberg procedure is never indicated in a patient with a unilateral deficiency. It has not been shown to improve function, and the appearance of the forearm treated with the Krukenberg procedure is strikingly abnormal.

Role of Prostheses

Children with unilateral forearm level transverse deficiency have few, if any, functional deficits. Prostheses do not improve performance of daily activities and are frequently abandoned.[21,22] However, prostheses may promote social acceptance by altering appearance. Specialized prostheses may be useful as tools for participation in some sports and playing musical instruments[21] (**Figure 6**).

Summary

Congenital transverse and intersegmental deficiencies are easily recognized. They may represent proximal continuums of symbrachydactyly and longitudinal deficiencies. Because bilateral upper

limb deficiencies may be part of a syndrome, a complete systemic workup for other congenital problems is warranted. Hand function may be augmented by reconstructive surgery, but this management option must be weighed against the attending donor-site morbidity. Prostheses may help with social acceptance and be useful in accomplishing specialized activities.

Acknowledgment

The authors thank Ms. Julia Serat, photographer, Shriners Hospital for Children, Northern California, for her assistance with the clinical photographs used in this chapter.

References

1. Tonkin MA, Tolerton SK, Quick TJ, et al: Classification of congenital anomalies of the hand and upper limb: Development and assessment of a new system. *J Hand Surg Am* 2013;38(9):1845-1853.

2. OMT Classification of Congenital Hand and Upper Limb Anomalies: Updated January 28, 2015. Available at: http://www.ifssh.info/2015_OMT_Classifiction_Congenital_Report.pdf. Accessed August 28, 2015.

3. Wynne-Davies R, Lamb DW: Congenital upper limb anomalies: An etiologic grouping of clinical, genetic, and epidemiologic data from 387 patients with "absence" defects, constriction bands, polydactylies, and syndactylies. *J Hand Surg Am* 1985;10(6):958-964.

4. Cheng JC, Chow SK, Leung PC: Classification of 578 cases of congenital upper limb anomalies with the IFSSH system: A 10 years' experience. *J Hand Surg Am* 1987;12(6):1055-1060.

5. Frantz CH, O'Rahilly R: Congenital skeletal limb deficiencies. *J Bone Joint Surg Am* 1961;43:1202-1224.

6. Kallemeier PM, Manske PR, Davis B, Goldfarb CA: An assessment of

the relationship between congenital transverse deficiency of the forearm and symbrachydactyly. *J Hand Surg Am* 2007;32(9):1408-1412.

7. Goldfarb CA, Sathienkijkanchai A, Robin NH: Amniotic constriction band: A multidisciplinary assessment of etiology and clinical presentation. *J Bone Joint Surg Am* 2009;91(suppl 4):68-75.

8. Goldfarb CA, Manske PR, Busa R, Mills J, Carter P, Ezaki M: Upper-extremity phocomelia reexamined: A longitudinal dysplasia. *J Bone Joint Surg Am* 2005;87(12):2639-2648.

9. Gover A, McIvor J: Upper limb deficiencies in infants and young children. *Infants Young Child* 1992;5(1):58-72.

10. Moore KL, Persaud TV, Torchia MG, et al: Development during weeks four to eight, in Moore KL, Persaud TVN, Torchia MG, eds: *Before We Are Born.* Ed 8. Philadelphia, PA, Elsevier Health Sciences, 2011, pp 49-61.

11. Goldberg NH, Watson HK: Composite toe (phalanx and epiphysis) transfers in the reconstruction of the aphalangic hand. *J Hand Surg Am* 1982;7(5):454-459.

12. Tonkin MA, Deva AK, Filan SL: Long term follow-up of composite non-vascularized toe phalanx transfers for aphalangia. *J Hand Surg Br* 2005;30(5):452-458.

13. Garagnani L, Gibson M, Smith PJ, Smith GD: Long-term donor site morbidity after free nonvascularized toe phalangeal transfer. *J Hand Surg Am* 2012;37(4):764-774.

14. James MA, Durkin RC: Nonvascularized toe proximal phalanx transfers in the treatment of aphalangia. *Hand Clin* 1998;14(1):1-15.

15. Seitz WH Jr, Shimko P, Patterson RW: Long-term results of callus distraction-lengthening in the hand and upper extremity for traumatic and congenital skeletal deficiencies. *J Bone Joint Surg Am* 2010;92(suppl 2):47-58.

16. Alekberov C, Karatosun V, Baran O, Günal I: Lengthening of congenital below-elbow amputation stumps by the Ilizarov technique. *J Bone Joint Surg Br* 2000;82(2):239-241.

17. Bernstein RM, Watts HG, Setoguchi Y: The lengthening of short upper extremity amputation stumps. *J Pediatr Orthop* 2008;28(1):86-90.

18. Kay SP, Wiberg M, Bellew M, Webb F: Toe to hand transfer in children: Part 2. Functional and psychological aspects. *J Hand Surg Br* 1996;21(6):735-745.

19. Kaplan JD, Jones NF: Outcome measures of microsurgical toe transfers for reconstruction of congenital and traumatic hand anomalies. *J Pediatr Orthop* 2014;34(3):362-368.

20. Chan KM, Ma GF, Cheng JC, Leung PC: The Krukenberg procedure: A method of treatment for unilateral anomalies of the upper limb in Chinese children. *J Hand Surg Am* 1984;9(4):548-551.

21. James MA, Bagley AM, Brasington K, Lutz C, McConnell S, Molitor F: Impact of prostheses on function and quality of life for children with unilateral congenital below-the-elbow deficiency. *J Bone Joint Surg Am* 2006;88(11):2356-2365.

22. Davids JR, Wagner LV, Meyer LC, Blackhurst DW: Prosthetic management of children with unilateral congenital below-elbow deficiency. *J Bone Joint Surg Am* 2006;88(6):1294-1300.

Chapter 69

Congenital Longitudinal Deficiencies of the Upper Limb

Michelle A. James, MD   Kathryn M. Peck, MD

Abstract

Radial and ulnar longitudinal deficiencies are the two most common congenital longitudinal deficiencies of the upper limbs and are characterized by a partially or completely absent radius or ulna, respectively. Radial longitudinal deficiency often is associated with abnormalities of other organ systems, including cardiac and renal systems, which can be potentially lethal and require a comprehensive medical evaluation. Ulnar longitudinal deficiency tends to be associated with other musculoskeletal abnormalities. Treatment aims to improve function and appearance and is best provided in a well-resourced setting in the context of a long-term relationship between the child, his or her family, and the hand surgeon.

Keywords: humeral hypoplasia; radial hypoplasia; radial longitudinal deficiency; thumb hypoplasia; ulnar longitudinal deficiency; upper limb hypoplasia

Introduction

Radial longitudinal deficiency (RLD) and ulnar longitudinal deficiency (ULD) are the two most common congenital longitudinal deficiencies of the upper limbs. These conditions historically were described as radial or ulnar "clubhand," but this term is no longer commonly used. The deficient bone may be partially or completely absent. In the original International Federation of Societies for Surgery of the Hand classification for congenital hand malformations, these deficiencies were considered failures of formation.[1] This classification was modified in 2013 by Kerby Oberg, Paul Manske, and Michael Tonkin and approved by the International Federation of Societies for Surgery of the Hand.[2] In this modification, these deficiencies are classified as malformations of the upper limb resulting from a failure of formation of the radial-ulnar (fetal anteroposterior) axis[2,3] (also known as preaxial [radius] or postaxial [ulna] longitudinal deficiencies).

Radial Longitudinal Deficiency

Clinical Features

RLD is characterized by partial or total absence of the radius and a short, bowed ulna that results in profound radial and palmar displacement of the hand and the carpus. The ulna is approximately two-thirds of its normal length. The humerus is often shorter than normal and, in rare cases, may be absent.[4] The elbow may be stiff, and the thumb may be absent or hypoplastic. The index and middle fingers also may be stiff; the ring and small fingers are usually flexible.

RLD often is bilateral and asymmetric. The wrist is unstable because of a lack of radial carpal support, and grip is weak because this instability is combined with finger stiffness. Children with RLD have difficulty reaching away from the body because of radial deviation of the wrist and bowing of the ulna. The severity of thumb deficiency is correlated with the severity of radial deficiency.[5] Children with manifestations of radial and thumb deficiencies may have difficulty attaining independence with activities of daily living, such as fastening buttons and performing personal hygiene.

Etiology

Two recent Northern European population studies showed that the incidence of RLD is 0.4 to 1.6 per 10,000 live births.[6,7] Golbfarb et al[8] found that 67% of children with RLD had an associated syndrome (**Table 1**) or a musculoskeletal condition. Scoliosis was the most common associated musculoskeletal condition. Other limb anomalies include humeral hypoplasia, radioulnar synostosis, radial head dislocation, and stiff digits.[9,10] The most common syndromes associated with RLD are VACTERL (vertebral malformations, imperforate anus, cardiac defects, tracheoesophageal fistula, renal abnormalities, and limb defects) and Holt-Oram syndrome; others that are less common but critical to diagnose preoperatively are thrombocytopenia absent radius syndrome, Diamond-Blackfan anemia (also known as congenital hypoplastic anemia), and Fanconi syndrome (also known as Fanconi anemia).

Dr. James or an immediate family member serves as a board member, owner, officer, or committee member of the American Board of Orthopaedic Surgery. Dr. Peck or an immediate family member has stock or stock options held in Eli Lilly.

Table 1 Most Common Syndromes Associated With Radial Longitudinal Deficiency

Syndrome	Inheritance Pattern	Associated Anomalies
VACTERL	Sporadic	Vertebral malformations, imperforate anus, cardiac defects, tracheoesophageal fistula, renal abnormalities, and limb defects
Holt-Oram syndrome	Autosomal dominant	Cardiac septal defects and radial dysplasia
Fanconi syndrome	Autosomal recessive	Pancytopenia and radial dysplasia
Thrombocytopenia absent radius syndrome	Autosomal recessive	Thrombocytopenia, absent radii, mildly hypoplastic thumbs present
Diamond-Blackfan anemia	Inherited, but heterogenous	Anemia and reticulocytopenia; growth retardation; craniofacial, upper limb, heart, and urinary system malformations

Table 2 Modified Bayne Classification of Radial Longitudinal Deficiency

Type	Thumb	Carpus	Distal Radius	Proximal Radius
N	Hypoplastic or absent	Normal	Normal	Normal
0	Hypoplastic or absent	Absence, hypoplasia, or coalition	Normal	Normal, radioulnar synostosis, or congenital dislocation of the radial head
1	Hypoplastic or absent	Absence, hypoplasia, or coalition	>2 mm shorter than the ulna	Normal, radioulnar synostosis, or congenital dislocation of the radial head
2	Hypoplastic or absent	Absence, hypoplasia, or coalition	Hypoplasia	Hypoplasia
3	Hypoplastic or absent	Absence, hypoplasia, or coalition	Physis absent	Variable hypoplasia
4	Hypoplastic or absent	Absence, hypoplasia, or coalition	Absent	Absent

VACTERL is a sporadic condition that includes anomalies of multiple different systems: vertebra, anus, cardiac, trachea/esophagus, renal, and limbs (including RLD).[11,12] Holt-Oram syndrome is an autosomal dominant condition that is characterized by cardiac septal defects as well as RLD.[7] Diamond-Blackfan anemia, Fanconi syndrome, and thrombocytopenia absent radius syndrome are bone marrow failure syndromes that may present as RLD. These conditions should be diagnosed preoperatively and treated by a pediatric hematologist because they are treatable and potentially lethal if not diagnosed and treated.[13]

Thalidomide, a teratogenic agent prescribed as a sedative in the late 1950s, resulted in various limb malformations, including RLD.[14] Other teratogens also may cause this malformation, depending on the timing of maternal exposure.

Diagnostic Studies

Children with RLD should undergo a complete physical examination, a thorough family history should be obtained, and a geneticist should be consulted. Radiographs of the entire upper limb (humerus, elbow, forearm, wrist, and hand—both sides) are essential to assess for associated abnormalities and classify the condition. A spine radiograph should be obtained to evaluate for congenital spine anomalies associated with VACTERL.

A complete blood count (bone marrow failure syndromes), a cardiac echocardiogram (VACTERL and Holt-Oram syndrome), a renal ultrasound (VACTERL), and a chromosomal breakage test (Fanconi syndrome) also are indicated.

Classification

Bayne and Klug[15] classified RLD into four types based on the extent of

radial hypoplasia demonstrated on radiographs. James et al[5] combined Bayne and Klug's classification with the modified Blauth classification for thumb hypoplasia to create a modified version that included children with carpal or thumb deficiencies in the presence of a normal radius[15] (**Tables 2** and **3**).

Treatment

The treatment of RLD is based on improving function and appearance. Functional impairments may be caused by thumb hypoplasia or absence, wrist instability with radial deviation and palmar flexion of the hand in relation to the forearm, and an overall shortened arm. Controversy still exists concerning the best way to surgically address the radially deviated wrist, although most pediatric hand surgeons agree that children fare better with surgical rather than nonsurgical treatment. Kotwal et al[16] reviewed 446 patients with RLD types

3 or 4 with a minimum follow-up of 5 years. Three hundred nine patients were treated surgically, and 137 patients were treated nonsurgically. Despite the high recurrence of deformity after centralization, improvements in the surgically treated group included the appearance and alignment of the wrist and hand, finger and wrist range of motion, and grip strength (**Figure 1**).

In addition to correcting ulnar bowing, centralization and radialization are two techniques for repositioning the hand onto the distal end of the ulna. Centralization aligns the long finger metacarpal and the ulna; radialization, as proposed by Buck-Gramcko,[17] placed the hand in ulnar deviation and aligned the index metacarpal with the ulna to diminish the recurrence of radial deviation. This technique, however, is no longer widely used. Both techniques are complicated by the recurrence of deformity and growth retardation from damage to the distal ulnar physis.

In addition to aligning the hand, surgical stabilization requires rebalancing of the tendon forces across the wrist. Stretching and splinting have been used to lengthen the soft tissues along the radial side of the ulna. Serial long arm, flexed-elbow casts can be used to stretch the radial and palmar soft tissue, and splints can be used to maintain correction. Splints can be applied to the radial side of the forearm to push or along the ulnar side to pull the hand ulnarly. In addition to splinting, parents should be taught how to stretch out a hand that exhibits radial deviation—a process that should be done several times per day.

If stretching exercises and splinting are insufficient, distraction can stretch the soft tissues to allow centralization. Goldfarb et al[18] described the use of a ring external fixator for soft-tissue distraction before centralization, gaining an average of 16 mm of distraction and enabling centralization without tension, thus minimizing the risk of damage to the ulnar physis. Nanchahal and

Table 3 Modified Blauth Classification of Hypoplastic Thumb

Type	Characteristic
I	Mild shortening or narrowing of the thumb
II	Thumb-index web space narrowing, hypoplastic intrinsic thenar muscles, and metacarpophalangeal joint instability
III	Type II hypoplasia plus: A: Extrinsic muscle abnormalities, hypoplastic metacarpal, and stable carpometacarpal joint B: Extrinsic muscle abnormalities, partial metacarpal aplasia, and unstable carpometacarpal joint
IV	Pouce flottant ("floating" thumb)
V	Absent thumb

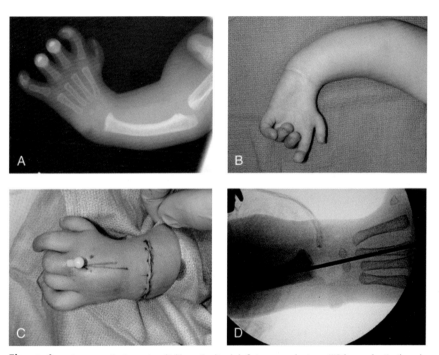

Figure 1   Images of a type 4 radial longitudinal deficiency and a type IIIB hypoplastic thumb in a child. **A,** AP radiograph. **B,** Clinical photograph of the limb. **C,** Postoperative photograph after centralization. **D,** AP radiograph after centralization, with intramedullary fixation in place.

Tonkin[19] showed that carpal realignment was possible in five of six patients who had soft-tissue distraction with an external fixator system before centralization, but if only centralization was performed, carpal realignment occurred in only one of six patients. However, a recent study reported that despite the ease of centralization after soft-tissue distraction, radial deviation was more likely to recur in those who underwent distraction versus the group who did not have distraction.[20]

After centralization, wrist motion is reduced;[15] thus, centralization is contraindicated when the ipsilateral elbow has an extension contracture because the child may need radial deviation and flexion to reach his or her mouth.

In addition to a high risk of recurrence of deformity, centralization places the distal ulnar physis at risk for early growth arrest, which is a devastating complication in an already shortened upper limb. Soft-tissue releases combined

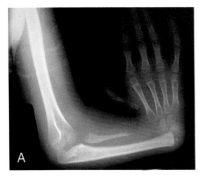 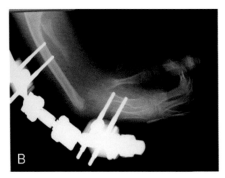 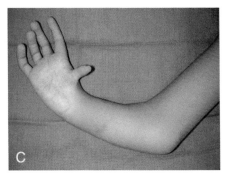

Figure 2 **A,** AP radiograph of a child with type 3 radial longitudinal deficiency and a type IIIB hypoplastic thumb. **B,** AP radiograph obtained after applying an external fixator for soft-tissue distraction. **C,** Clinical photograph obtained after soft-tissue distraction and centralization.

with tendon transfers and long-term splinting at night may improve wrist alignment while preserving wrist motion. For type 3 and 4 deficiencies, Wall et al[21] recommended the initiation of splinting and stretching, followed by releasing constricted radial soft tissues at the wrist with a volar bilobed flap for coverage of the radial side for a child aged 1 to 2 years. For a child aged 5 to 6 years, microvascular transplantation of the first metatarsophalangeal joint to the radial side of the wrist is considered, which was originally described by Vilkki;[22] however, most patients do not proceed further with the transfer because they are satisfied with both function and appearance. This approach maintains wrist motion and does not endanger the distal ulnar physis.

For adolescents with recurrent radial deviation, ulnocarpal arthrodesis is a salvage option. Pike et al[23] reported on 12 children with RLD who underwent ulnocarpal arthrodesis (11 patients underwent ulnocarpal epiphyseal arthrodesis, and 1 patient underwent traditional ulnocarpal arthrodesis). All achieved wrist stability and a decrease of 42° in radial deviation.

Ulnar lengthening has been used to treat RLD (**Figure 2**). Farr et al[24] reported eight ulnar lengthenings, noting an average increase of 75%, but correction of radial deviation and ulnar bowing was not maintained. Yoshida et al[25] reported on their experience of repeated

lengthenings of patients with type 4 RLD. With their initial lengthening, length increased 89% and then regressed to 70%; after the second lengthening, length increased to 102%, with the final length increase averaging 83%. Yoshida et al[25] recommended a second lengthening after skeletal maturity. Peterson et al[26] reported on 9 patients who underwent 13 ulnar lengthenings, achieving an average length of 4.4 cm with each lengthening. These authors commented that the process was long and arduous for both families and surgeons and fraught with complications. They recommended that this procedure be limited to the mature adolescent or teenager who has excellent family support.

Vascularized second metatarsophalangeal joint transfer has been used to stabilize the carpus and allow physeal growth. Vilkki[22] originally described this technique of transferring the second metatarsophalangeal joint along with the second ray to the radial aspect of the distal forearm. This technique provides structural support in addition to allowing growth resulting from the transposed toe phalanx physis. De Jong et al[27] reported 11-year follow-up, noting an average of 28° of radial deviation, average active wrist motion of 83°, and continued ulnar growth. The surgical procedure is technically demanding, and complications were reported in more than 50% of patients, resulting in subsequent procedures.

Another challenge with the surgical correction of RLD is soft-tissue coverage after the deviated wrist is corrected. The radial-side skin often is under substantial tension, and the ulnar-side skin often is redundant. Multiple techniques have been described to treat this, including the bilobed flap described by Evans et al,[28] which addresses the skin coverage issue by rotating the ulnar-side skin to the dorsum and the dorsal-side skin to the radial side. The bilobed flap can potentially lead to tip necrosis and cosmesis issues because of excessive ulnar skin. VanHeest and Grierson[29] and VanHeest[30] used a dorsal rotation flap that rotates the excessive ulnar skin radially. Subjective satisfaction with scar appearance was reported.[29]

Ulnar Longitudinal Deficiency
Clinical Features

The most important functional deficiencies in ULD involve the elbow and the forearm.[31] The ulna is partially or totally absent, and a cartilaginous anlage often is present.[32] The radius is typically shortened and bowed. The elbow is abnormal or fused (radiohumeral synostosis), and the entire arm is hypoplastic. The shoulder tends to be internally rotated. The carpus and the hand are almost always involved, with 90% of affected limbs missing digits, 70% demonstrating thumb abnormalities, and 30% demonstrating

Table 4 Modified Classification of Ulnar Longitudinal Deficiency

Type	Ulna	Radius	Elbow	Wrist/Hand
0	Normal	Normal	Stable	Absent or hypoplastic digits; carpal absence or coalition
1	Hypoplastic; distal and proximal epiphysis present	Mildly bowed	Stable	Mild ulnar wrist deviation; absent or hypoplastic digits
2	Partial aplasia; distal portion absent; ulnar anlage	Bowed	Variable stability; radial head may dislocate posterolaterally	Mild ulnar wrist deviation
3	Absent; no anlage	Straight	Unstable; posterolateral radial head dislocation; may have severe elbow flexion deformity	Less ulnar wrist deviation; severe carpal and digital deficiencies
4	Absent; ulnar anlage	Severely bowed	Radiohumeral synostosis; humeral internal rotation; forearm pronation	Ulnar wrist deviation
5	Absent	Straight	Radiohumeral synostosis; humeral bifurcation or large medial condyle	Less ulnar wrist deviation; severe carpal and digital deficiencies

syndactyly.[32] Unlike RLD, the hand is typically aligned with the wrist.

ULD is typically unilateral. Children with severe elbow contractures, radiohumeral synostosis, or bilateral ULD have limitations that are more related to function. They may have difficulty completing activities of daily living, especially personal hygiene and dressing. Children with radiohumeral synostosis and absent, deformed, or stiff fingers have the most limited function.[33,34]

Incidence and Etiology

Two recent epidemiologic studies of Northern European populations showed that the incidence of ULD is 0.2 to 0.4 per 10,000 live births.[6,7] Flatt[35] found that RLD is approximately four times as common as ULD. Unlike RLD, ULD is usually sporadic and not associated with systemic conditions.[32] It may be associated with other musculoskeletal malformations, including coxa vara, proximal femoral focal deficiency, fibular deficiency, phocomelia, scoliosis, absent digits, and radial ray deficiencies. Approximately 40% of children with ULD have associated contralateral upper limb abnormalities.[36] Syndromes associated with ULD include Weyers oligodactyly, Cornelia de Lange syndrome, ulnar mammary syndrome, Langer and

Reinhardt-Pfeiffer type mesomelic dysplasias, Pillay syndrome, ulnar fibular dysostosis, and femoral-fibular-ulnar deficiency syndrome.[34]

Diagnostic Studies

Radiographic imaging is necessary to determine the extent of ULD and classify the condition. Bilateral radiographs of the upper limbs are essential to evaluate for associated musculoskeletal anomalies, such as phocomelia, radiohumeral synostosis, absent digits, thumb hypoplasia, and syndactyly. Radiographs of the spine also should be obtained to evaluate for scoliosis.[37]

Classification

Multiple classification systems have been proposed for ULD, focusing on elbow and forearm anomalies. The classification system by Kummel[38] addressed the elbow joint and whether radiohumeral synostosis or dislocation of the radiocapitellar joint is present. Ogden et al[39] classified ULD based on the length of the ulna. The classification system by Bayne[40] combined ulnar length and elbow morphology[32] (**Table 4**). Cole and Manske[41] approached classification of ULD differently and based their system on the characteristics of the thumb and the first web (**Table 5**).

Table 5 Manske and Cole Classification of Thumb and First Web Space Anomalies Associated With Ulnar Longitudinal Deficiency

Type	Characteristic
A	Normal thumb and first web space
B	Mild first web space and thumb deficiency
C	Moderate to severe first web space and thumb deficiency (loss of opposition, malrotation, thumb index syndactyly, no extrinsic tendon function)
D	Absent thumb

Because the entire upper limb is involved, it is difficult to develop a classification system that addresses all associated anomalies. Therefore, most clinicians combine classification systems to develop a comprehensive plan to treat all the upper limb anomalies associated with ULD.

Treatment

The goals of treatment of children with ULD include improving the position and the function of the affected limb. Splinting of the wrist may prevent worsening of the ulnar deviation, but it has

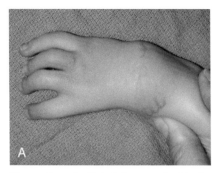 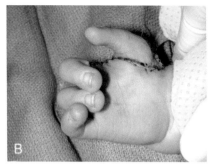

Figure 3 **A,** Clinical photograph of the hand of a child with type V absent thumb. **B,** Postoperative photograph of the hand after pollicization.

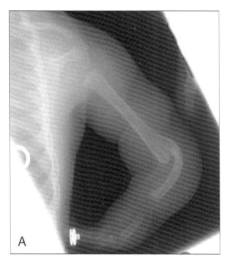 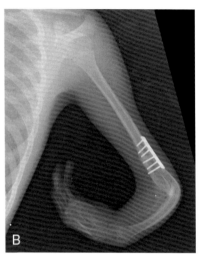

Figure 4 **A,** AP radiograph of a child with ulnar longitudinal deficiency. **B,** Postoperative AP radiograph of the same child taken several years later after humeral osteotomy.

Summary

RLD and ULD are failures of formation of the radius and the ulna, respectively. These conditions may be associated with other musculoskeletal conditions and syndromes. Treatment aims to improve function and appearance and is best provided in a well-resourced setting in the context of a long-term relationship between the child, his or her family, and the hand surgeon.

References

1. Swanson AB: A classification for congenital limb malformations. *J Hand Surg Am* 1976;1(1):8-22.

2. Tonkin MA, Tolerton SK, Quick TJ, et al: Classification of congenital anomalies of the hand and upper limb: Development and assessment of a new system. *J Hand Surg Am* 2013;38(9):1845-1853.

3. Ezaki M, Baek GH, Horii E, Hovius S: IFSSH Scientific Committee on Congenital Conditions. *J Hand Surg Eur Vol* 2014;39(6):676-678.

4. Goldfarb CA, Manske PR, Busa R, Mills J, Carter P, Ezaki M: Upper-extremity phocomelia reexamined: A longitudinal dysplasia. *J Bone Joint Surg Am* 2005;87(12):2639-2648.

5. James MA, McCarroll HR Jr, Manske PR: The spectrum of radial longitudinal deficiency: A modified classification. *J Hand Surg Am* 1999;24(6):1145-1155.

6. Koskimies E, Lindfors N, Gissler M, Peltonen J, Nietosvaara Y: Congenital upper limb deficiencies and associated malformations in Finland: A population-based study. *J Hand Surg Am* 2011;36(6):1058-1065.

7. Ekblom AG, Laurell T, Arner M: Epidemiology of congenital upper limb anomalies in Stockholm, Sweden, 1997 to 2007: Application of the Oberg, Manske, and Tonkin classification. *J Hand Surg Am* 2014;39(2):237-248.

not proved successful. Procedures to address hand anomalies include syndactyly release, first web space deepening, index pollicization (**Figure 3**), opponensplasty, and thumb metacarpal osteotomy.

Children with substantial internal rotation of the upper limb caused by ULD may have difficulty reaching their face and head with the ipsilateral hand. If they are able to perform activities of daily living, no treatment may be necessary. For persistent limitations, an external rotation osteotomy of the humerus places the hand in a more functional position (**Figure 4**).

Surgery for radiohumeral synostosis will not improve motion,[42] but a forearm rotational osteotomy may place the hand in a more functional position.[35] For children with partial ulnar deficiency, painful elbow instability, and limited forearm rotation, a one-bone forearm procedure can confer stability and reduce pain.[43-45]

Excision of the ulnar anlage, a fibrocartilaginous structure, is a controversial procedure for the treatment of ULD. Although some surgeons have hypothesized that the ulnar anlage fails to grow with the radius and acts as a tether, which leads to increased ulnar deviation and progressive wrist deformity,[34] progressive ulnar deviation deformity has not been consistently noted by others. Ulnar anlage resection appears most appropriate when progressive deformity of the wrist or elbow is present or if the bowing of the radius increases.[46]

8. Goldfarb CA, Wall L, Manske PR: Radial longitudinal deficiency: The incidence of associated medical and musculoskeletal conditions. *J Hand Surg Am* 2006;31(7):1176-1182.

9. Bauer AS, Bednar MS, James MA: Disruption of the radial/ulnar axis: Congenital longitudinal deficiencies. *J Hand Surg Am* 2013;38(11):2293-2302, quiz 2302.

10. James MA, McCarroll HR Jr, Manske PR: Characteristics of patients with hypoplastic thumbs. *J Hand Surg Am* 1996;21(1):104-113.

11. Quan L, Smith DW: The VATER association: Vertebral defects, anal atresia, T-E fistula with esophageal atresia, radial and renal dysplasia: A spectrum of associated defects. *J Pediatr* 1973;82(1):104-107.

12. Beals RK, Rolfe B: VATER association: A unifying concept of multiple anomalies. *J Bone Joint Surg Am* 1989;71(6):948-950.

13. Chirnomas SD, Kupfer GM: The inherited bone marrow failure syndromes. *Pediatr Clin North Am* 2013;60(6):1291-1310.

14. Lamb DW: Radial club hand: A continuing study of sixty-eight patients with one hundred and seventeen club hands. *J Bone Joint Surg Am* 1977;59(1):1-13.

15. Bayne LG, Klug MS: Long-term review of the surgical treatment of radial deficiencies. *J Hand Surg Am* 1987;12(2):169-179.

16. Kotwal PP, Varshney MK, Soral A: Comparison of surgical treatment and nonoperative management for radial longitudinal deficiency. *J Hand Surg Eur Vol* 2012;37(2):161-169.

17. Buck-Gramcko D: Radialization as a new treatment for radial club hand. *J Hand Surg Am* 1985;10(6 pt 2):964-968.

18. Goldfarb CA, Murtha YM, Gordon JE, Manske PR: Soft-tissue distraction with a ring external fixator before centralization for radial longitudinal deficiency. *J Hand Surg Am* 2006;31(6):952-959.

19. Nanchahal J, Tonkin MA: Preoperative distraction lengthening for radial longitudinal deficiency. *J Hand Surg Br* 1996;21(1):103-107.

20. Manske MC, Wall LB, Steffen JA, Goldfarb CA: The effect of soft tissue distraction on deformity recurrence after centralization for radial longitudinal deficiency. *J Hand Surg Am* 2014;39(5):895-901.

21. Wall LB, Ezaki M, Oishi SN: Management of congenital radial longitudinal deficiency: Controversies and current concepts. *Plast Reconstr Surg* 2013;132(1):122-128.

22. Vilkki SK: Vascularized joint transfer for radial club hand. *Tech Hand Up Extrem Surg* 1998;2(2):126-137.

23. Pike JM, Manske PR, Steffen JA, Goldfarb CA: Ulnocarpal epiphyseal arthrodesis for recurrent deformity after centralization for radial longitudinal deficiency. *J Hand Surg Am* 2010;35(11):1755-1761.

24. Farr S, Petje G, Sadoghi P, Ganger R, Grill F, Girsch W: Radiographic early to midterm results of distraction osteogenesis in radial longitudinal deficiency. *J Hand Surg Am* 2012;37(11):2313-2319.

25. Yoshida K, Kawabata H, Wada M: Growth of the ulna after repeated bone lengthening in radial longitudinal deficiency. *J Pediatr Orthop* 2011;31(6):674-678.

26. Peterson BM, McCarroll HR Jr, James MA: Distraction lengthening of the ulna in children with radial longitudinal deficiency. *J Hand Surg Am* 2007;32(9):1402-1407.

27. de Jong JP, Moran SL, Vilkki SK: Changing paradigms in the treatment of radial club hand: Microvascular joint transfer for correction of radial deviation and preservation of long-term growth. *Clin Orthop Surg* 2012;4(1):36-44.

28. Evans DM, Gateley DR, Lewis JS: The use of a bilobed flap in the correction of radial club hand. *J Hand Surg Br* 1995;20(3):333-337.

29. VanHeest A, Grierson Y: Dorsal rotation flap for centralization in radial longitudinal deficiency. *J Hand Surg Am* 2007;32(6):871-875.

30. VanHeest A: Wrist centralization using the dorsal rotation flap in radial longitudinal deficiency. *Tech Hand Up Extrem Surg* 2010;14(2):94-99.

31. Miller JK, Wenner SM, Kruger LM: Ulnar deficiency. *J Hand Surg Am* 1986;11(6):822-829.

32. Bednar MS, James MA, Light TR: Congenital longitudinal deficiency. *J Hand Surg Am* 2009;34(9):1739-1747.

33. Blair WF, Shurr DG, Buckwalter JA: Functional status in ulnar deficiency. *J Pediatr Orthop* 1983;3(1):37-40.

34. Johnson J, Omer GE Jr: Congenital ulnar deficiency: Natural history and therapeutic implications. *Hand Clin* 1985;1(3):499-510.

35. Flatt AE, ed: *The Care of Congenital Hand Anomalies*, ed 2. St. Louis, MO, Quality Medical Publishing Inc, 1994, pp 411-424.

36. Schmidt CC, Neufeld SK: Ulnar ray deficiency. *Hand Clin* 1998;14(1):65-76.

37. Kozin SH: Upper-extremity congenital anomalies. *J Bone Joint Surg Am* 2003;85(8):1564-1576.

38. Kummel W: Die Missbildungen der Extremitaeten durch Defekt, Verwachsung und Ueberzahl. *Bibliotheca Medica* 1895;3:1-83.

39. Ogden JA, Watson HK, Bohne W: Ulnar dysmelia. *J Bone Joint Surg Am* 1976;58(4):467-475.

40. Bayne LG: Ulnar club hand (ulnar deficiencies), in Green DP, ed: *Operative Hand Surgery*. New York, NY, Churchill Livingstone, 1982, pp 245-257, vol 11.

41. Cole RJ, Manske PR: Classification of ulnar deficiency according to the thumb and first web. *J Hand Surg Am* 1997;22(3):479-488.

42. Jacobsen ST, Crawford AH: Humeroradial synostosis. *J Pediatr Orthop* 1983;3(1):96-98.

43. Gogoi P, Dutta A, Sipani AK, Daolagupu AK: Congenital deficiency of distal ulna and dislocation of the radial head treated by single bone forearm procedure. *Case Rep Orthop* 2014;2014:526719.

44. Kitano K, Tada K: One-bone forearm procedure for partial defect of the ulna. *J Pediatr Orthop* 1985;5(3):290-293.

45. Sénès FM, Catena N: Correction of forearm deformities in congenital ulnar club hand: One-bone forearm. *J Hand Surg Am* 2012;37(1):159-164.

46. Broudy AS, Smith RJ: Deformities of the hand and wrist with ulnar deficiency. *J Hand Surg Am* 1979;4(4):304-315.

Chapter 70

Upper Limb Prostheses for Children

Robert D. Lipschutz, CP, BSME

Abstract

Fitting children with upper limb prostheses has many similarities to and many differences from adult prosthetic fittings. The components used in adult and pediatric devices are somewhat analogous in design, shape, and function. However, differences are seen in the size of the components, the etiology of the amputation or deficiency, the level of family involvement, and the required accommodations for future growth and component designs. Most adults with upper limb amputations are young men who have sustained traumatic injuries. Pediatric upper limb prostheses are more frequently fit in children who have congenital limb differences. All prosthetic fittings are unique to the situation and the individual. Common fitting principles for children are dependent on residual limb length, functional level, and age at the time of fitting.

Keywords: acquired amputation; acquired limb loss; body-powered prosthesis; congenital deficiency; externally powered prosthesis; limb deficiency; longitudinal deficiency; myoelectric control; passive prosthesis; prosthesis; transverse deficiency

Introduction

The decision of whether to fit children with upper limb prostheses has been a topic of controversy for many years. Compounding this dilemma is the ongoing development of prosthetic options for children and young adults.[1-7] Although some studies have reported no substantial benefits for fitting children with upper limb prostheses, others have demonstrated their usefulness in improving efficiency in manual activities.[8-12] Regardless of these conclusions, each child and family is unique and has its own reasons and desires concerning prosthetic fitting. Success in fitting a child with an upper limb prosthesis is subject to a multitude of variables, but it requires educating the family and the efforts of a dedicated healthcare team.

General Considerations

In preparing for prosthetic intervention, the family should have a thorough understanding and acceptance of the influence of amputation etiology, component options, functional benefits, cyclic wearing patterns, the child's motivation level, and the challenges associated with prosthetic use. At first, the parents will make the decision for their child; later in life, the child will be encouraged to become involved in the process of selecting a prosthesis and its components.

The primary etiology for upper limb amputations in children is congenital anomalies. In such patients, parents must understand and accept the differences in their child's upper limb. In a child with an acquired amputation caused by trauma, infection, tumor, or other injury, it may be even more difficult for the child and family to accept the amputation.

Information should be provided about the associated benefits and limitations of various prosthetic components, such as terminal devices and elbows. The child and family also need to clearly express their goals and desires for the prosthetic fitting (whether the device will be aesthetic, prehensile, or has some combination of aesthetic and prehensile attributes) and recognize that such preferences may change throughout the child's life. Periodically, children may express a reluctance to wear an upper limb prosthesis. This reluctance will often begin with nonverbal cues when the child is quite young and progress to complete rejection when the child has the ability to verbally communicate. Children and young adults have the ability to change their minds and often go through a cyclic pattern of use and rejection of upper limb prostheses. Throughout childhood and adolescence, patients will have the ability to try a variety of styles and components, allowing them to make a more educated decision on prosthetic design and use as they become adults.

The commitment of the family, the child, and the clinical team to the prosthetic fitting process is paramount in achieving success.[13,14] Over time, the attitudes of clinical teams and families toward the fitting and use of upper limb prostheses have changed[15]—with fewer absolutes and more gray zones. The clinical team should discuss the variables of prosthetic fitting, including voluntary nonuse by the child. If the child is fit with a prosthesis, a thorough effort

Neither Dr. Lipschutz nor any immediate family member has received anything of value from or has stock or stock options held in a commercial company or institution related directly or indirectly to the subject of this chapter.

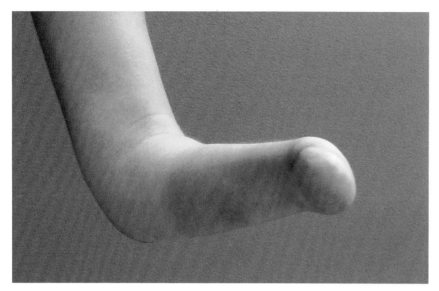

Figure 1   Clinical photograph of a transcarpal congenital limb deficiency with nubbins and physiologic wrist motion. (Courtesy of the Rehabilitation Institute of Chicago, Chicago, IL.)

must be made to train the child in its use. Families are often too busy to invest adequate time in the training process and expect that the child will accept the prosthesis without constant assistance in donning the device and reminders of how to incorporate it into his or her daily activities.

Along with family and peer support, professional training by an occupational therapist is also beneficial. Although many occupational therapists have limited training in working with upper limb prostheses, there are many centers that specialize in the care of children and have therapists with the required experience. When fitting a child with an upper limb prosthesis, the clinical team should seek the assistance of an experienced therapist to provide training and support.

The clinical characteristics of children with upper limb deficiencies vary widely. Longitudinal limb deficiencies are less common than transverse deficiencies; therefore, prosthetic fittings are more common in patients with transverse deficiencies.[16,17] In this chapter, the principles of prosthetic fitting will begin with the distal-most amputations and deficiencies and progress through more

proximal amputation levels. The components appropriate for different levels of limb absence in specific age groups are also detailed in this chapter.

Digital Absence

Congenital deficiencies are rarely the cause of isolated absences of a digit or digits. Syndromes such as Streeter dysplasia (often referred to as amniotic band syndrome), Möbius syndrome, or Poland syndrome may infrequently cause digital absence, but these disorders are uncommon, and prosthetic restoration of individual fingers is rare in affected patients. In the pediatric population, trauma is more likely the cause of digital amputations. Potential causes include injuries sustained from paper shredders, farming equipment, and fireworks.

The main prosthetic intervention for digit amputation is an aesthetic replacement of the finger for cosmetic and psychological reasons. The function of these digits is limited and often interferes with the child's ability to perform manual tasks. In addition, prostheses for this level of amputation that meet the aesthetic needs of the child and family often are very expensive and do not

last for long periods of time because of the child's continued growth. However, prosthetic intervention with an aesthetic prosthesis remains an available option, especially for older children and those with an acquired digital amputation.

Partial Hand With No Digits Remaining and Wrist Disarticulation

Partial hand amputations with no digits remaining (for example, transverse deficiency of the carpals) are much more common in children than adults. When an adult sustains a traumatic partial hand amputation, it is rare to have all five fingers completely absent, with a row of carpal bones remaining. In children, the limbs often have nubbins (small finger-like remnants on the distal end of the limb), along with movement through the carpal bones (**Figure 1**). Despite the differences between such amputations and wrist disarticulations, the prosthetic fitting principles will be addressed together in this chapter because of the similar limb lengths and overlapping prosthetic interventions, particularly when residual wrist and hand motion is limited.

A residual limb of this length allows the child to perform many tasks without a prosthesis in a physiologic position that is close to normal. Because the end of the affected limb is nearly the length of the contralateral limb, the manipulation of objects and the performance of bimanual tasks are only minimally affected (**Figure 2**).

Prosthetic fitting at this amputation level has both advantages and disadvantages. Creating reliance on the prosthesis allows the child to become accustomed to its use and encourages the child to incorporate the prosthesis into daily activities. However, covering the end of the residual limb decreases tactile feedback, which is an important aspect of manual dexterity and development. Some retention of tactile feedback may be accomplished by leaving

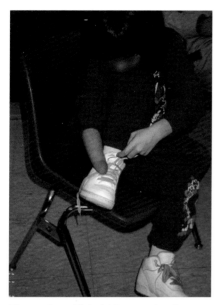

Figure 2 Clinical photograph of an approximately 5-year-old girl with a longer residual limb and minimal functional impairment. (Courtesy of the Rehabilitation Institute of Chicago, Chicago, IL.)

an opening at the end of the forearm of the prosthesis so that the distal residual limb is exposed (**Figure 3**). However, it is unclear whether this allowance benefits long-term prosthetic use and acceptance.

As with any longer residual limb, there are challenges for fitting components and maintaining prosthetic limb-length equality with the contralateral side. Epiphysiodeses of the radial and ulnar styloids have been suggested as a potential means of creating space for prosthetic components. However, opponents of this surgical approach cite the disadvantage of the exaggerated limb-length discrepancy if the individual chooses not to wear a prosthesis.

Fitting Infants

The age of a child at the first fitting with an upper limb prosthesis varies from clinic to clinic and according to the level of the limb deficit. At the partial hand and wrist disarticulation levels, it has been widely accepted that infants (younger than 1 year) can be fit with a prosthesis at approximately 6 months

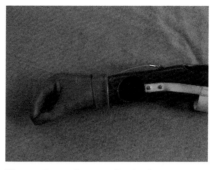

Figure 3 Photograph of a forearm prosthesis with a distal opening at the end of the forearm that exposes the distal residual limb to allow tactile feedback. (Courtesy of the Rehabilitation Institute of Chicago, Chicago, IL.)

of age when they are obtaining sitting balance and are beginning to explore their environment bimanually.[6,14,15,18] The optimal fitting age varies from child to child and may be affected by many variables, including the effect of having infants sleep on their backs to decrease the risk of sudden infant death syndrome. Limited "tummy time" may delay upper body development and coordination, thus delaying the benefits gained from using an upper limb prosthesis. For very young children, passive prostheses are the most widely accepted options for decreasing the difference in length between the residual and contralateral limbs, maintaining sitting balance, and encouraging bimanual activities. It has been suggested that the earlier prosthetic fitting begins, the more likely the child and family will be to accept the device; however, this topic is debatable.

In infants, the passive terminal devices may have the appearance of an open hand, a crawling hand, or a mitt. Standard terminal devices and wrist units are discouraged at these levels of limb absence because they make the prosthesis too long. Instead, proximally "hollowed" terminal devices and/or gloves filled with a flexible material are generally used. These options permit the socket to protrude into the proximal aspect of the terminal device to preserve limb-length equality.

At this early age, an infant's limbs have little bony definition and, thus, will not require the prosthetic accommodations for a bulbous distal end that will become necessary as the child matures. The shape of the socket is very generic, and reliance on sleeves or minimal harnessing for suspension is preferred. Socket construction for an infant's prosthesis often consists of a thin, lightweight lamination with a removable (onion-skin) layer to accommodate growth. A semiflexible thermoplastic material, such as Surlyn (Dupont), is often used for this removable layer (or inner socket) because it is hygienic and allows direct lamination of the rigid frame without a separator. Laminating directly over the semiflexible thermoplastic material permits the two sockets to temporarily bond together until such time that the prosthetist and the family deem it appropriate to remove the inner socket because of growth. When this transition occurs, the prosthetist should check the trim lines of the remaining laminated socket because the edges most likely will be sharp and require smoothing.

Additional volume management is often necessary because the child grows rapidly during this stage. Limb volume may be managed by initially oversizing the socket and using fitting socks that can be reduced in thickness and ultimately eliminated as the child grows. However, the thickness of the original sock should be limited because it further increases the size and bulk of the forearm, which is already larger because of the addition of the onion-skin layer. Although the preemptive use of an inner socket layer and additional fitting socks will ultimately prolong the useful life of the prosthesis, too large of a forearm may be unacceptable to the family.

Fitting Toddlers and Preschoolers

Similar components may be used when fitting a toddler (1 year to younger than 3 years) and a preschooler (aged 3 to

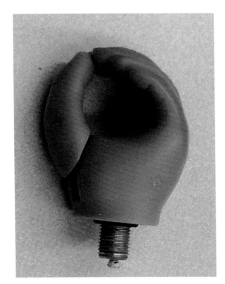

Figure 4 Photograph of a passive terminal device with prehensile capabilities. (Courtesy of the Rehabilitation Institute of Chicago, Chicago, IL.)

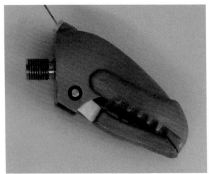

Figure 5 Photograph of the child-size CAPP terminal device, which has a wide palmar face and a friction cover for secure prehension. (Courtesy of the Rehabilitation Institute of Chicago, Chicago, IL.)

5 years). Although no exact age exists at which the child will be fit with a prosthesis that has grasping capabilities, the introduction of a child's first prehensile terminal device often is accomplished at the toddler stage. The main factors that necessitate the recommendation for most new prosthetic fittings at this developmental stage include anatomic changes to the limb and the child's capacity to use prosthetic designs with expanded capabilities. If designed appropriately with growth accommodations, the child's first prosthesis should last approximately 1 year, at which time the child will be approximately 18 months—an appropriate age for fitting a prosthesis with a prehensile terminal device.

At 18 months of age, toddlers with transverse deficiencies of the carpals may or may not have sufficient space for a prehensile terminal device in their prosthesis without having a length discrepancy of their forearm and hand. Congenital anomalies are rarely isolated to one structure, and these deficiencies are generally no exception. A discrepancy in the length of the ipsilateral humerus and/or radius and ulna is frequently associated with a transverse deficiency of the carpals. With this shortening, standard prosthetic components may be used without resulting in a longer prosthetic arm compared with the noninvolved arm.

Terminal devices for toddlers may be similar to the passive devices previously mentioned or passive devices with prehensile capabilities (**Figure 4**). They may have flexible, conformable fingers or true articulations with spring- or elastic-loaded closing force and the capabilities of cable activation later. These designs may be of various shapes, including hooks, hands, and the CAPP (Fillauer) terminal device (**Figure 5**). Arguments have been made for the functional abilities of one design compared with another; however, the most important aspect is acceptance by the family and actual use of the prescribed prosthesis.

Active, body-powered terminal devices also may be used and require a harness to provide cable activation of the prehensor. This transition will likely be new to the child and family and may require education and training for donning, use, and adjustments.

Arguments also have been made that toddlers do not have the cognitive ability and coordination for these types of devices, so an externally powered prosthesis is the most appropriate design for this age.[6] Externally powered options consist of electric hand terminal devices with one of two common input strategies that are both myoelectrically controlled. Toddlers are commonly fit with a single-site, voluntary-opening, automatic closing electronic scheme that is analogous to a body-powered voluntary opening terminal device. This often is referred to as a "cookie crusher" or St. Anthony's Circuit and was designed by T. Walley Williams III and Tom Haslam in the late 1980s.[19] This input design requires a single electrode, which is typically mounted in the socket over the child's wrist extensors, and requires muscle activation to signal opening of the hand. After the extensor signal falls below the open threshold, the hand is driven closed by means of either electric power or a spring, such as that used in the Scamp Hand (RSL-Steeper). The placement of the electrode over the extensors is not only intended for the current design and function but also anticipates future designs in which dual-site myoelectric systems will use wrist extensors for hand opening and wrist flexors for hand closing. If appropriate, this latter strategy may be planned for by incorporating an electrode dummy into the socket with the goal of later converting the prosthesis to dual-site control before a new device is applied. For a small percentage of toddlers, dual-site myoelectric prostheses may be used in the initial fitting because children with longer limbs have an innate ability to move the end of their residual limb by means of extensors and flexors, and they may have the cognitive abilities to use this strategy for their first prehensile design.

Regardless of the strategy for controlling the electric hand, a battery is required. Limbs of this length have adequate mechanical advantage and may well tolerate this added weight. The challenge, however, for these residual limb lengths is where to place the battery without compromising the aesthetics of the prosthesis. The battery must be either incorporated into the forearm, making the forearm more bulky and cylindric, or tethered on a cable, necessitating a more proximal attachment (**Figure 6**). Neither option is optimal.

If the child has substantial movement in his or her residual limb (wrist flexion and extension), opposition posts may be more beneficial than more traditional prostheses. Opposition posts are typically frame-type devices that fit over the forearm and have a distal extension that provides a platform about which the motion of the residual limb will oppose during wrist flexion. Adjustability of the platform position is generally provided to allow grasping of objects of varying sizes and shapes. The efficacy of these devices may be more pronounced in individuals with bilateral involvement.[20]

Fitting School-Age Children, Adolescents, and Young Adults

After a child reaches school age and beyond, if he or she has been previously fit with a prosthesis, a wearing pattern has typically been developed. The aforementioned component options (passive, body-powered, and externally powered) are still available and appropriate as the child grows. One difference that may become progressively apparent when examining the residual limb is the anatomic definition that has developed. For transverse deficiencies of the carpals, with partial amputations or wrist disarticulations, a bulbous distal end has now developed, which is both a benefit and a detriment. The benefit of these contoured limbs is the ability to provide suspension of the prosthesis by securing adequate purchase of the bulbous distal limb. Drawbacks include the difficulty of designing a prosthesis that permits easy donning. Various designs, including socket cutouts (doors) and expandable bladders, have been described. Self-suspension of any upper limb prosthesis has the benefit of reducing or

eliminating harnessing and potentially decreasing the amount of force being transmitted to the contralateral axilla by means of the harness.

An additional benefit of the limb definition may be the option of using alternative electronic means of input for an externally powered prosthesis for individuals with carpal motion. In myoelectric prostheses, electrodes must be in contact with muscle bellies. In traditional designs for this amputation level, electrodes are mounted over the wrist flexors and extensors at the proximal aspect of the forearm, requiring a socket that encompasses most of the forearm. If wrist motion is available, control is obtained by bending "flex strips" or initiating contact against opposing force-sensing resistors. The former may further permit the use of wrist articulation, preserving functional wrist motion within the prosthesis.

Transradial Level

A transradial amputation is usually the result of trauma, tumor, or (more likely) a congenital transverse deficiency of the forearm (predominantly in the upper one-third of the arm, leaving a short or very short limb). Children with transverse deficiencies often have residual nubbins, which are usually smaller than those on longer limbs and do not disrupt prosthetic fitting. Although fitting children with this level of limb absence may be somewhat controversial, differing opinions are less directed at the length and use of the prosthetic limb and more at the long-term use of a prosthesis and the improvement in the child's quality of life.[8,9] Despite not having a hand or long residual limb, children with this limb length will often find ways to use the residual limb for many tasks, such as opposing the residual limb against the other arm with an object captured between, catching an object in the cubital fold of the residual limb, or trapping an object under their axilla. However, these methods are generally used in positions

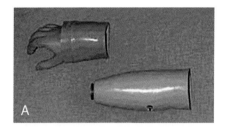

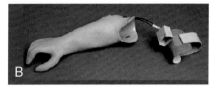

Figure 6 **A,** Photograph of a prosthesis with a bulky forearm with an incorporated battery. **B,** Photograph of a battery tethered on the triceps cuff of the prosthesis. (Courtesy of the Rehabilitation Institute of Chicago, Chicago, IL.)

in which visualization is less directed at the environment and is more within traditional lines of sight. Wearing a prosthesis will afford children the ability to manipulate objects further away from their body as well as provide prehensile capabilities in the terminal device that may be more beneficial to the task being performed. Contrary to the previously described levels of amputation, these limbs often are quite short and could conceivably benefit from orthopaedic lengthening techniques. However, evidence has shown that this is rarely performed; when lengthening is performed, complications often arise.[21]

Fitting Infants

In addition to moving bimanual tasks toward more functional lines of sight, additional reasons for fitting a prosthesis to an infant with a transradial-level deficit are analogous to reasons for fittings at longer limb levels and will be pertinent throughout the remainder of this chapter. Early fittings begin at approximately 6 months of age and consist of passive terminal device options. Fabrication often consists of removable inner sockets for growth and lightweight, laminated outer sockets that are pigmented to

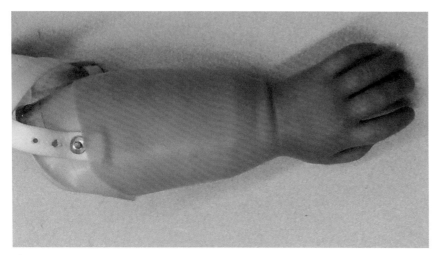

Figure 7   Photograph of a passive transradial prosthesis for an infant of approximately 6 months of age. The prosthesis has a removable inner socket for growth and a lightweight, laminated outer socket that is pigmented to match the child's skin. These prostheses often result in a proximal section that is larger than the forearm, thus creating an abrupt transition from the socket to the forearm. (Courtesy of the Rehabilitation Institute of Chicago, Chicago, IL.)

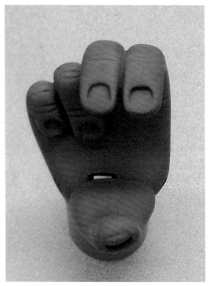

Figure 8   Photograph of a voluntary closing terminal device with sculpted fingers for a toddler or preschool-age child. (Courtesy of the Rehabilitation Institute of Chicago, Chicago, IL.)

match the child's skin. These prostheses often result in a proximal section that is larger than the forearm or glove that is being applied, thus creating an abrupt transition from the socket to the forearm (**Figure 7**). Because of material limitations associated with the vinyl used in many glove types, it is challenging to stretch the prefabricated glove over this circumference.

These prostheses are suspended by means of a small sleeve or lightweight figure-of-8 or chest strap harness. Because children have a way of wiggling out of their prostheses (especially when the residual limb is short), it is beneficial to have a harness in place to prevent loss of the device. Applying the prosthesis and the harness to an infant often is challenging, with parents, therapists, and prosthetists alike finding it difficult to keep the infant's limb in the socket while simultaneously securing the harness in place. This situation can be a source of frustration for parents and caretakers and an impetus for trying a sleeve for suspension.

A more recent suspension strategy that is being incorporated into pediatric fittings is the use of high-density silicone sockets with integrated silicone sleeves. This flexible material may be reflected proximally, donned onto the limb, and rolled back over the child's limb, where it provides compressive forces to suspend the device. In these designs, the entire outer surface, including the socket, is fabricated from silicone and is customarily a one-piece design. Although the appearance is more satisfactory than laminated sockets and vinyl gloves, these designs are not easily modified.

Fitting Toddlers and Preschoolers

The decision to either keep the current design or try an alternative prosthetic approach is generally made when a child achieves the milestone of either outgrowing the current device or beginning to investigate his or her environment to the degree that the child's family feels a new design is warranted. As with the previously described limb levels, passive, passive with prehensile capabilities, cable-activated, or myoelectric prostheses may be chosen. In contrast, however, adequate room generally exists between the distal end of the residual limb and the final length of the terminal device in all of these prosthetic strategies.

A child's cognitive ability to use a body-powered prostheses may present a challenge, but training by an occupational therapist usually remedies problems.[5,6] Parental acceptance of the aesthetics of a cable-driven prosthesis tends to be the greater challenge. Regardless of the degree of function permitted with a given terminal device, if it is not acceptable in appearance to the family, they will not be motivated to put it on the child, and the fitting will likely fail.

Voluntary-opening terminal devices are limited to the split-hook design, the CAPP terminal device, or mechanical hands. Voluntary-closing terminal devices for children are available in a variety of shapes and colors, including those with sculpted fingers (**Figure 8**). Because parents often desire a more lifelike prosthesis for their child, they often choose devices with a hand-like appearance. More conventional mechanical hands with voluntary opening or voluntary closing activation patterns are an available option but are much more difficult for the child to operate, largely because of the gloves that cover them.

When a glove is applied over a mechanical hand, it dramatically decreases the mechanical efficiency of the system by increasing the forces required for operation.[22] Spring tension in the hands may be reduced for easier opening; however, this also affects the grasping force of the hands, especially voluntary-opening hands.

Myoelectric prostheses are another popular option because they provide a hand-like terminal device with a glove that does not require gross body movements for use. The motor, which is housed within the hand, provides the necessary force to open and close the device against the resistance of the glove. However, the weight of the electric hand must be considered because most children with transradial limbs have transverse deficiencies in the proximal one-third of their anatomic forearm length, which puts their short residual limbs at a mechanical disadvantage relative to the mass of the hand and the forearm. In addition, as described previously, such systems require a battery, which adds more weight to the prosthesis distal to the residual limb. Although these batteries have become substantially smaller in recent years, they still add weight that must be overcome by the residual limb.

Cookie-crusher strategies are the most popular for a first electric prosthesis, especially in children younger than 4 years. At this limb level, a single-control (voluntary opening) pattern may be elicited much more easily than a dual-control (voluntary opening and closing) pattern. Because there is less preserved movement at the end of the residual limb, training a child with a short transradial deficiency to contract antagonistic muscles is much more difficult than for a child with a longer residual limb. Asking the child to "wiggle" the end of his or her arm is a typical training prompt, but it does not always elicit a consistent response in a child younger than 3 years.

Prosthetic sockets are much more invasive for shorter residual limbs than for longer limbs. They often cross the elbow joint proximally to provide stability and obtain purchase on the limb. Proximal extensions of the socket also distribute forces over a larger surface area, thus decreasing pressure. Many prosthetists choose self-suspending sockets when designing prostheses for children of this age. Traditional Münster socket designs are appropriate for this limb length. They incorporate high and tight anteroposterior trim lines that straddle the biceps tendon and extend above the olecranon, respectively. Because of this design, they require a donning technique in which the soft tissues are drawn into the socket by means of a "pull sock," a technique that is often difficult to master for both the parents and the child. In addition, because of its proximal extension and containment, the Münster socket reduces range of motion (both flexion and extension) at the elbow when worn. In response, a hybrid socket design that incorporates principles of tight anteroposterior and mediolateral trim lines may be used. This design will facilitate easier donning (although a donning aid may still be needed), but it will not limit range of motion of the prosthesis as dramatically, and the aesthetics of the static and dynamic use of the prosthesis will not be affected. Lower trim lines allow greater range of flexion for midline and cephalic activities.

The dramatic difference in children's limb shapes when the elbow is extended, also makes socket fit more difficult. Many of these children have substantial ligamentous laxity about the elbow and are capable of hyperextending their elbows (**Figure 9**). When doing so, the radial head frequently subluxates anteriorly, causing a bulge in the anterolateral aspect of their cubital fold. This change in limb shape must be considered to create a comfortably fitting socket.

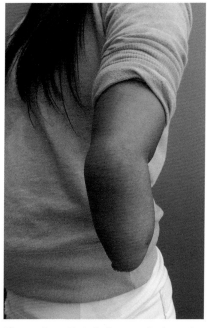

Figure 9 Clinical photograph shows hyperextension of a transradial limb. (Courtesy of the Rehabilitation Institute of Chicago, Chicago, IL.)

Fitting School-Age Children, Adolescents, and Young Adults

As mentioned for other amputation levels, if a child has developed a wearing pattern with a particular style of prosthesis, he or she is likely to continue with that design. However, as children grow older they may want a prosthesis that is more accepted by their peers (hand-like terminal devices). All of the aforementioned prosthetic control options (passive, body-powered, and externally powered) are available for children of school age or older who have amputations at the transradial level. Externally powered hands are a good option for these children because they add aesthetic value, require minimal movement to activate, and maintain prehensile capabilities. At these ages, the child would most likely prefer to have volitional control of both opening and closing; therefore, a cookie-crusher circuit often is abandoned for a dual-site control strategy. It may be challenging to educate the child to perform these movements and accurately capture them

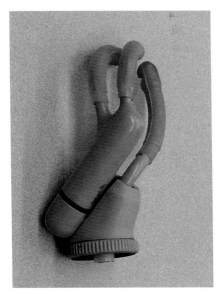

Figure 10 Photograph of a pediatric, externally powered hand with oppositional grasp. (Courtesy of the Rehabilitation Institute of Chicago, Chicago, IL.)

in a myoelectric control strategy. The residual limb is often quite short, and when the muscles on the medial aspect of the forearm (those assumed to be wrist and finger flexors) are contracted, the residual limb becomes even shorter, often pulling away from the socket walls. It is imperative that the medial electrode be well situated on the limb to capture this surface electromyographically. Unfortunately, this electrode begins to encroach on the medial epicondyle because it must be located more proximally to maintain skin contact during muscle contraction.

An additional challenge with electronic hands for school-aged children may be changes in the grasp patterns of the hand. The two main hand grasp patterns for children's electronic hands are palmar prehension (three-jaw-chuck) and oppositional grasp.[4,23] Several manufactures, including Variety Ability Systems and RSLSteeper, make prosthetic hands with the palmar prehension pattern, and the hands are available in a variety of age-correlated sizes, ranging from 0 to 3 for infants and toddlers and 7 to 11 for adolescents. The Electrohand

2000 line from Ottobock also is available in a range of similar sizes; however, this line provides a more oppositional-type grasp (**Figure 10**). When transitioning to larger hands, this grasp pattern is no longer available, so a young adult must adapt to a palmar prehension pattern. Prehensile patterns may be further altered as young adult users continue to grow, with the availability of newer multifunctional hands that provide a variety of grasp patterns through various means of mode selection.

Transhumeral Level
Limb lengths at the transhumeral level of amputation or deficiency vary quite dramatically. Children with a very short ulna may be fit prosthetically as if they have an elbow disarticulation. Relatively long congenital transhumeral deficiencies also are frequently observed. The most challenging patients are those with midlength to short transhumeral limbs because of the fairly substantial mechanical disadvantage along with the frequent need for revisions that further shorten the limb segment. Such revisions often are necessary because of the absence of the distal humeral epiphysis, making the limb prone to bony overgrowth, which is often referred to as spiking. As this distal bone is removed to relieve spiking and damage to the internal soft tissue, the residual limb becomes shorter, thus losing more leverage for controlling a prosthesis.

Fitting Infants
Children with deficiencies through the humerus may also be fit early. However, a lack of consensus exists as to when to introduce components that are more complex and when to expect the child to gain the ability to control the prosthesis entirely with the involved limb.[1,3,13,18] First fittings for these children include passive prostheses, most of which do not have articulating joints or prehensile terminal devices. Prosthetic elbows are usually omitted because they would

require a prohibitively sophisticated feature that could vary the amount of friction between loading and unloading during crawling. The resistance to elbow movement in the sagittal plane would need to be low when pre-positioning the hand for activity; however, resistance to the weight of the child when leaning on the device would need to be high to prevent inadvertent elbow flexion. In many instances, this first prosthesis will resemble a "banana arm"—a transhumeral prosthesis with no elbow articulation but with a severe flexion "bow" that permits the child to easily reach midline with the terminal device. The aforementioned terminal device may be a passive hand or a spring-loaded component that permits objects (for example, bottles and rattles) to be held.

Fitting Toddlers and Preschoolers
Articulating joints often are incorporated into prostheses for children older than 20 months. The activation, however, will depend on the child's cognitive abilities, the family's willingness to participate in the functional use of the device, and the clinical team's experience in fitting and training the child with these added components. Passive friction elbows permit positioning against some resistance, which is helpful for some bimanual tasks. However, if substantial weight is placed through the terminal device or on the forearm of the prosthesis, the elbow may inadvertently move, which is a source of frustration for the young prosthesis user.

Instead of a passive frictional component, a component with a positive locking feature may be used (either outside locking hinges or an internal locking elbow). Outside hinges with a "step-lock" style mechanism may be used, especially for longer limbs (**Figure 11**). Step-lock mechanisms permit the user to manually flex the joints to a greater degree of flexion, which then blocks the joints from going into extension. To bring the arm back into extension, the

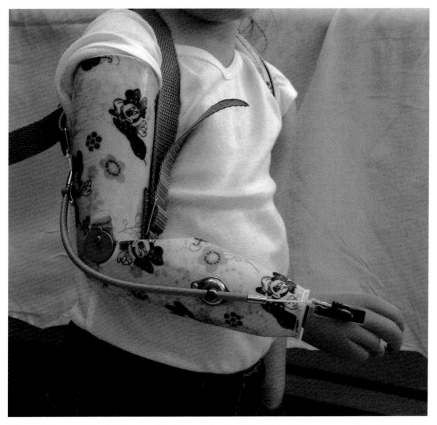

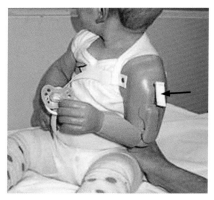

Figure 12   Clinical photograph of a prosthesis with an alternating locking mechanism that is manually activated by pulling and releasing the webbing (arrow) attached to the elbow cable lock. (Courtesy of the Rehabilitation Institute of Chicago, Chicago, IL.)

Figure 11   Clinical photograph of a prosthesis with outside hinges and a "step-lock" style mechanism. (Courtesy of the Rehabilitation Institute of Chicago, Chicago, IL.)

joints must be maximally flexed, which then releases the lock and permits full extension of the elbow.

In elbows with a mechanism that allows alternating locking and unlocking, the mechanism should be easily activated by attaching a loop or other form that is readily grasped by the parent or the child's contralateral hand (**Figure 12**). The aforementioned elbows may be successfully combined with a body-powered terminal device if a Bowden cable system is used.

Activating the elbow locking and unlocking mechanism with the typical combined motions of glenohumeral extension, glenohumeral abduction, and shoulder depression is a sophisticated task that is reserved for experienced, older children. Most children cannot complete this complex combination of motions until they are at least age 5 years.[5,18] Devices that use a fairlead

cable and housing approach require that, after the child has the elbow locked in the desired position of flexion, he or she must have enough remaining body excursion to open the terminal device. Because of the cabling configuration, such a process is challenging for a young child and is proportionately more difficult for those with shorter limbs.

Active control of the prosthetic elbow and the terminal device may be facilitated when an electronic hand is used within a hybrid prosthesis. Electronic elbow choices for children of this age are no longer available because the only suitable pediatric electronic elbows have been discontinued by their manufacturers. The use of larger pediatric electronic elbows is reserved for older children, children with bilateral limb loss above the elbow, or those with shoulder disarticulations. If active use of the elbow and the hand is desired in a toddler or

a preschool-age child, a hybrid prosthesis consisting of a body-powered elbow combined with an externally powered hand must be chosen.

Fitting School-Age Children, Adolescents, and Young Adults

School-age children have the cognitive ability to perform some of the more complex body movements required to activate transhumeral body-powered and externally powered prostheses. In school-age children with recently acquired amputations resulting from trauma or tumor, there may be greater motivation to use prostheses with more complex controls compared with their age-matched counterparts with congenital deficiencies because those with a recent amputation have been accustomed to living with an active elbow. At this age, the elbow locking/unlocking functions generally may be controlled by means of the previously described ipsilateral shoulder movements. In addition, powered prosthetic components, such as electronic elbows and terminal devices, may be introduced to provide function without the limitations of insufficient body excursion. Electronic elbows for children are limited to the VASI 8-12 Elbow[4] (Liberating Technologies; **Figure 13**). Electronic terminal devices are

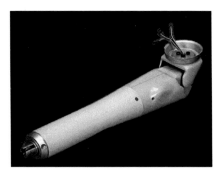

Figure 13 Photograph of a VASI 8-12 elbow, which is the only electric prosthetic elbow available for children and preteens. (Courtesy of the Rehabilitation Institute of Chicago, Chicago, IL.)

analogous to those described previously in this chapter and may be combined with electronic elbows in an externally powered prosthesis or a hybrid design.

Shoulder Disarticulation Level

Congenital shoulder disarticulation levels for an infant are either true shoulder disarticulations (for example, transverse deficiency of the arm), complete limb absence (often referred to as amelia), or a variety of longitudinal deficiencies in which most or all of the humerus is absent, with only a phocomelic hand or digits present. Other anomalies are frequently concomitant with these limb deficiencies and often take precedence in the care and treatment of the very young child. Acquired shoulder disarticulations are uncommon in children, but they can result from traumatic events such as electrical and farm equipment injuries.[24]

Fitting Infants

In children with amelia or phocomelia, prosthetic fittings are frequently delayed because an entire shoulder disarticulation prosthesis for an infant is cumbersome and ineffective. Although early fitting contributes to successful prosthesis use, in these patients, prosthetic fittings are impractical because they may inhibit the achievement of infant developmental milestones by preventing

rolling and mobility. It may be feasible to begin prosthetic fitting when sitting balance is achieved; however, this milestone may be delayed if the child's body asymmetry makes it difficult for him or her to balance when sitting.

If a prosthesis is provided for these children, it often will have a passive friction shoulder (or no shoulder joint), a friction elbow, and a passive terminal device. A passive elbow would be used for infants at the shoulder disarticulation level because of the inability of the infant to actively position the prosthetic arm in space. The therapist and parents must show the child how to use the prosthesis. Friction settings on these elbows tend to be set quite high because the infant is not expected to preposition the elbow at such a young age.

Fitting Toddlers and Preschoolers

If a child with a congenital shoulder disarticulation and his or her family have successfully adopted the prosthesis at the toddler to preschool stage, they will most likely continue with prosthetic fittings. In addition to the components mentioned for the infant user, the toddler may have a prehensile terminal device that is either passively prehensile or activated by cable excursion. Because glenohumeral flexion is not an option for controlling the cable system, excursion is quite limited. It may be worth considering an externally powered terminal device combined with electrical activation schemes through a harness (scapular protraction) to control the terminal device. Electronic control of the terminal device decreases the amount of excursion necessary compared with a body-powered component. Such externally powered prostheses may be configured with volitional control of opening with automatic closing or with volitional opening and closing of the terminal device. Although myoelectric control would eliminate the need for excursion to activate a component, it is very difficult to teach such control

to a child of this age with a shoulder disarticulation.

Fitting School-Age Children, Adolescents, and Young Adults

In addition to children with congenital shoulder disarticulation limb absence, school-age children, adolescents, or young adults may have sustained a traumatic event that necessitated a shoulder disarticulation. Depending on the size of the child, component selection may vary.

Prosthetic shoulders include friction-regulated flexion-abduction joints. However, adolescents and young adults may benefit from a shoulder joint that offers both locking and free-swinging positions in the sagittal plane. A free-swinging arm feature may improve comfort while walking and may translate to improved wear and compliance.

The available components distal to the shoulder are the same as those described for the transhumeral amputation level. Because excursion for shoulder disarticulations is even more limited, it is essential to use either a hybrid control (**Figure 14**) or a completely externally powered prosthesis if an active elbow and a terminal device are required. The VASI 8-12 Elbow would be required for an externally powered prosthesis until the child reached a size at which he or she could benefit from another commercially available elbow such as the Boston Digital Arm (Liberating Technologies), the Utah Arm (Motion Control), or the Dynamic Arm (Ottobock).

Bilateral Shoulder Disarticulation

Bilateral upper limb absence is primarily seen in individuals who have congenital deficiencies.[2,18,25] It has been well documented that prosthetic use is quite challenging in these patients. If available, individuals with bilateral shoulder disarticulation should be trained to use other parts of their anatomy (such as feet and legs) for grasping and manipulating

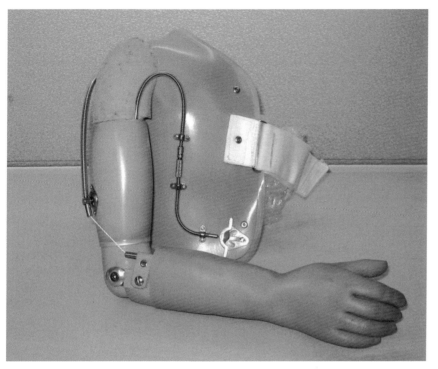

Figure 14 Photograph of a shoulder disarticulation prosthesis with hybrid control. (Courtesy of the Rehabilitation Institute of Chicago, Chicago, IL.)

objects. Individuals may be quite successful at using their feet like hands and can develop excellent coordination and dexterity. Prostheses fittings in these children may be attempted but are frequently unsuccessful because the benefits often do not outweigh the drawbacks.[26]

Summary

Successful fitting of upper limb prostheses for pediatric patients involves a team effort, with the child and family at the core of this team. All team members need to be educated on the pros and cons of prosthetic fitting and the functional benefits and limitations of available devices. Infants will often use their prostheses for very different functions than toddlers, school-age children, and young teens. Regardless of the child's age, the level of limb absence or amputation has a great influence on the use of prostheses. As in all prosthetic fittings, the shorter the residual limb and the higher the level of the limb difference or amputation, the more challenging is

fitting, the achievement of good function, and prosthesis acceptance.

References

1. Supan T: Prosthetic and orthotic management, in Bowker JH, Michael JW, eds: *Atlas of Limb Prosthetics: Surgical, Prosthetic, and Rehabilitation Principles,* ed 2. St. Louis, MO, Mosby Year Book, 1992, pp 761-766.

2. Clark MW, Atkins DJ, Hubbard SA, Patton JG, Shaperman J: Prosthetic devices for children with bilateral upper limb deficiencies: When and if, pros and cons, in Herring JA, Birch JG, eds: *The Child With a Limb Deficiency.* Rosemont, IL, American Academy of Orthopedic Surgeons, 1998, pp 397-403.

3. Patton J: Prosthetic components for children and teenagers, in Meier R, Atkins D, eds: *Comprehensive Management of the Upper-Limb Amputee.* New York, NY, Springer-Verlag, 1989, pp 99-120.

4. Sauter W: Electric pediatric and adult prosthetic components, in Meier R, Atkins D, eds: *Comprehensive Management of the Upper-Limb Amputee.* New York, NY, Springer-Verlag, 1989, pp 121-136.

5. Brenner C: Electric limbs for infants and pre-school children. *J Prosthet Orthot* 1992;4:184-190.

6. Schuch CM: Prosthetic principles in fitting myoelectric prostheses in children, in Herring JA, Birch JG, eds: *The Child With a Limb Deficiency.* Rosemont, IL, American Academy of Orthopedic Surgeons, 1998, pp 405-416.

7. Hubbard SA, Kurtz I, Heim W, Montgomery G: Powered prosthetic intervention in upper extremity deficiency, in Herring JA, Birch JG, eds: *The Child With a Limb Deficiency.* Rosemont, IL, American Academy of Orthopedic Surgeons, 1998, pp 417-431.

8. James MA, Bagley AM, Brasington K, Lutz C, McConnell S, Molitor F: Impact of prostheses on function and quality of life for children with unilateral congenital below-the-elbow deficiency. *J Bone Joint Surg Am* 2006;88(11):2356-2365.

9. Wagner L, Bagley A, James M: Reasons for prosthetic rejection by children with unilateral congenital forearm total deficiency. *J Prosthet Orthot* 2007;19(2):51-54.

10. Davids JR, Wagner LV, Meyer LC, Blackhurst DW: Prosthetic management of children with unilateral congenital below-elbow deficiency. *J Bone Joint Surg Am* 2006;88(6):1294-1300.

11. Wright FV, Hubbard S, Naumann S, Jutai J: Evaluation of the validity of the prosthetic upper extremity functional index for children. *Arch Phys Med Rehabil* 2003;84(4):518-527.

12. Lerman JA, Sullivan E, Barnes DA, Haynes RJ: The Pediatric Outcomes Data Collection Instrument (PODCI) and functional assessment of patients

with unilateral upper extremity deficiencies. *J Pediatr Orthop* 2005;25(3):405-407.

13. Patton J: Training the child with a unilateral upper-extremity prosthesis, in Meier R, Atkins D, eds: *Functional Restoration of Adults and Children With Upper Extremity Amputation*. New York, NY, Demos Medical Publishing, 2004, pp 297-315.

14. Gaebler-Spira D, Lipschutz R: *Pediatric Limb Deficiencies in Pediatric Rehabilitation*, ed 4. New York, NY, Demos Medical Publishing, 2010, pp 334-360.

15. Blakeslee B: *The Limb-Deficient Child*. Berkeley, CA, University of California Press, 1963.

16. Frantz C, O'Rahilly R: Congenital skeletal limb deficiencies. *J Bone Joint Surg Am* 1961;43(8):1202-1224.

17. Schuch M, Pritham C: International Standards Organization terminology: Application to prosthetics and orthotics. *J Prosthet Orthot* 1994;4:29-33.

18. Patton J: Developmental approach to pediatric prosthetic evaluation and training, in Meier R, Atkins D, eds: *Comprehensive Management of the Upper-Limb Amputee*. New York, NY, Springer-Verlag, 1989, pp 137-149.

19. Fairley M: T. Walley Williams III. The O&P EDGE, March 2013. Available at: http://www.oandp.com/articles/2013-03_09.asp. Accessed November 5, 2015.

20. Mahoney T, Frankovitch K: Use of opposition posts in children. *J Assoc Child Prosthet-Orthot Clin* 1991;26(1):33.

21. Bernstein RM, Watts HG, Setoguchi Y: The lengthening of short upper extremity amputation stumps. *J Pediatr Orthop* 2008;28(1):86-90.

22. Smit G, Bongers RM, Van der Sluis CK, Plettenburg DH: Efficiency of voluntary opening hand and hook prosthetic devices: 24 years of development? *J Rehabil Res Dev* 2012;49(4):523-534.

23. Trost F, Rowe D: Externally powered prostheses, in Bowker JH, Michael JW, eds: *Atlas of Limb Prosthetics: Surgical, Prosthetic, and Rehabilitation Principles*, ed 2. St. Louis, MO, Mosby Year Book, 1992, pp 767-778.

24. McClure SK, Shaughnessy WJ: Farm-related limb amputations in children. *J Pediatr Orthop* 2005;25(2):133-137.

25. Friedmann L: Functional skills in multiple limb anomalies, in Meier R, Atkins D, eds: *Comprehensive Management of the Upper-Limb Amputee*. New York, NY, Springer-Verlag, 1989, pp 150-164.

26. Setoguchi Y, Patton J, Shida-Tokeshi J: Pediatric case studies of upper extremity limb deficiencies, in Meier R, Atkins D, eds: *Functional Restoration of Adults and Children With Upper Extremity Amputation*. New York, NY, Demos Medical Publishing, 2004, pp 322-324.

Chapter 71

Pediatric Hand Deficiencies

Jakub Stuart Langer, MD

Abstract

Congenital hand deficiencies and abnormalities present unique diagnostic and therapeutic challenges. A holistic approach, including aesthetic and psychological considerations and surgical techniques for restoring normal kinesiology and function of the deficient limb, is necessary to treat children with such deficiencies. Common deficiencies include symbrachydactyly, syndactyly, longitudinal deficiencies, and polydactyly. Improved basic knowledge of pediatric hand deficiencies will aid surgeons and clinicians in choosing the best treatment strategy for their patients.

Keywords: congenital hand deficiency; longitudinal deficiency; polydactyly; symbrachydactyly; syndactyly

Introduction

The birth of a child with an upper limb deficiency elicits a myriad of confusing parental emotions. Medical professionals should address parental concerns and expectations in an optimistic, compassionate, honest, and forthright manner. Parents may grieve that their infant is not the perfect child that they had anticipated through the course of the pregnancy. Some will voice anger that prenatal evaluations did not detect their child's abnormality. Many parents feel an intense need to "do something," either surgical or prosthetic, to make their child "normal" and whole. Conflicting advice from well-meaning friends and relatives may contribute to parental stress. When the child's condition is potentially hereditary, conflicts between the father's and mother's families may be heightened.

Despite frequently voiced parental concerns, a recent self-concept scale study demonstrated that overall, children with congenital anomalies possessed equal self-concept to healthy children.[1] Interestingly, children with more mild anomalies had worse scores than children with more severe anomalies.

Some parents initially elect a cosmetic prosthesis to conceal their child's abnormality without regard to the functional effect of the prosthesis. The lack of success when a purely aesthetic prosthesis covers the sensate skin of an anomalous hand should be openly discussed. Although an aesthetic upper limb prosthesis may facilitate rehabilitation in a child with a traumatic amputation, it is usually a hindrance to a child with congenital amputation who possesses a mobile hand and wrist, even when fingers are absent. Aesthetic prostheses may become a source of conflict between parent and child if the child regards the prosthesis as a hindrance

to function. The child may feel that the prosthesis is to be worn merely to please parents who are embarrassed by his or her appearance. If an active prosthesis is to be successfully integrated into the child's life, it must help the child either accomplish otherwise impossible activities or perform meaningful activities with greater facility.

A recent advancement in prosthetic care is three-dimensional prosthetic printing, which provides a low-cost alternative to traditional aesthetic or functional prosthetic devices.[2] This patient- and family-driven modality gives the child or family the ability to easily customize and alter the prosthesis to meet the child's needs and wants, and may aid in the emotional adjustment to his or her disability.

Upper Limb Kinesiology

The hand allows children to explore their environment and to manipulate objects within that environment. The hand should be able to maneuver in space under volitional control and should be able to reach the body and the area in front of the body. Using both visual and tactile clues, a child must be able to aim the hand so that it can precisely approach an object. The object is then grasped by the closing fingers and adducting the thumb. The hand must also be capable of releasing the object from its grasp.

The two major types of grasp are precision prehension and power prehension.[3] Precision prehension is used to hold relatively small objects with modest force, whereas power prehension is used to hold larger objects, often with greater force. In precision prehension, the object

Neither Dr. Langer nor any immediate family member has received anything of value from or has stock or stock options held in a commercial company or institution related directly or indirectly to the subject of this chapter. This chapter is adapted from Light TR: Hand deficiencies, in Smith DG, Michael JW, Bowker JH, eds: Atlas of Amputations and Limb Deficiencies: Surgical, Prosthetic, and Rehabilitation Principles, ed 3. Rosemont, IL, American Academy of Orthopaedic Surgeons, 2004, pp 853-861.

is secured between the distal phalanx of the thumb and the index finger or within the thumb, index, and middle fingers. The fingers are usually extended at the interphalangeal (IP) joints, and the metacarpophalangeal (MCP) joints are partially flexed. The object itself usually does not contact the palm.

The three most common forms of precision grasp or pinch are palmar pinch, lateral pinch, and tip pinch. With palmar pinch, the flat palmar pads of the thumb and fingers secure opposite sides of the object being grasped. With lateral pinch, the palmar surface of the thumb's distal phalanx is brought against the radial border of the index finger. Because this posture is often used to grasp and twist a key, this pattern is also known as key pinch. Tip pinch provides contact with the distal end of the distal phalanx of the thumb with the distal phalanx of the index or of the index and middle fingers. Tip pinch is used to pick up small objects such as a pin or a dime from a tabletop.

Power prehension involves the ulnar digits (most often the ring and little fingers), whereas the radial digits (the index and middle fingers) are used primarily in precision prehension. Power grasp usually results in contact of the object against three surfaces: (1) the palmar aspects of the flexing fingers, (2) the palm of the hand, and (3) the thumb metacarpal or proximal phalanx. Although the distal phalanx of the thumb may wrap around the object, most thumb power is contributed by the stabilizing effect of the adductor pollicis, which buttresses the pressure transmitted from the fingers through the object.

The hand also plays an important role in nonprehensile activities. These activities usually involve the transmission of force through the terminal portion of the limb to another object. Nonprehensile activities include keyboarding or button pushing, pushing open a swinging door, throwing a punch, or striking a karate blow.

The hand may also be used to cradle or hold objects against the chest or to support objects such as a tray. Congenitally anomalous hands without prehensile capability are often used with great dexterity to perform these nonprehensile functions.

Other Considerations

As infants begin to explore their environment, they learn to use their unique physical capabilities to the best advantage. The young child's goal is to reach the cookie, grasp it, and bring it to his or her mouth. If this is most easily accomplished with one hand, the closest or most efficient hand will be used. If the object is large or if single-hand prehension is impossible, then both hands will be used together, or the child will secure the object against the chest. When upper limb prehension is severely compromised, a child may become facile using foot prehension.

The child's growing awareness of his or her abnormality is usually the result of comments from playmates, siblings, or well-meaning adults. The child usually does not become self-conscious until approximately the age of 6 or 7 years. Peer pressure may cause the child with a unilateral abnormality to conceal the hand in a pocket or to reject an otherwise successful prosthesis.

Other points of psychological stress occur during adolescence when concerns arise over attractiveness. Feelings may be further complicated by impending marriage and the prospect of offspring with similar abnormalities. Access to knowledgeable genetic counseling is essential, particularly at that time.

Aesthetic considerations are important when weighing therapeutic alternatives in the management of congenital hand abnormalities. The hand and face are the unclothed areas of skin most often exposed to scrutiny. When anomalous parts have an abnormal appearance and do not contribute to function, they

may be removed. In the perception of many, conversion of a malformed part to an amputation may result in an aesthetic improvement.

On occasion, the removal of a functionless part may facilitate prosthetic fitting. Approximately 50% of individuals with congenital lower limb amputations require surgical revision before prosthetic fitting, whereas only approximately 10% of congenital anomalous upper limbs fit for prostheses require surgical revision.[4] Consultation between the surgeon and prosthetist helps the surgeon understand which anomalies will obstruct prosthetic donning and wear. Portions of the affected limb that are useful for prehension without a prosthesis should never be amputated. A prosthesis can be fit around a short phocomelic limb to allow the child to maintain functional capabilities without the prosthesis.

Clinical Presentation

Although congenital upper limb abnormalities are increasingly diagnosed by prenatal ultrasound, they typically are first diagnosed at birth. Parents often have a deep need to understand the nature of their child's abnormality and the potential treatments available. Early consultation with experienced physicians and therapists is helpful for most families.

Classification

The Oberg, Manske, and Tonkin (OMT) classification of congenital anomalies of the hand and upper limb (**Table 1**) was proposed in 2010 as a replacement for the Swanson International Federation of Societies for Surgery of the Hand classification system (**Table 2**). The OMT system uses recent increasing knowledge of molecular and developmental pathways, and relates them to clinically relevant anomalies. It separates malformations from deformations and dysplasias. Malformations are subdivided according to the axis of formation and differentiation

Table 1 Oberg, Manske, and Tonkin Classification of Congenital Anomalies of the Hand and Upper Limb

Malformations

A. Failure of axis formation/differentiation—entire upper limb
  1. Proximal-distal outgrowth
  Brachymelia with brachydactyly
  Symbrachydactyly
  Transverse deficiency
  Intersegmental deficiency
  2. Radial-ulnar (anteroposterior axis)
  Radial longitudinal deficiency
  Ulnar longitudinal deficiency
  Ulnar dimelia
  Radioulnar synostosis
  Humeroradial synostosis
  3. Dorsal-ventral axis
  Nail-patella syndrome

B. Failure of axis formation/differentiation—hand plate
  1. Radial-ulnar (anteroposterior) axis
  Radial polydactyly
  Triphalangeal thumb
  Ulnar polydactyly
  2. Dorsal-ventral axis
  Dorsal dimelia (palmer nail)
  Hypoplastic/aplastic nail

C. Failure of axis formation/differentiation—unspecified axis
  1. Soft tissue
  Syndactyly
  Camptodactyly
  2. Skeletal deficiency
  Brachydactyly
  Clinodactyly
  Kirner deformity
  Metacarpal and carpal synostoses
  3. Complex
  Cleft hand
  Synpolydactyly
  Apert hand

Deformations

A. Constriction ring sequence
B. Arthrogryposis
C. Trigger digits
D. Not otherwise specified

Dysplasias

A. Hypertrophy
  1. Macrodactyly
  2. Upper limb
  3. Upper limb and macrodactyly
B. Tumorous conditions

Table 2 Modified Swanson/International Federation of Societies for Surgery of the Hand Classification

Type	Description
I	Failure of formation of parts (arrest of development)
II	Failure of differentiation (separation) of parts
III	Duplication
IV	Overgrowth (gigantism)
V	Undergrowth (hypoplasia)
VI	Congenital constriction band syndrome
VII	Generalized skeletal abnormalities

and involvement of the whole limb or the hand plate alone.

Conditions in which body parts are absent are referred to as failures of formation. In most patients, the anatomic border between normal tissue and absent elements is indistinct and gradual; a blend of dysplastic and hypoplastic tissue typically forms a transition zone that may extend the entire length of the limb. Constriction ring sequence, also termed congenital constriction band syndrome or amniotic bands, is the result of highly localized intrauterine trauma to the growing limb, and it is one condition in which there may be an abrupt transition from normal tissue to absent elements (**Figure 1**). In these limbs, the anatomy proximal to the area of abnormality is usually perfectly normal.

Anomalies that extend the entire length of the limb are termed longitudinal deficiencies. When the preaxial border of the limb is involved, the condition is termed a radial deficiency, and when the postaxial border of the limb is involved, the condition is referred to as an ulnar deficiency. Absence or hypoplasia of the thumb is often a component of radial deficiency. In some patients, thumb absence may be a component of ulnar deficiency.

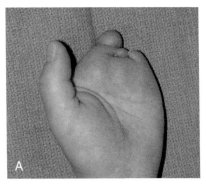 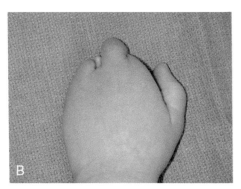 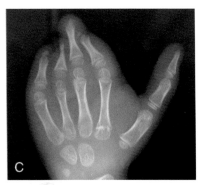

Figure 1 Photographs demonstrate early congenital amniotic rupture sequence with amputation and syndactylization of the index, middle, ring, and little fingers. **A,** Palmar view demonstrates interdigital sinuses. **B,** Dorsal view. **C,** AP radiograph shows tapering of the distal end of the proximal phalanx of the ring finger.

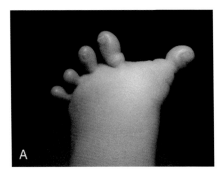 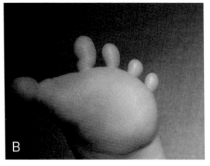

Figure 2 Dorsal (**A**) and palmar (**B**) photographs of a terminal transverse deficiency characterized by persistent digital nubbins without bony phalangeal elements.

Conditions in which the absence is most intense in the distal portion of the limb are usually referred to as terminal deficiencies (**Figure 2**). The entire limb, including the chest, must be evaluated to fully understand these abnormalities. Distal anomalies involving the hand, such as syndactyly, may be associated with chest abnormalities in children with Poland syndrome.

Symbrachydactyly

The most common forms of terminal limb deficiency are related to the symbrachydactyly sequence of abnormalities.[5-7] The term symbrachydactyly literally refers to a hand with syndactyly of short fingers. The use of the expression symbrachydactyly sequence is confusing initially because many of the children grouped into this malformation sequence have neither syndactyly nor fingers. Symbrachydactyly represents the prototypic form for this group of terminal failure of formation abnormalities. Many limbs with syndactylization have primitive digits, often termed nubbins. These bud-like, incompletely formed digits often include small finger nails. In many instances, digital flexor and extensor tendons insert into the nubbin, enabling children to pucker or withdraw the tip of the digit proximally into the residual limb. Manifestations may be as mild as slightly shortened middle phalanges or as severe as a very short forearm segment with digital nubbins protruding from its distal end (**Figure 3**). Children with intermediate forms may have only a thumb or only a thumb and little finger with small nubbins representing the undeveloped fingers. Mild hypoplasia of the ipsilateral humerus is common, as is dysplasia or hypoplasia of the forearm. When multiple digits are involved, the central three digits are usually the most profoundly affected. The symbrachydactyly

sequence abnormalities are usually unilateral and nonhereditary. The left upper limb is involved more often than the right upper limb. Boys are more frequently affected than girls.

The term hypodactyly has recently been coined to describe an entity of digital absence distinct from symbrachydactyly or amniotic disruption sequence where digits are truncated without evidence of terminal ectodermal elements or amniotic bands.[8] This entity is thought to occur by a different developmental mechanism.

Imaging Studies

Radiographs of the entire upper limb should be obtained. Comparison views of the opposite hand may be useful in predicting the ultimate size of the affected part because its size in proportion to the unaffected side will likely not change even as the child grows. Radiographs of young children may underestimate the extent of bone formation, particularly in thin syndactylized fingers. Portions of the anomalous fingers and carpus often include unossified cartilage.

Classification

Digital absence may be simply described as thumb absence, index finger absence, middle finger absence, ring finger absence, or little finger absence. In many patients with a terminal limb deficiency, the deficiency involves only part of

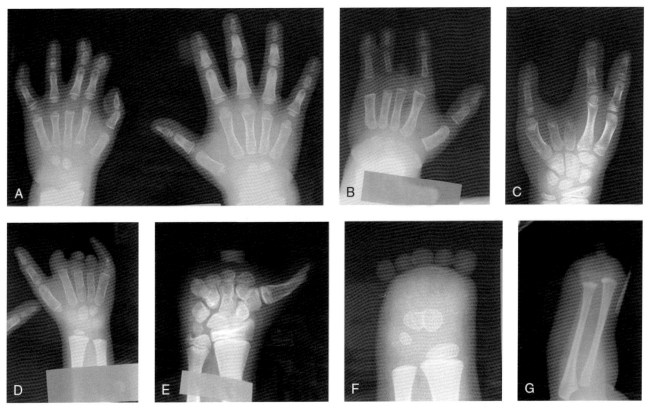

Figure 3   Radiographs demonstrate the variable morphology of unilateral symbrachydactyly. **A,** Five-digit–type hand with biphalangeal thumb and biphalangeal fingers (left) is smaller than the contralateral, normal hand. **B,** Four-digit–type hand with four biphalangeal digits and one digital nubbin. **C,** Three-digit–type hand includes a narrowed syndactylized web between the biphalangeal thumb and biphalangeal ring finger. **D,** Two-digit–type hand shows limited ossification of the distal phalanx within the nubbin index, middle, and ring fingers. **E,** Monodigital-type hand consists of a widely abducted thumb metacarpal. **F,** Carpal-type hand with five soft-tissue nubbins. **G,** Wrist disarticulation-type hand with a single digital nubbin.

the digit. The phalangeal elements may be absent, but the corresponding metacarpal is present. The extent of dysplasia in each ray should be assessed. A brief description of the more common forms of this condition is presented in **Table 3**.

Associated Findings

Poland syndrome is the ipsilateral finding of symbrachydactyly and chest abnormality.[5-7,9-14] Interestingly, the proximal chest abnormality is more common with the milder, more distal forms of symbrachydactyly than with more profound limb abnormalities. The most frequently associated chest abnormality is absence of the sternocostal head of the pectoralis major muscle. More profound chest abnormalities include total absence of the pectoralis major muscle and rib abnormalities.

Asymmetric nipple location may occasionally be seen. As girls mature, ipsilateral breast hypoplasia may be evident.

Functional Deficits

The functional deficits in children with symbrachydactyly are a direct consequence of the degree of involvement as detailed in **Table 3**. In the more distal forms, prehension with digital independence is possible. Individual digital function may be compromised by syndactyly, IP joint instability, or angulation.

The absence of central digits may compromise hand dexterity and limit the child's ability to play certain musical instruments. Stable grasp and manipulative ability are diminished in a hand that has only two or three fingers. A two-digit hand is capable of

prehension if the two digits can actively touch one another. Prehension requires that at least one of the digits is mobile and actively controlled. Hands with only a single digit are capable of nonprehensile activity such as pushing buttons or striking a letter on a keyboard.

Adactylous hands with wrist motion are used to cradle objects against the trunk and to hold objects in place for manipulation by the unaffected hand. The adactylous hand can hold a piece of paper in place while the other hand holds the pen or pencil to draw or write on the paper.

Differential Diagnosis

A hand that possesses only the thumb and little finger has, in the past, been referred to as an atypical cleft hand.[15,16] It is important to recognize, however,

Table 3 Classification of Common Types of Digital Absence

Type of Hand	Characteristics
Symbrachydactyly	
Five digits with biphalangeal thumb	All fingers triphalangeal Incomplete simple syndactyly of the index, middle, and ring fingers
Five digits with biphalangeal thumb	Biphalangeal index, middle, and ring fingers Triphalangeal little finger Incomplete simple syndactyly of the index, middle, and ring fingers
Five digits with biphalangeal thumb	Monophalangeal index, middle, and ring fingers
Three digits with biphalangeal thumb	Nubbin index and middle fingers Monophalangeal ring finger Biphalangeal little finger
Two digits with monophalangeal thumb	Nubbin index, middle, and ring fingers Monophalangeal little finger
Monodigital with monophalangeal thumb	Nubbin index, middle, ring, and little fingers
Aphalangeal	
Adactylous with five metacarpals	Five nubbins
Adactylous with two metacarpals	Thumb metacarpal Little finger metacarpal Digital nubbins
Carpal	Digital nubbins No metacarpals or phalanges Mobile carpus
Wrist disarticulation level	Digital nubbins No wrist motion No carpal, metacarpal, or phalangeal elements
Short transradial level	Extremely short forearm Digital nubbins

Reproduced from Light TR: Hand deficiencies, in Smith DG, Michael JW, Bowker JH, eds: *Atlas of Amputations and Limb Deficiencies: Surgical, Prosthetic, and Rehabilitation Principles*, ed 3. Rosemont, IL, American Academy of Orthopaedic Surgeons, 2004, p 857.

that these two-digit hands are unrelated to cleft hand, an autosomal dominant condition often with bilateral hand and foot involvement.

Surgical Treatment

Because symbrachydactyly is almost always unilateral, most affected children are remarkably facile at performing activities of daily living. The extent of involvement determines the extent of function in the affected limb. Involved digits may be short and unstable. In some patients, an empty digital skin sleeve or nubbin is evident. Release of syndactyly between fingers with local skin flaps and full-thickness skin grafts increases digital independence.

Nonprehensile activities such as typing may be improved by the stabilization of unstable IP joints by capsulodesis, chondrodesis, or arthrodesis (**Figure 4**). Angulation of digits, usually the result of a trapezoidal middle phalanx, may be treated by a simple closing wedge osteotomy.

When a soft-tissue digital sleeve is redundant and devoid of skeletal elements, puckering of the tip will demonstrate the insertion of extrinsic flexor and extensor tendons. In such digits, it is often possible to reconstruct a short, mobile digit by a simple nonvascularized proximal phalanx transfer from the foot to the hand (**Figure 5**).

The monodactylous hand consisting of only a mobile, actively motored thumb is capable of nonprehensile activities such as stabilizing a shoelace but incapable of either power or precision grasp. Construction of an ulnar-sided buttressing digit by distraction lengthening, toe-phalanx transfer, or free toe transfer may allow the hand to achieve meaningful prehension. A recent review of nonvascularized toe phalangeal transfers reported on the potential substantial morbidity of this procedure, including gait abnormality, abnormal appearance, and toe instability.[17] A prosthesis that provides a passive ulnar-sided buttress may also make prehension possible.

When a mobile carpus is devoid of fingers, the microvascular transfer of both second toes has been suggested.[18] Although this procedure is technically possible, the results are often disappointing because of the limited mobility of the transferred digits, making meaningful prehension unpredictable after a technically demanding intervention. Alternatively, Vilkki[19] and Foucher[20] suggested placing a single microvascular toe transfer on the distal radius in a position in which the mobile carpal segment can flex and extend in relation to the transferred toe. This unconventional digital position creates a more predictable prehension.

Syndactyly
Clinical Presentation and Classification

Syndactyly is the physical joining or tethering of fingers or toes. When syndactylization extends the entire length of a digit, the condition is termed complete syndactyly. When the web involves only part of the length of the digit, it is termed an incomplete syndactyly. When skeletal and nail elements of the syndactylized digits are separate, the syndactyly is said to be simple. When digital skeletal and/or nail elements are fused, the syndactyly is termed complex (**Figure 6**). Acrosyndactyly refers to syndactyly in which the ends of the fingers are joined, often as a result of early amniotic rupture sequence (formerly termed congenital constriction band syndrome). Syndactyly of the digits containing angulated phalanges is termed complicated syndactyly.[21]

Surgical Treatment

Surgical release of syndactylized digits will enhance digital independence, an important element of keyboarding. Even short digits consisting of only a proximal phalanx may benefit from separation. Index finger radial abduction may be increased and pinch improved when a short index finger is released from the middle finger. Syndactyly release must provide skin coverage of the adjacent lateral surfaces of the released digits and also create a proper web space floor. Because the surface area of two syndactylized digits is far less than the skin surface area of two separated digits, a full-thickness skin graft is necessary to supplement local flaps.

Many skin flap techniques have been advocated for the separation of syndactylized digits.[22-28] Successful surgical procedures cover the surface of both digits with durable skin, create an appropriate web space floor, and accommodate growth of the digit without secondary contracture (**Figure 7**). Effective techniques use skin flap tissue to create a sloping web space floor of true anatomic proportions both in width and depth. This flap tissue may be derived either from the dorsum of the hand,

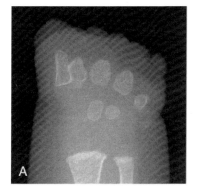
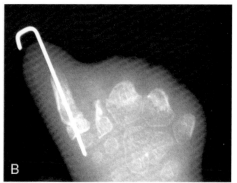
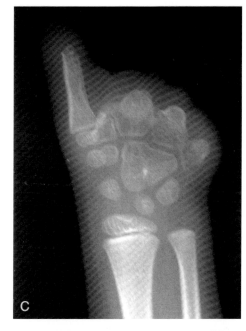

Figure 4 Radiographs of an adactylous hand treated with a transverse osteotomy. **A,** Preoperative radiograph shows the five small metacarpal elements, which had limited thumb metacarpal motion. **B,** Transverse osteotomy of the thumb metaphysis allowed insertion of intercalated bone graft from the adjacent index metacarpal. **C,** Additional length allowed improved monodigital function.

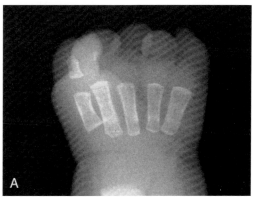
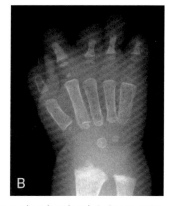

Figure 5 Radiographs show the reconstruction of a monodactylous hand. **A,** Preoperative radiograph of the hand with a monophalangeal thumb and empty finger skin sleeves. **B,** Nonvascularized toe phalangeal grafts from the third and fourth toe proximal phalanges enhance digital stability, length, and dexterity.

from the palmar aspect of the hand, or from a combination of both palmar and dorsal tissue. Dorsal flaps provide the best skin color match when the web space is viewed from the dorsum but may result in a hypertrophic scar across the interdigital commissure. A palmar flap provides a better commissure contour but results in the shifting of pink palmar skin into the web space. Because the web space is usually viewed from the dorsum, the difference in color is particularly noticeable in dark-skinned individuals.

The web space floor normally begins just distal to the MCP joint and slopes to the edge of the palmar commissure, approximately one-third the length of the proximal phalangeal segment. The web palmar commissure is supple enough to allow interdigital abduction of up to 45°.

Skin incisions on the palmar and dorsal surfaces of the syndactylized digits should be planned to avoid longitudinal scars crossing digital flexion creases because these scars tend to contract with growth. Zigzag incisions may be planned to interdigitate skin flaps to either achieve full closure of one digit or partial closure of two adjacent digits. Skin grafts are sutured in place. Interdigital dressings are maintained until all wounds have healed.[29,30]

When multiple digits are syndactylized, surgeries should be staged to avoid releasing both sides of a digit during a single operation.

Early Amniotic Rupture Sequence

Clinical Presentation

Early amniotic rupture sequence, formerly referred to as congenital constriction band syndrome, amniotic bands, or annular bands, is a condition often characterized by upper and lower limb involvement and, in some patients, facial involvement.[31-33] Manifestations may include areas of ring-like narrowing of a digit or limb, amputation of the part distal to an encircling area of band formation, acrosyndactyly, and enlargement of the segment distal to the area of constriction. Because this condition represents an intrauterine injury that disrupts normal limb formation, the level of amputation is often through the diaphysis of a phalanx.

Surgical Treatment

Areas of band indentation may be effectively treated by excision of indented skin and constricting underlying fascia. A layered closure combined with local rotation flaps will improve contour of the limb or digit. When deep bands compress underlying nerves, compromising distal neurovascular function, decompression and nerve grafting may be helpful. Acrosyndactyly may be addressed using traditional syndactyly release techniques. If an interdigital sinus is present, it should be excised at the time of syndactyly release.

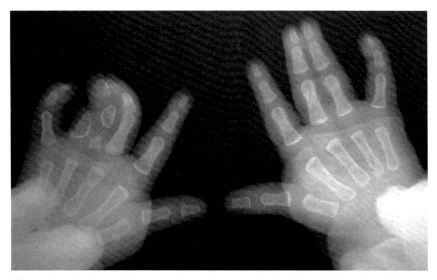

Figure 6 Radiograph shows a patient with syndactyly of both hands. The left hand demonstrates, a complete, complex central synpolydactyly, whereas the right hand demonstrates a complete simple syndactyly.

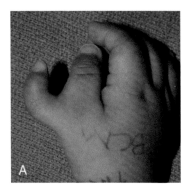
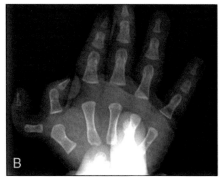
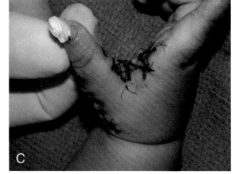

Figure 7 Images show thumb polydactyly, consisting of two biphalangeal digits and a narrow first web space. **A,** Clinical photograph. **B,** Radiograph. **C,** Reconstruction includes removal of the skeletal elements of the radial digit, reconstruction of the collateral ligament of the metacarpophalangeal joint, first web space release, and Z-plasty.

Complications

Because the level of amputation through the forearm or phalangeal bones often passes through the bone's diaphysis, bony overgrowth frequently occurs. Diaphyseal bony overgrowth results in tapered ends of fingers. The most distal bone grows faster than the soft-tissue coverage, resulting in tender, poorly padded finger tips or recurrent problems with prosthesis fit. Revision of the ends of these digits or limb ends should be generous to minimize the likelihood of recurrent overgrowth.

Polydactyly

Clinical Presentation

Polydactyly takes many forms. In black children, postaxial (ulnar) polydactyly is the most common form, whereas in white children, preaxial (radial) polydactyly is more frequent. Central polydactyly is less common than either preaxial or postaxial polydactyly.[34] Polydactylous digits are rarely supernumerary, that is, they rarely represent parts additional to a normal hand.[26] Most often, digits with polydactyly are structurally abnormal.[35] The challenge of surgery is not simply to remove sufficient tissue but rather to retain tissue sufficient to optimally reconstruct the retained digits.[36-39]

Surgical Treatment

Simply amputating one of the duplicate digits may result in an inadequate residual digit that is smaller than its counterpart on the opposite side. This effect can be decreased by soft-tissue coaptation (**Figure 8**). Incisions are planned to facilitate the coapting of soft tissues from both digits to provide optimal soft-tissue bulk. Angular deformity in either phalanx or metacarpal should be corrected by osteotomy. Surgical reconstruction aims to achieve a digit in which the carpometacarpal, MCP, and IP joints are parallel. The longitudinal axis of the metacarpals and phalanges should be perpendicular to the three joints.

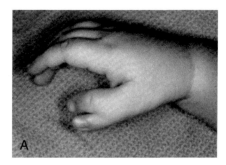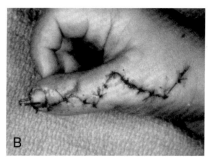

Figure 8   Photographs of a Wassel type IV thumb duplication. **A,** Preoperative photographs demonstrate angulation of the larger ulnar thumb metacarpophalangeal (MCP) and the interphalangeal joint levels. **B,** Surgical reconstruction of the thumb included a soft-tissue coaptation flap from the excised radial digit, a closing wedge osteotomy of the thumb metacarpal, and an opening wedge osteotomy of the proximal phalanx to achieve appropriate longitudinal alignment of the digit. The radial collateral ligament of the MCP joint was reconstructed, and the abductor pollicis brevis muscle reinserted in the retained digit.

Correction of angulation is usually achieved by a closing wedge osteotomy and secured with Kirschner wires. An opening wedge osteotomy using a segment of excised bone as intercalated graft is occasionally indicated. Correction of angulation is usually achieved by osteotomy or tendon rerouting or rebalancing, with reconstructed thumbs demonstrating excessive late angulation and yielding the worst patient satisfaction scores.[40-42]

Classification

Preaxial polydactyly takes many forms. Wassel[43] classified these abnormalities into seven categories, six of which involve biphalangeal thumbs (**Figure 9**). Type I deformities may present as simply a wide distal phalanx and nail, in which case no treatment is indicated. If two nails are present, two treatment alternatives may be considered: (1) excision of one nail with the underlying bone or (2) central resection of adjacent nail borders and underlying bone, combined with longitudinal phalangeal osteotomies, to narrow the distal phalanx. The latter technique, known as the Bilhaut-Cloquet procedure, requires care in nail matrix repair, articular surface alignment, and physeal alignment to avoid creating a stiff IP joint with a longitudinal nail ridge. Osteotomies

should be performed distal to the physis to avoid growth disturbance.

Type II duplications consist of two undersized (compared to normal) distal phalanges seated atop a somewhat widened proximal phalangeal distal articular surface. The more radial digital element has a collateral ligament along its radial border, whereas the ulnar digit has a collateral ligament along its ulnar border. The two digits abut with adjacent articular facets and are bound by pericapsular tissue. In most instances, it is preferable to excise the more radial digit because it is usually less well developed. The broad distal articular surface of the proximal phalanx may need to be tapered to a size appropriate to the distal phalanx. The collateral ligament that initially secured the radial aspect of the deleted radial digit must be retained to securely stabilize the radial aspect of the new IP joint. Retained flexor and extensor tendons must be examined to ensure that the course and insertion of residual tendons are centered.

Type III abnormalities are usually treated by deleting the radial digit. Type IV abnormalities usually require deletion of the radial digit, narrowing of the metacarpal head, and reconstruction of the collateral ligament. The intrinsic muscles that originally inserted into the more radial thumb are reinserted into

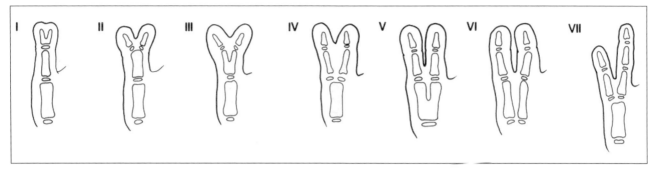

Figure 9   Illustration of Wassel's original classification scheme for thumb polydactyly, which has been modified to demonstrate the most common form of thumb polydactyly (type IV), in which two proximal phalanges each possess separate secondary ossification centers.

the hood of the residual ulnar thumb component. Type V abnormalities usually require deletion of the more radial digit and reinsertion of the intrinsic muscle insertion into the residual ulnar digit. Type VI abnormalities may require shifting of the more distal portion of the radial digit onto the more proximal portion of the ulnar digit.

Central polydactyly often presents in combination with syndactyly.[34] Frequently, an anomalous central digit lacks normal metacarpal development and is bound to the middle or ring finger. In these patients, the skeletal elements of the unsupported digit are excised, and skin flaps are designed to preserve or reconstruct normal web space contour and digital bulk. When formal ray resection is required, web space–preserving incisions should be used.

Postaxial polydactyly of the digit joined only by soft tissue may be treated by simple excision. When the most ulnar digit articulates with the metacarpal head in a fashion similar to that in the Wassel type IV thumb duplication, simple digital excision will result in an inadequate residual digit. It may be necessary to narrow the metacarpal head, but it should be recognized that the metacarpal head of the little finger, unlike that of the thumb, contains a physis and that care must be taken to preserve physeal growth. If the hypothenar musculature inserts into the more ulnar little finger, its insertion must be detached from the skeletal elements

being resected and reinserted into the retained radial little finger. Similarly, the ulnar collateral ligament of the deleted digit must be retained and reconstructed to stabilize the ulnar aspect of the residual little finger MCP joint.

Ulnar dimelia (mirror hand) is an unusual abnormality characterized by duplication of the postaxial border of the hand with seven or eight fingers.[44] Neither the thumb nor the radius is present. Surgery on the preaxial proximal ulna is useful in expanding the arc of elbow flexion and extension but does not provide forearm rotation. Because there is an overabundance of flexor musculature and relative paucity of extensor musculature, release of the wrist flexion contracture may be necessary. Deletion of two or three digits with pollicization of one of the digits along the preaxial border will improve the aesthetic appearance of the hand and modestly improve function.[45]

Wrist Disarticulation

The Krukenberg procedure has been suggested as a reconstructive alternative for children with congenital absence of the hand, particularly in those with profound contralateral abnormalities, associated blindness, or a lack of access to prosthetic care.[46,47] The distal radius and ulna are surgically separated by division of the interosseous membrane and resurfacing the radial aspect of the ulna and the ulnar aspect of the radius. This creates a prehensile limb that will

also allow prosthetic fitting. Because the cosmetic disadvantage of this procedure is substantial, its use in patients with unilateral absence is controversial.

Short Transradial Amputation

This common level of terminal deficiency is effectively treated with prosthetic management. Surgical reconstruction is rarely necessary, although Seitz[48] reported distraction lengthening of a very short ulna to facilitate suspension of a conventional myoelectric prosthesis. Initial prosthetic management begins with a passive hand. The sophistication of the prosthesis can be increased as the child matures.

Timing of Management

Although surgical reconstruction of an anomalous hand can begin during the first year of life, recent literature supports a delay in surgical intervention until the child is at least 2 years of age to avoid any risk to child's cognitive development.[49]

Some procedures, such as nonvascularized toe-phalanx transfer, must be performed early for optimal revascularization and subsequent growth.[6,50] Children undergoing digit-shifting procedures, such as pollicization or cleft hand reconstruction, may benefit from early integration of the shifted digit into evolving patterns of grasp.

Systemic consideration may cause surgery to be delayed until children are older. For example, children with thrombocytopenia with absent radius (TAR) syndrome have low platelet counts at birth, but these usually gradually increase with age. Surgical reconstruction usually should be delayed until the child's platelet count is at least 60,000/mm³. Centralization of the wrist, which is typically done within the first year of life, may sometimes be delayed in these children until 3 or 4 years of age.

Decisions regarding the reconstruction or deletion of digits or digital nubbins are best made when children are young. It is inappropriate to place the burden for deciding whether a digit is to be deleted on an adolescent. Parents should not be encouraged to allow children to "decide for themselves when they are older" because this serious decision places inappropriate pressure on adolescents.

Summary

When treating a child with a congenital hand deficiency, the surgeon is tasked with providing an accurate diagnosis, assessing function, offering a prognosis, and counseling the patient and family about potential surgical and nonsurgical treatments. Most children with congenital hand differences and deficiencies will adapt to their environment and situation in creative and efficient ways. The role of surgeons is to identify situations and difficulties that may be improved by either targeted use of prostheses and assistive devices or specific goal-oriented surgical reconstructions to improve aesthetics and function.

References

1. Andersson GB, Gillberg C, Fernell E, Johansson M, Nachemson A: Children with surgically corrected hand deformities and upper limb deficiencies: Self-concept and psychological well-being. *J Hand Surg Eur Vol* 2011;36(9):795-801.

2. Gretsch KF, Lather HD, Peddada KV, Deeken CR, Wall LB, Goldfarb CA: Development of novel 3D-printed robotic prosthetic for transradial amputees. *Prosthet Orthot Int* 2015; May 1 [Epub ahead of print].

3. Light TR: Kinesiology of the upper limb, in *Atlas of Orthotics,* ed 2. St. Louis, MO, Mosby-Year Book, 1985, pp 126-138.

4. Aitken GT, Pellicore RJ: Introduction to the child amputee, in *Atlas of Limb Prosthetics: Surgical and Prosthetic Principles.* St. Louis, MO, Mosby Year-Book, 1981, pp 493-500.

5. Blauth W, Gekeler J: Symbrachydactylias. *Handchirurgie* 1973;5(3):121-174.

6. Buck-Gramcko D: The role of nonvascularized toe phalanx transplantation. *Hand Clin* 1990;6(4):643-659.

7. De Smet L, Fabry G: Characteristics of patients with symbrachydactyly. *J Pediatr Orthop B* 1998;7(2):158-161.

8. Knight JB, Pritsch T, Ezaki M, Oishi SN: Unilateral congenital terminal finger absences: A condition that differs from symbrachydactyly. *J Hand Surg Am* 2012;37(1):124-129.

9. Beals RK, Crawford S: Congenital absence of the pectoral muscles: A review of twenty-five patients. *Clin Orthop Relat Res* 1976;119:166-171.

10. Goldberg MJ, Mazzei RJ: Poland syndrome: A concept of pathogenesis based on limb bud embryology. *Birth Defects Orig Artic Ser* 1977;13(3D):103-115.

11. Ireland DC, Takayama N, Flatt AE: Poland's syndrome. *J Bone Joint Surg Am* 1976;58(1):52-58.

12. Poland A: Deficiency of pectoralis muscle. *Guys Hosp Rep* 1841;6:191-193.

13. Wilson MR, Louis DS, Stevenson TR: Poland's syndrome: Variable expression and associated anomalies. *J Hand Surg Am* 1988;13(6):880-882.

14. Catena N, Divizia MT, Calevo MG, et al: Hand and upper limb anomalies in Poland syndrome: A new proposal of classification. *J Pediatr Orthop* 2012;32(7):722-726.

15. Barsky AJ: Cleft hand: Classification, incidence and treatment. Review of the literature and report of nineteen cases. *J Bone Joint Surg Am* 1964;46:1707-1720.

16. Miura T, Suzuki M: Clinical differences between typical and atypical cleft hand. *J Hand Surg Br* 1984;9(3):311-315.

17. Garagnani L, Gibson M, Smith PJ, Smith GD: Long-term donor site morbidity after free nonvascularized toe phalangeal transfer. *J Hand Surg Am* 2012;37(4):764-774.

18. Kay SP, Wiberg M: Toe to hand transfer in children: Part 1. Technical aspects. *J Hand Surg Br* 1996;21(6):723-734.

19. Vilkki SK: Advances in microsurgical reconstruction of the congenitally adactylous hand. *Clin Orthop Relat Res* 1995;314:45-58.

20. Foucher G: The "stub" operation: Modification of the Furnas and Vilkki technique in traumatic and congenital carpal hand reconstruction. *Ann Acad Med Singapore* 1995; 24(4, suppl):73-76.

21. Dobyns JH, Wood VE, Bayne LG: Congenital hand deformities, in Green DP, ed: *Operative Hand Surgery.* New York, NY, Churchill Livingston, 1988.

22. Bauer TB, Tondra JM, Trusler HM: Technical modification in repair of syndactylism. *Plast Reconstr Surg (1946)* 1956;17(5):385-392.

23. Eaton CJ, Lister GD: Syndactyly. *Hand Clin* 1990;6(4):555-575.

24. Ashmead D, Smith PJ: Tissue expansion for Apert's syndactyly. *J Hand Surg Br* 1995;20(3):327-330.

25. Flatt AE: Treatment of syndactylism. *Plast Reconstr Surg Transplant Bull* 1962;29:336-341.

26. Light TR: Congenital anomalies: Syndactyly, polydactyly and cleft hand, in Peimer CA, ed: *Surgery of the Hand and Upper Extremity.* New York, NY, McGraw-Hill, 1996.

27. Toledo LC, Ger E: Evaluation of the operative treatment of syndactyly. *J Hand Surg Am* 1979;4(6):556-564.

28. Upton J: Congenital anomalies of the hand and forearm, in McCarthy JG, May JW Jr, Littler JW, eds: *Plastic Surgery: The Hand. Part 2.* Philadelphia, PA, WB Saunders, 1990, vol 8.

29. Miyamoto J, Nagasao T, Miyamoto S: Biomechanical analysis of surgical correction of syndactyly. *Plast Reconstr Surg* 2010;125(3):963-968.

30. Goldfarb CA, Steffen JA, Stutz CM: Complex syndactyly: Aesthetic and objective outcomes. *J Hand Surg Am* 2012;37(10):2068-2073.

31. Foukes GD, Reinker K: Congenital constriction band syndrome: A seventy year experience. *J Pediatr Orthop* 1994;19:973-976.

32. Jones KL: *Smith's Recognizable Patterns of Human Malformation.* Philadelphia, PA, WB Saunders, 1988.

33. Ogino T, Saitou Y: Congenital constriction band syndrome and transverse deficiency. *J Hand Surg Br* 1987;12(3):343-348.

34. Tada K, Kurisaki E, Yonenobu K, Tsuyuguchi Y, Kawai H: Central polydactyly: A review of 12 cases and their surgical treatment. *J Hand Surg Am* 1982;7(5):460-465.

35. Marks TW, Bayne LG: Polydactyly of the thumb: Abnormal anatomy and treatment. *J Hand Surg Am* 1978;3(2):107-116.

36. Cheng JC, Chan KM, Ma GF, Leung PC: Polydactyly of the thumb: A surgical plan based on ninety-five cases. *J Hand Surg Am* 1984;9(2):155-164.

37. Ezaki M: Radial polydactyly. *Hand Clin* 1990;6(4):577-588.

38. Miura T: Duplicated thumb. *Plast Reconstr Surg* 1982;69(3):470-481.

39. Tada K, Yonenobu K, Tsuyuguchi Y, Kawai H, Egawa T: Duplication of the thumb: A retrospective review of two hundred and thirty-seven cases. *J Bone Joint Surg Am* 1983;65(5):584-598.

40. Tonkin MA: Thumb duplication: Concepts and techniques. *Clin Orthop Surg* 2012;4(1):1-17.

41. Xu YL, Shen KY, Chen J, Wang ZG: Flexor pollicis longus rebalancing: A modified technique for Wassel IV-D thumb duplication. *J Hand Surg Am* 2014;39(1):75-82.e1.

42. Goldfarb CA, Patterson JM, Maender A, Manske PR: Thumb size and appearance following reconstruction of radial polydactyly. *J Hand Surg Am* 2008;33(8):1348-1353.

43. Wassel HD: The results of surgery for polydactyly of the thumb: A review. *Clin Orthop Relat Res* 1969;64(64):175-193.

44. Barton NJ, Buck-Gramcko D, Evans DM: Soft-tissue anatomy of mirror hand. *J Hand Surg Br* 1986;11(3):307-319.

45. Barton NJ, Buck-Gramcko D, Evans DM, Kleinert H, Semple C, Ulson H: Mirror hand treated by true pollicization. *J Hand Surg Br* 1986;11(3):320-336.

46. Bora FW Jr, Nicholson JT, Cheema HM: Radial meromelia: The deformity and its treatment. *J Bone Joint Surg Am* 1970;52(5):966-979.

47. Swanson AB: The Krukenberg procedure in the juvenile amputee. *J Bone Joint Surg Am* 1964;46:1540-1548.

48. Seitz WH Jr: Distraction osteogenesis of a congenital amputation at the elbow. *J Hand Surg Am* 1989;14(6):945-948.

49. Wang X, Xu Z, Miao CH: Current clinical evidence on the effect of general anesthesia on neurodevelopment in children: An updated systematic review with meta-regression. *PLoS One* 2014;9(1):e85760.

50. Goldberg NH, Watson HK: Composite toe (phalanx and epiphysis) transfers in the reconstruction of the aphalangic hand. *J Hand Surg Am* 1982;7(5):454-459.

Chapter 72

Transverse Deficiencies of the Lower Limb

Michael J. Forness, DO

Abstract

Transverse deficiencies of the lower limb have multiple etiologies in the pediatric population. The level of amputation has a dramatic effect on energy consumption and function, and knowledge of optimal management techniques is helpful in ensuring the best long-term outcomes. Pain and the psychologic aspects of limb differences also may need to be addressed in the growing child. A team approach to care that empowers the patient and his or her family is encouraged.

Keywords: complications; congenital; energy consumption; gait analysis; infection; ischemia; limb; pain; psychology; transverse deficiencies; trauma

Introduction

Transverse deficiency is a term used in the International Society of Prosthetics and Orthotics classification of limb deficiencies. It describes a limb where the missing part of the extremity involves the entire cross-sectional volume of the limb. This contrasts with a longitudinal deficiency that involves either the medial or the lateral aspect of the limb.

A transverse deficiency can be either terminal (the most common type) or intercalary, in which the distal part of the limb is present but the more proximal portion is missing. An example is phocomelia. The level of the amputation can have a dramatic effect on the ability of a patient to participate in certain activities and on the process of energy consumption. The level also affects the need for secondary procedures as a child grows. The clinician must be clearly aware of potential remaining growth and prosthetic issues to optimize both the initial surgical treatment and later residual limb management.

Both the etiology and the extent of the deficiency on initial presentation are major influences on the outcome of surgical management. However, optimal management (or, contrarily, mismanagement or less-than-optimal management) can substantially influence a child's function both during the growth years and into adulthood. General principles of amputation in children are shown in **Table 1**.

Etiology
Acquired
Trauma

Trauma accounts for a large percentage of acquired transverse deficiencies of the lower limb. Lawnmower injuries alone account for nearly 50% of all amputations performed in children younger than 10 years.[1-3] Small children who are sitting in the lap of a riding mower operator may accidentally fall and land under the mower; in other cases, the operator may inadvertently back over a child, unaware that the child is in the

Table 1   General Principles of Amputation in Children

Preserve proximal joints (hip, knee) whenever possible.

Preserve length (both actual and potential growth plates).

Amputate through the joint if the bone distal to it cannot be saved.

Tissues in children are quite resilient and, as a rule, heal very well. A variety of techniques can be used to preserve joints and length.

Proximal osteotomies or external fixator techniques may be needed in growing children to accomplish ideal biomechanical limb alignment and optimal residual limb length.

vicinity. These injuries often involve substantial bone loss, soft-tissue destruction, and contamination. Aggressive surgical débridement is necessary. Vacuum-assisted closure systems have been used effectively for wounds that cannot be closed initially.[4] Injuries to and the frank loss of growth centers result in the need for multiple secondary procedures as a child develops.

High-energy injuries, such as train–pedestrian or motor vehicle–pedestrian crashes, often result in amputations. Multiple débridements are necessary before definitive closure. These injuries may require revision amputation to higher levels than expected because of soft-tissue and bony destruction.[5] As with lawnmower injuries, further interventions often are needed as a child grows.

Blast injuries to the lower limbs also can result in transverse ablations. Edwards et al[6] reviewed interventions for pediatric blast injuries in Afghanistan

Neither Dr. Forness nor any immediate family member has received anything of value from or has stock or stock options held in a commercial company or institution related directly or indirectly to the subject of this chapter.

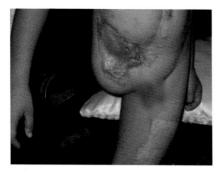

Figure 1 Clinical photograph of a child with an intra-abdominal injury that resulted from shelling and shrapnel. The injury resulted in a hip disarticulation.

and Iraq between 2002 and 2010. They found that of the more than 1,600 children reviewed, all amputations occurred in children older than 4 years (**Figure 1**). Younger children appeared to sustain only central injuries (that is, injuries to the trunk rather than injuries to a limb). In a review of traumatic amputations at a regional level I US trauma center hospital, gunshot wounds and dog bites (**Figure 2**) also were noted as sources of amputation.[3] A study by Loder[7] reported that most pediatric amputations that were related to motor-vehicle crashes occurred in adolescents, perhaps caused by either inexperience or immaturity of younger drivers.

Electrical injuries can be problematic. Two mechanisms of electrical action damage tissue: Electric current disrupts cell membranes, and heat causes tissue necrosis. Tarim and Ezer[8] reported that 75% of electrical burns were high-voltage injuries that resulted in high mortality and morbidity rates. The body is more of a conductor than a resistor, and tissue destruction is often underestimated initially. In a severely thermally burned patient, amputation often is a life-saving decision.[9] Tissue necrosis and sepsis are the driving factors for decision making for both thermal and electrical burns. Adjacent growth plates can be affected in an occult fashion, causing long-term limb-length discrepancies and/or angular deformities.

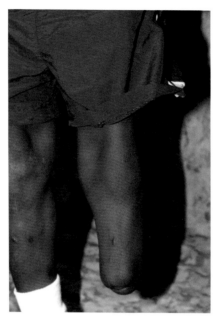

Figure 2 Clinical photograph of a child who had a mangling injury to the left limb from a dog bite. The limb was not salvageable, and a transtibial amputation was performed.

Neoplasms
Prior to the advent of modern chemotherapeutic agents, amputation for a limb malignancy was common. During the past 35 years, newer protocols have supported limb salvage techniques. Rotationplasty and endoprosthetic replacement are now the mainstays of treatment after the lesion is resected. When adequate margins are not possible in limb salvage surgery for osteogenic sarcoma or other malignancy, transfemoral or transtibial amputation is required (**Figure 3**). Substantial neurovascular involvement, poor distal limb function, failed attempts at limb salvage, or persistent local recurrence of disease also are indications for amputation.[10] Rotationplasty, a limb salvage procedure that is particularly used in very young children, is itself a transverse intercalary amputation.

Sepsis
Nearly 50% of all meningococcemia infections in children occur in those younger than 2 years; the peak number of cases occurs in those younger than

4 months.[11] These children often have rapidly progressive disease. Their limbs are cool with delayed capillary refill, and tachycardia is present. According to a series by Powars et al,[12] patients with serogroup C or purpura fulminans had a 50% fatality rate. Of the survivors, 70% had amputations (**Figure 4**). Mozzo et al[13] described a case of meningococcemia and heparin-induced thrombocytopenia that resulted in bilateral lower limb ischemia and subsequent amputations. In a review of patients with purpura fulminans, Canavese et al[14] described the incidence of amputations and other limb deformities associated with meningococcemia. Limb ischemia in the perinatal period can result in limb compromise. Thromboembolic events and hypercoagulable states can lead to arterial occlusions, including sepsis, polycythemia, and protein C deficiency. The immature fibrinolytic system in newborns may put them at higher risk.[15] Arterial catheterization also can lead to complete thrombosis. Blank et al[16] found this to be true in 50% of the ischemic limbs reviewed in their series.

Congenital Longitudinal Deficiencies
Transverse ablations are the time-honored treatment of two congenital longitudinal deficiencies, complete tibial hemimelia and fibular hemimelia, with joint disarticulations performed through the knee and the ankle, respectively. Other treatment options have been discussed. Depending on the severity of the deformity, these other options are controversial. Centralization techniques of the fibula for tibial hemimelia have been described. Complications such as knee instability, knee flexion contractures, and extensor mechanism deficiency have been noted, and mixed outcomes have been reported.[17] Patel et al[18] proposed the use of a super ankle procedure for fibular hemimelia rather than a Syme ankle disarticulation. Osteotomies to realign the tibial and subtalar deformities along with soft-tissue balancing

at a young age are recommended; these procedures are then followed by tibial lengthening.

Increasingly severe deformities often require more aggressive interventions, which can result in increased stiffness in the subtalar region and deformed ball-and-socket ankle joints; these complications can decrease function. In both tibial and fibular hemimelia, extensive discussion with the child's family should occur before treatment to determine the family's preference for limb-preserving treatment; options include multiple surgical procedures and the risks of surgical morbidity versus one index amputation procedure that requires a lifetime of prosthetic upkeep.

More severe forms of proximal femoral focal deficiency often are treated with a knee fusion and rotationplasty or a Syme ankle disarticulation on the affected side. If a Syme disarticulation and a knee fusion are the chosen procedures, an effort is made to carry out the procedures at an appropriate age in early childhood so that the fused and shortened femur and tibia are ultimately slightly shorter than the femur on the opposite side. This allows for the placement of a prosthetic knee at the same level as the unaffected contralateral side at the end of skeletal growth.

Syndromes

A Syme ankle disarticulation is a salvage option for the treatment of congenital pseudarthrosis with or without underlying neurofibromatosis. Despite efforts with bone grafting, vascularized fibular grafting, and bone transport, healing does not always ensue; thus, ablation is the best option, especially when performed early in a child's life. Klippel-Trénaunay-Weber syndrome is a mixed vascular malformation in which the deep venous and lymphatic structures often are deficient.[19] Conservative treatment is the primary approach to care. Ultimately, in patients with severe gigantism or vascular compromise,

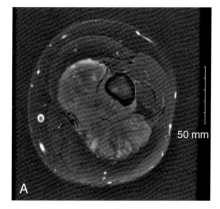 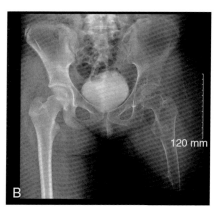

Figure 3   Images of the femur in a patient with osteosarcoma. **A,** Cross-sectional axial MRI of the femur with associated lesion. **B,** Postoperative AP radiograph after the patient independently decided to have a transfemoral amputation.

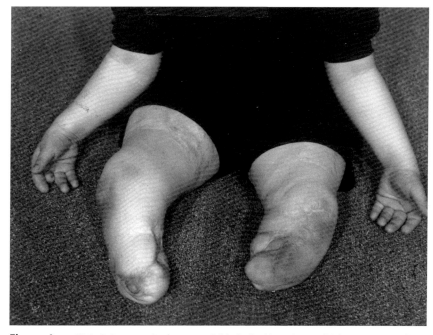

Figure 4   Clinical photograph of a young child who had lateral transtibial amputations after a severe meningococcemia infection.

amputation is necessary. This also can be true in patients with Proteus syndrome.[20]

Congenital Deficiencies

The etiology for most congenital transverse deficiencies is poorly understood. As with many disease entities, the underlying mechanism for the individual defects may be a combination of genetic,[21] vascular, and environmental causes. One gene that has been identified is *ECSO2* on the eighth chromosome,

which causes phocomelic defects in Roberts syndrome.[22] Historically, it has been well documented that phocomelic defects are directly linked to thalidomide, a sedative used to treat morning sickness. Since then, data from the National Birth Defects Prevention Study have been carefully reviewed, and correlations have been found with other possible teratogens. Caspers et al[23] studied maternal exposure to active or passive cigarette smoke during pregnancy. They found that cigarette smoke is a

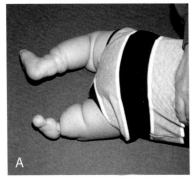 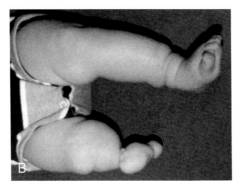

Figure 5 Clinical dorsal (**A**) and anterior (**B**) photographic views of a child with amniotic banding of both lower limbs. The left leg has soft-tissue involvement that was easily treated. The right leg had transtibial autoamputation. Because of the very narrow residuum, prosthetic fitting was problematic.

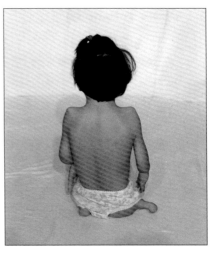

Figure 6 Clinical photograph of a child with bilateral lower limb phocomelia.

potential agent that affects limb and digit formation. Terminal transverse limb deficiencies were correlated with smoke exposure. In addition, Hernandez et al[24] reported a small to moderate increased risk of transverse limb deficiencies with the maternal use of ibuprofen, aspirin, and naproxen in the first trimester.

Amniotic band syndrome (Streeter dysplasia) is another source of transverse amputation. The lesions can vary from a simple band around the limb, which causes no substantial deficit, to complete vascular obstruction that necessitates the removal of the compromised distal segment or even the entire limb (**Figure 5**). Amniotic band syndrome can be detected in utero by ultrasound. Javadian et al[25] reported cases from their own center and a review of the literature. With fetoscopic surgery, they found a limb function rate of preservation equal to 50%.

Categories

In 1961, Frantz and O'Rahilly[26] devised a classification system for congenital limb anomalies. The nomenclature from this system is still used in longitudinal deficiencies but has not been as well accepted in transverse lesions. In the early 1970s in Dundee, Scotland, a group met to develop a system that would gain wider acceptance. Out of this work, the International Organization for Standardization (ISO) system

for congenital limb anomalies was developed. This system has been adopted in Europe and may be more appropriate for transverse deficiencies.[27] However, the terms phocomelia (flipper-like limb) and intercalary are still currently used in many practices.

Transverse Terminal

A transverse terminal limb is essentially a normal limb; it has a discrete end, beyond which are no more skeletal components. There may be soft-tissue nubbins but no bone. The ISO system describes total transverse loss at the pelvis, thigh, or leg. The thigh and leg are subdivided into upper, middle, and lower third deficiencies.

Transverse Intercalary

Using both old and new terminology, a transverse intercalary limb represents a missing segment of a limb between the proximal and distal portions. Phocomelia is a deficiency defined as the absence of the leg, with the foot attached directly to the pelvis (**Figure 6**). Intercalary deficiencies involve absence of the thigh, with the leg and foot attached to the pelvis, or absence of the leg, with the foot attached to the end of the thigh (**Figure 7**). A rotationplasty involves a form of acquired transverse intercalary deficiency. The knee, including the distal femur and the proximal tibia, is removed in an oncologic procedure,

after which the femur and the tibia are reapproximated in the newly rotated position.

Level
Foot

Congenital transverse amputations can occur at the forefoot, the Lisfranc, or the Chopart levels. After trauma, it is appropriate to maintain as much viable tissue as possible. In a growing child, there is a tremendous capacity for healing and remodeling. Immediate revision to the traditional adult midtarsal or tarsal metatarsal levels may be counterproductive to achieving maximal function. Revision surgery can be considered at a later date when the entire treatment team, including the patient, can be involved in the decision-making process.

Syme Ankle Disarticulation

The Syme disarticulation involves removing the foot through the ankle while retaining the heel pad for weight bearing. This procedure often is used for the treatment of congenital longitudinal deficiency of the fibula (fibular hemimelia) or recalcitrant pseudarthrosis of the tibia. Posterior slippage of the heel pad can be problematic. The advantage of a Syme ankle disarticulation is that it is end-bearing. In a child, the Syme

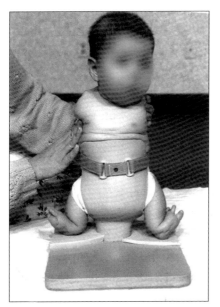

Figure 7 Clinical photograph of an infant with bilateral intercalary defects of the lower limbs. The feet are attached to the end of the thighs.

amputation is a true disarticulation, with both the distal tibial and fibular growth plates left intact. This allows normal subsequent growth and, importantly, prevents stump overgrowth. It also allows for excellent prosthetic fit and function. A Boyd amputation involves fusing a portion of the calcaneus to the tibia. It allows for more length, but malunion can be an issue. In addition, this amputation level limits the space available for prosthetic components, unless further limb shortening is anticipated with differential growth.

Transtibial Amputation

A transtibial amputation often is performed in a nonelective situation, such as trauma, or for the treatment of disease when a more distal level is not possible. In a child, a transtibial amputation should be avoided because of multiple issues, such as bony overgrowth and difficulty in prosthetic fitting. Osseous overgrowth has been well described.[28,29] Compared with diaphyseal amputations, overgrowth is slightly more likely to develop in a metaphyseal amputation (45%

versus 50%, respectively). Endosteal bone combined with periosteum-derived bone creates the overgrowth.[30] Bursae, cysts, and frank ulcerations can develop at the overgrowth site.

Ranade et al[31] described angular deformity. In their study, deformity in either the coronal or sagittal planes or both developed in more than one-third of the patients. Treatment often consisted of osteotomies or lengthening and realignment. Patella alta and even patellar dislocation associated with transtibial amputations have been reported in the literature.[32,33] One-third of the children in a study by Mowery et al[33] had patella alta, a positive apprehension test, and dislocations. The authors postulated that the patellar tendon weight-bearing prosthesis may eventually cause the patellar tendon to stretch out and predispose the patient to subluxation or dislocation. Mowery et al[33] recommended distributing the weight bearing area of the prosthesis over a larger area of the knee to prevent this problem. In terms of energy consumption, increased proximal muscle activity has been shown to compensate for the loss of plantar flexion power in a transtibial amputation, specifically hip extensor strength.[34]

Knee Disarticulation

A knee disarticulation allows for end-bearing weight with a prosthetic limb. The growth plate is intact, which decreases limb-length discrepancy at maturity. Bony overgrowth is therefore not an issue. Fitting with a prosthetic knee may be more difficult in a unilateral situation. Careful timing with an epiphysiodesis of the distal femur of the involved limb or even a shortening osteotomy (removing a section of the diaphysis) may be important to keep the intact knee and the prosthetic knee at the same height at the end of growth.

Function and energy consumption are affected by the level of amputation. Waters et al[35] demonstrated that

performance decreases but oxygen consumption increases with each proximal level of amputation. The authors also showed that the rate of oxygen consumption did not depend on the amputation level, which is an apparent paradox. They found that amputees decrease their customary walking speed with each higher level of amputation in an effort to keep oxygen consumption constant. This finding correlated well with a study by James[36] that concluded that amputees seem to spontaneously choose a gait with the same power cost as a nonamputee—hence a slower speed. A study specifically in children by Herbert et al[37] demonstrated that oxygen consumption was 15% greater in a child with a transtibial amputation than in a child without an amputation. Despite this fact, the customary walking speed in children with a transtibial amputation was not slower than that of their peers. Furthermore, the heart rate of these children did not increase. Jeans et al,[38] however, demonstrated that children with a Syme ankle disarticulation, a transtibial amputation, or a knee disarticulation walked with essentially the same speed and oxygen cost as children with two intact lower limbs.

Transfemoral Amputation

A transfemoral amputation is performed when a more distal level of resection is not possible. Bony overgrowth and prosthetic fitting can be issues. The latter is made worse the more proximal the ablation. In addition, in a growing child, loss of the distal femoral growth plate may make limb-length discrepancy much worse at maturity, resulting in a shorter femoral lever arm than expected. Every effort should be made to preserve the distal femoral growth plate in very young children and infants; otherwise, a very short femoral segment at skeletal maturity would allow for only a hip disarticulation–like prosthetic fitting.

Patients with transfemoral amputations recruit trunk musculature in gait.

Upper body angular range of motion increases as velocity decreases.[39] Bell et al[40] found that patients with longer residual femurs after amputation had a faster self-selected walking velocity. In a study of 13 young amputees, Baum et al[41] found that if the length of the remaining femur was at least 57% of the unaffected femur, length did not dramatically affect gait.

In a 2011 study, Jeans et al[38] reported that children with transfemoral amputations and hip disarticulations had a reduction of normal walking speed equal to 80% and 72%, respectively, and a VO$_2$ cost of 151% and 161%, respectively. Hip disarticulation further compromises gait efficiency. Compared with a control group, Nowroozi et al[42] demonstrated a further decrease in comfortable walking speed to 61%. The patients with hip disarticulation were able to maintain a relatively constant energy cost. Transfemoral amputations increase energy consumption and decrease function. Stability and proprioception are compromised.[43] The unaffected leg in a unilateral amputee must assume compensatory tasks in both the stance and swing phases of gait. Aerobic conditioning has been shown to decrease oxygen consumption and improve the overall economy of walking in those with lower limb amputation.[44]

Hip Disarticulation

Hip disarticulation is seen in the treatment of severe traumatic situations, life-threatening infections, and oncologic lesions. Prosthetic fitting is much more challenging and often uncomfortable. Energy consumption is nearly twice that of normal consumption. Gait analysis can play an important role in clarifying pathologic factors in prosthetic gait and subsequently help select from among available interventions for treatment.[45] For example, following the placement of the prosthesis, decreased stance phase time and increased swing phase duration are noted to a greater extent in patients with transfemoral amputations and hip disarticulations.[46] Two studies have demonstrated increased abduction moments in the hip and the knee of the unaffected leg or decreased moments on the affected side.[47,48] Nadollek et al[49] reported that increasing hip abductor strength on the side of the amputation could increase weight bearing or stance phase time on that side.

Other Considerations
Pain and Phantom Sensation

Pain and phantom sensation after amputation are common problems. To offer effective treatment in any patient, three types of sensory phenomena need to be differentiated: phantom sensation; phantom limb pain; and residual limb pain, including reflex sympathetic dystrophy. Phantom sensation is a patient's sense that the amputated limb is still present and includes nonpainful sensations such as itching or pressure. It occurs in nearly all patients with amputations and tends to resolve with time.[50] Phantom pain is pain in the limb that is not there. Proximal amputations have a higher rate of phantom pain than distal amputations. Melzack et al[51] reported a 42% rate of phantom limb pain at long-term follow-up. In a more recent study involving children and young adults, pain was prevalent 76% of the time in the first year after oncologic amputation but only 10% of the time thereafter.[52] Patients with electrical burn injuries have had a higher rate of phantom pain than patients with amputations secondary to thermal burns.[53] In nontraumatic situations, an epidural block initiated before elective amputation has been helpful in reducing phantom pain.[54] Residual limb pain originates from the remaining portion of the limb. The etiology for this type of pain can be scarring; bursal pain; pain generated from the prosthesis; neurogenic causes, including neuromas; and other sources.[55] Reflex sympathetic dystrophy in children also can be an issue. The overwhelming causes of pain in the residual limb are distal bone overgrowth or poor prosthetic fitting.

Psychological Concerns

More attention has been paid during the past few decades to the psychological aspect of limb deficiency in the growing child. Children tend to understand that they are different before they understand the disability itself. Discussions at home are noted to be very important to a child's understanding of his or her disability. Interestingly, in a study by Dunn et al,[56] 27% of families reported no such discussions. Adolescence can be a particularly difficult time for dealing with limb absence. Clinical follow-up visits at this age may have less orthopaedic relevance because growth is leveling off, but psychological issues may have greater importance. Wallace et al[57] noted a high degree of resiliency in response to patient experiences. The focus of their study was related to appearance changes in postmeningococcal septicemia, in which amputations and substantial extremity scarring occurs. The authors also noted the importance of long-term support for emotional and psychological adjustment to a new body image.

Summary

Transverse deficiencies have several etiologies that must be clearly understood in a growing child. It is important to consider the potential for growth disparity, pain management, energy consumption, and prosthetic fitting. As much limb length as possible should be maintained. Preserving the distal femoral growth plate in the young child is paramount to decrease long-term limb-length discrepancy. Saving the knee joint preserves function, proprioception, and energy. End-bearing amputations rather than transosseous amputations avoid issues such as bony overgrowth and improve end–weight bearing.

It is critical to keep the family informed and to progressively educate the child on the best methods of dealing with his or her limb deficiency. Including the family and child on the treatment team empowers the family when difficult decisions arise. Sports and recreational activities can foster overall development and help achieve the goals of assisting the child to become as active and functional as possible.

References

1. Love SM, Grogan DP, Ogden JA: Lawn-mower injuries in children. *J Orthop Trauma* 1988;2(2):94-101.

2. Smith GA; Committee on Injury and Poison Prevention: Technical report: Lawn mower-related injuries to children. *Pediatrics* 2001;107(6):E106.

3. Trautwein LC, Smith DG, Rivara FP: Pediatric amputation injuries: Etiology, cost, and outcome. *J Trauma* 1996;41(5):831-838.

4. Shilt JS, Yoder JS, Manuck TA, Jacks L, Rushing J, Smith BP: Role of vacuum-assisted closure in the treatment of pediatric lawn-mower injuries. *J Pediatr Orthop* 2004;24(5):482-487.

5. Blazar PE, Dormans JP, Born CT: Train injuries in children. *J Orthop Trauma* 1997;11(2):126-129.

6. Edwards MJ, Lustik M, Carlson T, et al: Surgical interventions for pediatric blast injury: An analysis from Afghanistan and Iraq 2002 to 2010. *J Trauma Acute Care Surg* 2014;76(3):854-858.

7. Loder RT: Demographics of traumatic amputations in children: Implications for prevention strategies. *J Bone Joint Surg Am* 2004;86(5):923-928.

8. Tarim A, Ezer A: Electrical burn is still a major risk factor for amputations. *Burns* 2013;39(2):354-357.

9. Winkley JH, Gaspard DJ, Smith LL: Amputation as a life-saving measure in the burn patient. *J Trauma* 1965;5(6):782-791.

10. Marulanda GA, Henderson ER, Johnson DA, Letson GD, Cheong D: Orthopedic surgery options for the treatment of primary osteosarcoma. *Cancer Control* 2008;15(1):13-20.

11. Kirsch EA, Barton RP, Kitchen L, Giroir BP: Pathophysiology, treatment and outcome of meningococcemia: A review and recent experience. *Pediatr Infect Dis J* 1996;15(11):967-978, quiz 979.

12. Powars D, Larsen R, Johnson J, et al: Epidemic meningococcemia and purpura fulminans with induced protein C deficiency. *Clin Infect Dis* 1993;17(2):254-261

13. Mozzo E, Vidal E, Pettenazzo A, Amigoni A: Meningococcemia and heparin-induced thrombocytopenia: A dangerous combination. *Paediatr Anaesth* 2013;23(2):197-199.

14. Canavese F, Krajbich JI, LaFleur BJ: Orthopaedic sequelae of childhood meningococcemia: Management considerations and outcome. *J Bone Joint Surg Am* 2010;92(12):2196-2203.

15. Askin SR, Sullivan G, Dave K, Zubrow A, Razi N: Limb gangrene secondary to thromboembolic disease of the newborn. *Orthop Rev* 1992;21(1):49-51.

16. Blank JE, Dormans JP, Davidson RS: Perinatal limb ischemia: Orthopaedic implications. *J Pediatr Orthop* 1996;16(1):90-96.

17. Christini D, Levy EJ, Facanha FA, Kumar SJ: Fibular transfer for congenital absence of the tibia. *J Pediatr Orthop* 1993;13(3):378-381.

18. Patel M, Paley D, Herzenberg JE: Limb-lengthening versus amputation for fibular hemimelia. *J Bone Joint Surg Am* 2002;84(2):317-319.

19. McCarron JA, Johnston DR, Hanna BG, et al: Evaluation and treatment of musculoskeletal vascular anomalies in children: An update and summary for orthopaedic surgeons. *Univ Pennsyl Ortho J* 2001;14:15-24.

20. Guidera KJ, Brinker MR, Kousseff BG, et al: Overgrowth management in Klippel-Trenaunay-Weber and Proteus syndromes. *J Pediatr Orthop* 1993;13(4):459-466.

21. Klaassen Z, Shoja MM, Tubbs RS, Loukas M: Supernumerary and absent limbs and digits of the lower limb: A review of the literature. *Clin Anat* 2011;24(5):570-575.

22. Downer J: Fifteen-year hunt uncovers gene behind pseudothalidomide syndrome. Available at: http://www.hopkinsmedicine.org/Press_releases/2005/04_11_05.html. Accessed June 11, 2015.

23. Caspers KM, Romitti PA, Lin S, Olney RS, Holmes LB, Werler MM; National Birth Defects Prevention Study: Maternal periconceptional exposure to cigarette smoking and congenital limb deficiencies. *Paediatr Perinat Epidemiol* 2013;27(6):509-520.

24. Hernandez RK, Werler MM, Romitti P, Sun, Anderka M; National Birth Defects Prevention Study: Nonsteroidal antiinflammatory drug use among women and the risk of birth defects. *Am J Obstet Gynecol* 2012;206(3):228.

25. Javadian P, Shamshirsaz AA, Haeri S, et al: Perinatal outcome after fetoscopic release of amniotic bands: A single-center experience and review of the literature. *Ultrasound Obstet Gynecol* 2013;42(4):449-455.

26. Frantz CH, O'Rahilly R: Congenital skeletal limb deficiencies. *J Bone Joint Surg Am* 1961;10:24-35.

27. International Organization for Standardization: *IS0 8548-1: Prosthetics and Orthotics. Limb Deficiencies: Part 1. Method of Describing Limb Deficiencies Present at Birth*. Geneva, Switzerland, International Organization for Standardization, 1989, pp 1-6.

28. Aitken GT: Osseous overgrowth in amputations in children, in Swinyard CW, ed: *Limb Development and*

Deformity Problems in Evaluation and Rehabilitation. Springfield, IL, Charles C Thomas, 1969, pp 448-456.

29. Pellicore RJ, Sciora J, Lambert CN, Hamilton RC: Independence of bone overgrowth in the juvenile amputee population. *Interclin Info Bull* 1974;13:1.

30. O'Neal ML, Bahner R, Ganey TM, Ogden JA: Osseous overgrowth after amputation in adolescents and children. *J Pediatr Orthop* 1996;16(1):78-84.

31. Ranade A, McCarthy JJ, Davidson RS: Angular deformity in pediatric transtibial amputation stumps. *J Pediatr Orthop* 2009;29(7):726-729.

32. McIvor JB, Gillespie R: Patellar instability in juvenile amputees. *J Pediatr Orthop* 1987;7(5):553-556.

33. Mowery CA, Herring JA, Jackson D: Dislocated patella associated with below-knee amputation in adolescent patients. *J Pediatr Orthop* 1986;6(3):299-301.

34. Powers CM, Boyd LA, Fontaine CA, Perry J: The influence of lower-extremity muscle force on gait characteristics in individuals with below-knee amputations secondary to vascular disease. *Phys Ther* 1996;76(4):369-377, discussion 378-385.

35. Waters RL, Perry J, Antonelli D, Hislop H: Energy cost of walking of amputees: The influence of level of amputation. *J Bone Joint Surg Am* 1976;58(1):42-46.

36. James U: Oxygen uptake and heart rate during prosthetic walking in healthy male unilateral above-knee amputees. *Scand J Rehabil Med* 1973;5(2):71-80.

37. Herbert LM, Engsberg JR, Tedford KG, Grimston SK: A comparison of oxygen consumption during walking between children with and without below-knee amputations. *Phys Ther* 1994;74(10):943-950.

38. Jeans KA, Browne RH, Karol LA: Effect of amputation level on energy expenditure during overground walking by children with an amputation. *J Bone Joint Surg Am* 2011;93(1):49-56.

39. Goujon-Pillet H, Sapin E, Fodé P, Lavaste F: Three-dimensional motions of trunk and pelvis during transfemoral amputee gait. *Arch Phys Med Rehabil* 2008;89(1):87-94.

40. Bell JC, Wolf EJ, Schnall BL, Tis JE, Potter BK: Transfemoral amputations: Is there an effect of residual limb length and orientation on energy expenditure? *Clin Orthop Relat Res* 2014;472(10):3055-3061.

41. Baum BS, Schnall BL, Tis JE, Lipton JS: Correlation of residual limb length and gait parameters in amputees. *Injury* 2008;39(7):728-733.

42. Nowroozi F, Salvanelli ML, Gerber LH: Energy expenditure in hip disarticulation and hemipelvectomy amputees. *Arch Phys Med Rehabil* 1983;64(7):300-303.

43. Eberhart HD, Elftman H, Inman VT: The locomotor mechanism of the amputee, in Klopsteg PE, Wilson PD, eds: *Human Limbs and Their Substitutes: Presenting Results of Engineering and Medical Studies of the Human Extremities and Application of the Data to the Design and Fitting of Artificial Limbs and to the Care and Training of Amputees.* New York, NY, Haffner, 1968, pp 472-480.

44. Pitetti KH, Snell PG, Stray-Gundersen J, Gottschalk FA: Aerobic training exercises for individuals who had amputation of the lower limb. *J Bone Joint Surg Am* 1987;69(6):914-921.

45. Esquenazi A: Gait analysis in lower-limb amputation and prosthetic rehabilitation. *Phys Med Rehabil Clin N Am* 2014;25(1):153-167.

46. Schnall BL, Baum BS, Andrews AM: Gait characteristics of a soldier with a traumatic hip disarticulation. *Phys Ther* 2008;88(12):1568-1577.

47. Royer TD, Wasilewski CA: Hip and knee frontal plane moments in persons with unilateral, transtibial amputation. *Gait Posture* 2006;23(3):303-306.

48. Molina Rueda F, Alguacil Diego IM, Molero Sánchez A, Carratalá Tejada M, Rivas Montero FM, Miangolarra Page JC: Knee and hip internal moments and upper-body kinematics in the frontal plane in unilateral transtibial amputees. *Gait Posture* 2013;37(3):436-439.

49. Nadollek H, Brauer S, Isles R: Outcomes after trans-tibial amputation: The relationship between quiet stance ability, strength of hip abductor muscles and gait. *Physiother Res Int* 2002;7(4):203-214.

50. Finnoff J: Differentiation and treatment of phantom sensation, phantom pain, and residual-limb pain. *J Am Podiatr Med Assoc* 2001;91(1):23-33.

51. Melzack R, Israel R, Lacroix R, Schultz G: Phantom limbs in people with congenital limb deficiency or amputation in early childhood. *Brain* 1997;120(9):1603-1620.

52. Burgoyne LL, Billups CA, Jirón JL Jr, et al: Phantom limb pain in young cancer-related amputees: Recent experience at St Jude Children's Research Hospital. *Clin J Pain* 2012;28(3):222-225.

53. Thomas CR, Brazeal BA, Rosenberg L, Robert RS, Blakeney PE, Meyer WJ: Phantom limb pain in pediatric burn survivors. *Burns* 2003;29(2):139-142.

54. Danshaw CB: An anesthetic approach to amputation and pain syndromes. *Phys Med Rehabil Clin N Am* 2000;11(3):553-557.

55. Davis RW: Phantom sensation, phantom pain, and stump pain. *Arch Phys Med Rehabil* 1993;74(1):79-91.

56. Dunn NL, McCartan KW, Fuqua RW: Young children with orthopedic handicaps: Self-knowledge about their disability. *Except Child* 1988;55(3):249-252.

57. Wallace M, Harcourt D, Rumsey N: Adjustment to appearance changes resulting from meningococcal septicaemia during adolescence: A qualitative study. *Dev Neurorehabil* 2007;10(2):125-132.

Chapter 73

Congenital Longitudinal Deficiency of the Fibula

Michael Schmitz, MD   Brian J. Giavedoni, MBA, CP, LP

Abstract

Fibular deficiency is a spectrum of disease manifested as congenital longitudinal abnormality of the fibula with associated abnormalities of the surrounding joints and musculature. The etiology is unknown. The clinical status of the foot and overall limb-length discrepancy, which are expressed as a percentage, are predictive for treatment pathways of amputation and reconstruction for prosthesis wear or limb salvage with lengthening and reconstruction.

Keywords: classification; congenital longitudinal fibular deficiency; fibular deficiency; fibular hemimelia

Introduction

Congenital longitudinal deficiency of the fibula, or fibular hemimelia (as the condition is frequently called), is also described as postaxial deficiency of the lower limb. The latter term most accurately describes the actual condition because the entire lateral (postaxial) aspect of the limb is affected to various degrees (**Figures 1** and **2**). At a minimum, the limb manifests a mild degree of fibular dysplasia, a ball-and-socket ankle joint, a lax (dysplastic) anterior cruciate ligament, and a mildly hypoplastic lateral femoral condyle. On the other end of the spectrum is femoral deficiency; a hypoplastic lateral femoral condyle with knee valgus; femoral retroversion; complete absence of the cruciate ligaments; complete absence of the fibula; a shortened, bowed tibia; equinovalgus deformity of the ankle; and a dysplastic foot with absent lateral rays and hindfoot and tarsal coalitions.

This chapter focuses on the various presentations of congenital fibular deficiencies, including classification systems; factors that influence the choice and types of treatment; and prosthetic consideration for patients treated with foot ablation.

Incidence

Fibular deficiency is the most common hemimelia, with an incidence of 5.7 to 20 cases per 1 million births.[1-3] The deficiency is twice as common in males as in females, and it can be unilateral (usually right side) or bilateral.[4]

Etiology

Various mechanisms, including absence of the anterior tibial artery, defects in muscle development, disruption of the apical ectodermal ridge expression, and developmental field defects have been proposed as etiologic factors.[1,5-7] At present, however, the etiology remains unknown. Most cases of fibular deficiency are sporadic, but in some instances a syndrome is associated with the deficiency.[3] Fibular aplasia, tibial camptomelia, and oligodactyly syndrome (FATCO); Fuhrmann syndrome; and femur-fibula-ulna complex are syndromes with multifocal skeletal abnormalities, including variable fibular deficiency.[8-10]

Associated Abnormalities

The spectrum of fibular deficiency includes varying degrees of musculoskeletal abnormalities that can involve the pelvis, femur, knee, tibia, ankle, and foot.[11] It is important for the clinician to look for and identify all the associated deficiencies, because they can often have a substantial influence on treatment decisions.[12-15] The most common femoral abnormalities are proximal femoral focal deficiency, congenital short femur, and congenital coxa vara.[13,14] Distal femoral valgus can lead to genu valgum, which can be associated with lateral patellar subluxation.[14] The cruciate ligaments are often absent, with laxity demonstrable on physical examination but rarely resulting in functional instability.[14] Foot abnormalities include a ball-and-socket ankle joint, tarsal coalitions, and absent lateral rays.[16,17] The tibia can be dysplastic or bowed, possibly secondary to a residual fibrotic fibula that has restricted normal growth.[1]

In addition, the upper limb may be involved, with disorders ranging from syndactyly to a hypoplastic or dysplastic ulna.[12,18,19] Although upper limb abnormalities do not affect ambulation, they can limit donning and doffing capability of lower limb prostheses. In patients with bilateral upper limb abnormalities, the feet may be required for prehension.

Dr. Schmitz or an immediate family member serves as a paid consultant to or is an employee of Stryker and serves as a board member, owner, officer, or committee member of the Pediatric Orthopaedic Society of North America. Neither Mr. Giavedoni nor any immediate family member has received anything of value from or has stock or stock options held in a commercial company or institution related directly or indirectly to the subject of this chapter.

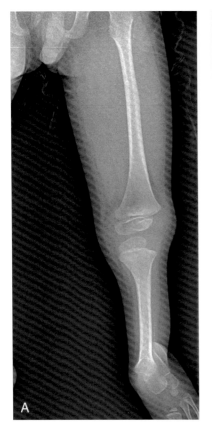
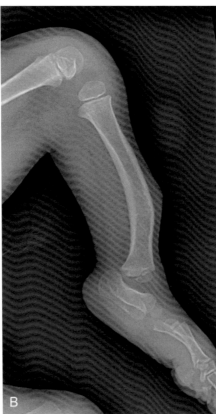

Figure 1 Radiographs from a child with a longitudinal deficiency of the fibula. **A,** AP view of the fibular length deficiency and ankle abnormality. **B,** The lateral view shows the anterior tibial bow and complete tarsal coalition.

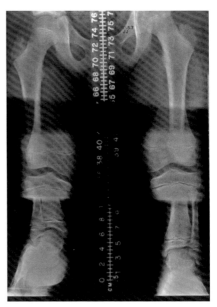

Figure 2 AP radiograph of the lower limbs of a child with a mild limb-length discrepancy and a ball-and-socket ankle joint, which is typical in patients with mild deficiencies.

Classification

A good classification system should aid the clinician in choosing the most effective interventions for a given problem, provide information useful for counseling the patient and parents regarding the diagnosis, and serve as a basis for future studies of the patient population. Ideally, the classification system should further define the deficiency with variables that are known to affect outcomes and help identify effective interventions. The identification of these determinant variables must be reproducible to allow researchers to appropriately define populations for study. The variables that have the greatest effect on outcome in fibular deficiency are limb-length discrepancy, ankle function, foot function, and the presence and extent of upper limb abnormalities.

The classification system of Coventry and Johnson,[20] which does not address function, is based on the radiographic appearance of the fibula and the presence of associated abnormalities. Congenital deficiencies of the fibula are divided into three main types. Type I involves a unilateral deficiency with a hypoplastic fibula, no foot involvement, and a substantial limb-length discrepancy. Type II is a unilateral abnormality, with nearly complete or complete absence of the fibula. Type III, is a bilateral abnormality, with complete absence of the fibula and a proximal femoral focal deficiency or upper limb involvement or involvement of the contralateral foot or tibia.[20]

Achterman and Kalamachi[21] presented a simplified classification system based only on the radiographic appearance of the fibula. It is most applicable in retrospective evaluations when only radiographs are available for review. In type IA abnormalities, the entire fibula is present but dysplastic, and in type 1B there is a partial absence of the proximal fibula, and the distal fibula does not support the ankle. A type II abnormality is characterized by complete absence of the fibula. The authors recommend limb-length equalization for nearly normal fibulae (type IA) and early amputation for fibular absence or deficiency associated with an unstable ankle (types IB and II).

Birch et al[22] reported on a retrospective review of 104 patients with fibular deficiencies treated at one institution between 1971 and 2005. The authors concluded that both the Coventry and Johnson and the Achterman and Kalamachi systems had poor predictive value regarding treatment. In addition, the authors found that femoral shortening affected the overall treatment plan in more than 80% of the patients. As surgeons became more proficient at lengthening procedures and reconstruction, classification systems based

Table 1 Classification of Congenital Longitudinal Deficiency of the Fibula by Birch et al[22]

Type	Description
I	Foot with three or more rays capable of providing a stable weight-bearing base with or without reconstructive procedures
A	Limb-length inequality 0% to <6%
B	Limb-length inequality 6% to 10%
C	Limb-length inequality 11% to 30%
D	Limb-length inequality >30%
II	Foot is unsalvageable
A	Intact upper limbs
B	Bilateral lower limb involvement and upper limb dysfunction that may require foot substitution for function

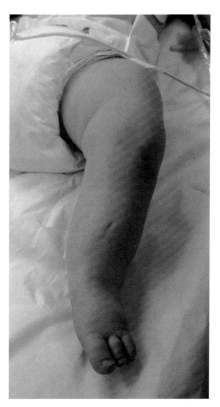

Figure 3 Clinical photograph of an infant with a fibular deficiency. Note dimpling of skin over the apex of the anterior tibial bow, the equinovalgus foot, and the absent lateral rays.

on functional determinants were needed. Birch et al[22] proposed a simplified classification system based on the clinical status of the foot, with the overall limb-length discrepancy expressed as a percentage (**Table 1**). This system allows classification of a fibular deficiency at birth and was found to more accurately predict management of the condition in patients treated at the Texas Scottish Rite Hospital for Children in Dallas, Texas.

Clinical Findings

The deficiency is usually apparent at birth and manifests as variable shortening of the fibula and an equinovalgus foot with a stiff hindfoot. There may be associated shortening of the femur and the tibia with apex anterior angulation and an anterior skin dimple over the apex. Frequently, lateral rays of the foot are missing and there is syndactylization of the toes (**Figure 3**). The patient should be fully examined to assess upper limb abnormalities as well as contralateral deficiencies. Radiographs of the bilateral lower limbs should be obtained, with a ruler placed to allow assessment of the percentage of total limb-length inequality and angular deformity.

Treatment

Treatment of a fibular deficiency is directed toward optimizing the function of the affected limb to allow the child's development to parallel that of an unaffected child to the extent possible. An accurate assessment of the determinate variables of total limb-length discrepancy, ankle function, foot function, hip and knee stability and function, bilateral involvement, and upper limb function will allow the clinician to develop a management plan. Treatment options include no treatment or only a shoe lift or foot orthosis in very mild cases; surgical restoration of the limb using foot stabilization and limb equalization techniques; and restoring use of the limb with the aid of a prosthesis, usually after foot ablation.

The treatment options, indications, risks, and benefits should be discussed early with the child's parents, because some decisions may be necessary before the child is able to participate in the decision-making process.[23]

Factors in Decision Making

Historically, treatment decisions were based on the radiographic appearance of the fibula and the presence of associated abnormalities.[20,21,23] Relative preservation of the fibula was seen as an indication for lengthening and reconstruction, whereas an absent fibula was an indication for foot ablation and prosthetic fitting. Bilateral involvement often did not require limb-length equalization, but it could necessitate treatment to create a functional foot (**Figure 4**). The potential for foot substitution for absent hand prehension was seen as a relative contraindication for foot ablation. In a 2011 study, Birch et al[22] demonstrated that the radiographic appearance of the fibula was not a good factor for determining a treatment plan. The presence of a salvageable foot (defined as a painless, plantigrade foot able to support weight bearing with or without reconstructive procedures) and the percentage of the total limb-length discrepancy were more appropriate factors to consider in the choice of amputation or limb salvage treatment for children with congenital fibular deficiency.

Advancements in limb-lengthening and reconstruction techniques offer viable limb salvage options for patients

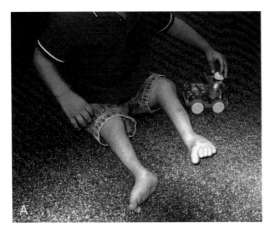
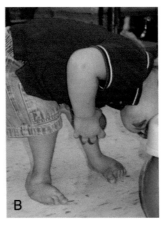

Figure 4   Postoperative sitting (**A**) and standing (**B**) photographs of a child with bilateral fibular deficiency. After Achilles lengthening, the child had functional, braceable, plantigrade feet.

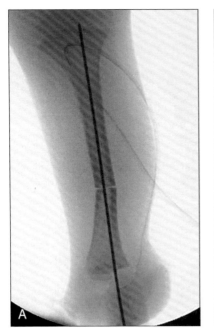
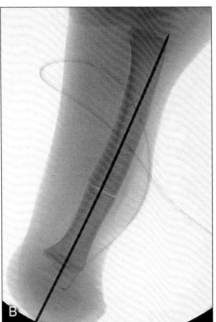

Figure 5   AP (**A**) and lateral (**B**) intraoperative fluoroscopic images of a complete fibular deficiency treated with a Syme ankle disarticulation and a tibial osteotomy secured with a temporary percutaneous Kirschner wire. The wire will be removed after the osteotomy has healed.

and considerable variation exists in reconstruction techniques. Generally, the indications or contraindications for reconstruction or amputation are based on relative factors. Good fibular length and foot preservation suggest reconstruction, whereas the lack of a fibula or poor fibular length or the lack of a functional foot are relative indications for amputation.[22,25,29] If the patient has associated upper limb functional deficits requiring foot substitution for prehensile function, early amputation should be avoided.

Surgical Procedures

Foot ablation can be accomplished with either a Syme ankle disarticulation or Boyd amputation.[15,26,29] Tibial angular deformity can be addressed at the time of the procedure with an osteotomy, and a removable pin can be used for fixation (**Figure 5**). A Syme ankle disarticulation can be associated with migration of the heel pad and growth of an inadvertently retained calcaneal apophysis that requires subsequent resection.[15] Because the Syme procedure is a true disarticulation, the whole calcaneus, including the apophysis, must be removed, and the distal Achilles tendon must be widely sectioned to avoid heel pad migration. Comparisons of patients treated with Syme disarticulations and Boyd amputations show fewer complications with the Boyd procedure.[15] However, a Syme ankle disarticulation offers excellent long-term outcomes, allows greater variability in prosthetic design, and is more easily performed in patients with extreme hindfoot equinus.[30,31] Angular deformities of the tibia or femur at the knee may require later treatment with hemiepiphyseal stapling or osteotomy.[14,15,22]

Limb salvage requires procedures to create a plantigrade, painless foot and equalized limb lengths and to correct angular deformities. These procedures may include Achilles lengthening, peroneal lengthening, a hindfoot osteotomy

with congenital fibular deficiencies.[23-28] A plantigrade, painless foot that can function as a support, a limb length that can be equalized, and a stable hip and knee are requirements when considering limb salvage. If surgical reconstruction is the best option, foot ablation and prosthetic fitting involves only one surgical procedure and one hospital stay to correct the foot, ankle, and limb-length deformity, which is then followed at an appropriate time by a prosthetic fitting. Comparisons of reconstruction and amputation outcomes show that the treatment options achieve nearly equivalent functional results, but patients treated with limb lengthening require more surgical procedures and hospitalizations, incur higher medical costs, and have more complications.[26,29] However, randomized or matched group comparisons have not been completed, to neutralize the hindfoot, and metatarsal osteotomies to allow shoe wear. Lengthening can be accomplished through the tibia, femur, or both, and can be performed concurrently with angular correction of both the tibia and femur. Complications increase as the magnitude of the lengthening increases.[32] Complications range from minor difficulties, such as pin tract infections, to major problems such as hip and knee subluxation and dislocation, nonunion, and substantial joint stiffness.[33] Limb-length discrepancies of less than 6% can be treated with a lift or epiphysiodesis, whereas discrepancies of 6% to 10% require an epiphysiodesis or single-stage lengthening.[22] Limb-length discrepancies of 11% to 30% require at least one lengthening procedure and may require two procedures or a bifocal lengthening. Patients with a discrepancy of more than 30% will require extensive lengthening, and they may be best treated with amputation and prosthetic fitting.[13,15,22,24,25]

Prosthetic Considerations

The common adage that "children are not small adults" should be recognized when considering the design of a prosthesis for a child. Function and the ability to undergo change to accommodate growth are the two most important prosthetic considerations for pediatric amputees.

The first prosthetic socket, which often uses a sleeve for suspension, should be easy for the parents to put on the child; comfortable; and not overly modified, so that the child's pending physiologic growth can be accommodated. To allow the socket design to take advantage of the difference between the widest aspect of the malleoli and the area just proximal to it for suspension purposes, surgical shaving or remodeling of the malleoli is strongly discouraged. The circumferential difference between these two landmarks determines the design of the socket. The smaller the difference in these two dimensions, the more likely that the prosthesis will require secondary suspension. The greater the difference in the dimensions, the more likely that the design will involve some sort of anatomically self-suspending socket, with an extreme design using an obturator, an opening, or a door that will allow passage of the residual limb.

A child treated with a Syme ankle disarticulation may be able to bear weight distally; however, achieving space for a prosthetic foot is challenging. Many prosthetic feet will fit using either a Syme plate to attach to the socket or a very short lamination core. Generally, 6 cm is the minimum amount of clearance needed for a basic prosthetic foot. The greater the technology and functional ability of a prosthetic foot, the more space that is required for the foot. In a Boyd amputation, the calcaneus remains intact and is fused to the tibia. This results in an amputation that is longer than a Syme disarticulation and much more challenging to accommodate with a prosthetic foot because there is almost no clearance.

Anterior tibial bowing found in longitudinal deficiency of the fibula usually must be accommodated because most children and adults have a relatively low pain threshold for pressure on the tibial crest. In many patients, mild bowing can be accommodated with the prosthesis. If bowing is more severe, bone straightening should be considered. A tibial osteotomy to straighten the bone can be performed during the foot ablation procedure at the pull-to-stand stage of development in a child. Placement of the prosthetic foot is very challenging in a patient with severe tibial bowing. As the tibia grows, the aspect distal to the apex of the bow continues to grow or migrate posteriorly, making correct placement of the foot more difficult.

One type of prosthetic design incorporates a full foam liner with inner diameters matching the contours of the limb anatomy and a uniform outer diameter that has been built up to the same circumference as the distal bulbous heel. A laminated shell is then formed over this insert (**Figure 6, A**). The patient dons the liner first. When required, a slit in the liner can facilitate adequate defection of the material to allow the passage of the bulbous distal aspect of the limb through the narrow bottleneck of the liner. When the liner is fully donned, it is slipped into the laminated outer receptacle. An atrophied residual limb with a small heel pad is best suited for this type of design, and a good degree of cosmetic restoration can be expected.

Another design is a silicone or bladder prosthesis that uses an inner elastic area that stretches to permit passage of the bulbous end of the residual limb (**Figure 6, B**). A third type of design, a prosthesis with an obturator or a medial opening, is recommended only when absolutely necessary (**Figure 6, C**). This design is appropriate when the distal end of the residual limb is large and the medial malleolus is prominent. Because of the inherent weaknesses in the design, catastrophic failure along the distal aspect of the opening is a common occurrence. Although these various designs are not uniquely used for pediatric patients, they are used to a greater extent in pediatric prosthetic designs than in adult designs.

As a child's longitudinal growth continues, the limb generally tends to become slimmer. The design of the socket for pediatric patients must be able to change with their physiologic growth.[34] Because pediatric socket designs must allow for continued adjustments to compensate for the growing limb, component choices are restricted to feet that will allow reasonable vertical growth compensation so that a level pelvis can be maintained throughout the period of routine height adjustments. For example, the prosthetic foot shown in **Figure 7** contains an inner carbon section and an outer shell that replicates

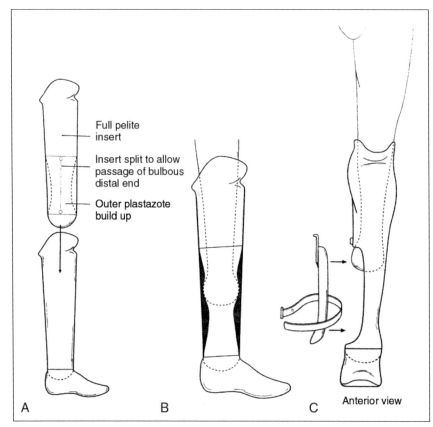

Full pelite insert

Insert split to allow passage of bulbous distal end

Outer plastazote build up

A   B   C   Anterior view

Figure 6 Illustrations of different types of Syme-level prostheses. **A,** Prothesis with segmented pelite liner that allows donning of the liner over the bulbous end, which is then inserted into the outer socket to lock the residual limb into the prosthesis. **B,** Prothesis with bladder design that allows insertion of the bulbous end into the prosthesis, with the silicone bladder expanding into a hollow air chamber and then constricting back onto the residual limb. **C,** Prothesis with lateral obturator (door) that is removed to allow passage of the bulbous end and then is locked back into place to secure the limb. (Adapted from Morrissy RT, Giavedoni B, Coulter C: The limb deficiency child, in Morrissy RT, Weinstein SL: *Pediatric Orthopaedics*. Philadelphia, PA, Lippincott, 2001, vol 2, pp 1218-1272.)

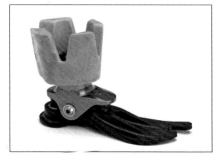

Figure 7 The Truper (College Park Industries) multiaxial foot accommodates spacer disks that allow the prosthesis to be lengthened in increments.

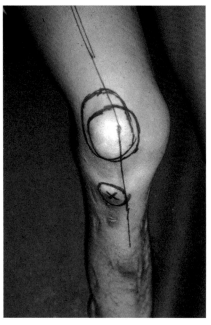

Figure 8 Clinical photograph of the limb of a patient with a fibular deficiency. The clearly marked patella alta with lateral patellar subluxation and severe genu valgum pose increased challenges to prosthetic socket design.

an anatomic foot. The shell can be exchanged up to three foot sizes before it is necessary to change the inner carbon section. In addition, longitudinal growth is accommodated by placing "growth" plates between the foot and the socket, up to several centimeters. This facilitates all possible growth challenges and extends the time a child can remain in the same prosthesis, provided that the socket fit is comfortable and protective.

The prosthesis has a high medial and lateral proximal brim, similar to the supracondylar suspension design. The contours of the proximal brim are equal in height to a supracondylar brim without

the contouring required for suspension. This helps to better control medial and lateral instability of the knee and affords added protection. This design also allows the proximal brim to better contain a growing limb and maximizes the amount of time the child can use the same socket. In most cases, a well-designed prosthesis can remain functional from 12 to 14 months, depending on the child's rate of growth. Component failure caused by normal wear and tear is more common in pediatric prostheses than in comparable adult devices.

Genu valgum and knee laxity are two common comorbidities that pose a

considerable challenge to prosthetic fitting in a child with a longitudinal fibular deficiency who has undergone a foot ablation (**Figure 8**). Prosthesis alignment must follow biomechanical principles for optimal functional outcomes. Increasing the height of the medial and lateral socket walls will afford additional control and protection to the knee. Foot placement (**Figure 9**) is routinely inset so that the ground reaction force falls through the center of the knee to reduce

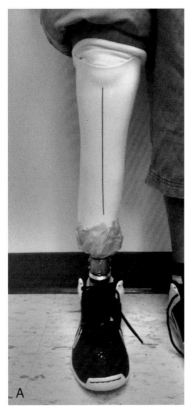
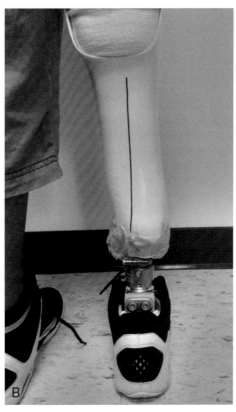

Figure 9 Anterior (**A**) and posterior (**B**) clinical photographs demonstrate that proper foot alignment can accommodate angular issues in a patient with a fibular deficiency. Note that foot placement for the child with a fibular deficiency should always reduce or eliminate any mediolateral moments around the knee to help preserve and protect an otherwise vulnerable structure.

any additional stresses that otherwise would be present.[35]

By understanding the anatomic differences of congenital longitudinal fibular deficiencies contrasted to the traumatic Syme ankle disarticulations, the prosthetist can better fit and adjust alignment expectations for optimal outcomes. Medial whips in the prosthesis are unavoidable because of the valgus deformity of the knee, and femoral hypoplasia must be taken into consideration for attaining a level pelvis in the prosthesis. Prosthetic fit should be comfortable while maintaining a balance between intimate fit and reasonable growth potential before the child or teen requires a new prosthesis. Above all, anticipating future needs and maximizing outcomes prior to skeletal maturity is an ongoing challenge with the pediatric patient.

Summary

Fibular deficiency is a spectrum of disease affecting limb length, knee stability, and ankle and foot function. These factors, in addition to other associated abnormalities, including bilaterality and upper limb dysfunction, must be considered before embarking on the treatment pathways of amputation and prosthetic fitting or lengthening and reconstruction. Treatment goals are the achievement of equal limb lengths, painless and functional knee and ankle joints, a plantigrade foot, and an appropriate mechanical axis. Amputation and prosthetic fitting is an excellent option to attain these goals but requires reliance on a prosthetic device. Limb lengthening and reconstruction can obtain these goals and obviate the need for a prosthesis but usually do not result in a better functioning limb.

References

1. Fordham LA, Applegate KE, Wilkes DC, Chung CJ: Fibular hemimelia: More than just an absent bone. *Semin Musculoskelet Radiol* 1999;3(3):227-238.

2. Froster UG, Baird PA: Congenital defects of lower limbs and associated malformations: A population based study. *Am J Med Genet* 1993;45(1):60-64.

3. Ghanem I: Epidemiology, etiology, and genetic aspects of reduction deficiencies of the lower limb. *J Child Orthop* 2008;2(5):329-332.

4. Reed MH: Normal and abnormal development, in Reed MH, ed: *Pediatric Skeletal Radiology*. Baltimore, MD, Williams and Wilkins, 1992, pp 349-392.

5. Levinsohn EM, Hootnick DR, Packard DS Jr: Consistent arterial abnormalities associated with a variety of congenital malformations of the human lower limb. *Invest Radiol* 1991;26(4):364-373.

6. Baek GH, Kim JK, Chung MS, Lee SK: Terminal hemimelia of the lower extremity: Absent lateral ray and a normal fibula. *Int Orthop* 2008;32(2):263-267.

7. Lewin SO, Opitz JM: Fibular a/hypoplasia: Review and documentation of the fibular developmental field. *Am J Med Genet Suppl* 1986;2(S2):215-238.

8. Hecht JT, Scott CI Jr: Limb deficiency syndrome in half-sibs. *Clin Genet* 1981;20(6):432-437.

9. Lipson AH, Kozlowski K, Barylak A, Marsden W: Fuhrmann syndrome of right-angle bowed femora, absence of fibulae and digital anomalies: Two further cases. *Am J Med Genet* 1991;41(2):176-179.

10. Lenz W, Zygulska M, Horst J: FFU complex: An analysis of 491 cases. *Hum Genet* 1993;91(4):347-356.

11. Pavone L, Viljoen D, Ardito S, et al: Two rare developmental defects of the lower limbs with confirmation of the Lewin and Opitz hypothesis on the fibular and tibial developmental fields. *Am J Med Genet* 1989;33(2):161-164.

12. Birch J, Lincoln T, Mack P: Functional classification of fibular deficiency, in Herring JA, Birch JG, eds: *The Child With a Limb Deficiency.* Rosemont, IL, American Academy of Orthopaedic Surgeons, 1998, 161-170.

13. Miller LS, Bell DF: Management of congenital fibular deficiency by Ilizarov technique. *J Pediatr Orthop* 1992;12(5):651-657.

14. Stevens PM, Arms D: Postaxial hypoplasia of the lower extremity. *J Pediatr Orthop* 2000;20(2):166-172.

15. Fulp T, Davids JR, Meyer LC, Blackhurst DW: Longitudinal deficiency of the fibula: Operative treatment. *J Bone Joint Surg Am* 1996;78(5):674-682.

16. Takakura Y, Tamai S, Masuhara K: Genesis of the ball-and-socket ankle. *J Bone Joint Surg Br* 1986;68(5):834-837.

17. Grogan DP, Holt GR, Ogden JA: Talocalcaneal coalition in patients who have fibular hemimelia or proximal femoral focal deficiency: A comparison of the radiographic and pathological findings. *J Bone Joint Surg Am* 1994;76(9):1363-1370.

18. Holmes L: *Common Malformations.* New York, NY, Oxford University Press, 2011.

19. Bohne WH, Root L: Hypoplasia of the fibula. *Clin Orthop Relat Res* 1977;125:107-112.

20. Coventry MB, Johnson EW Jr: Congenital absence of the fibula. *J Bone Joint Surg Am* 1952;34 A(4):941-955.

21. Achterman C, Kalamchi A: Congenital deficiency of the fibula. *J Bone Joint Surg Br* 1979;61-B(2):133-137.

22. Birch JG, Lincoln TL, Mack PW, Birch CM: Congenital fibular deficiency: A review of thirty years' experience at one institution and a proposed classification system based on clinical deformity. *J Bone Joint Surg Am* 2011;93(12):1144-1151.

23. Epps CH Jr, Schneider PL: Treatment of hemimelias of the lower extremity: Long-term results. *J Bone Joint Surg Am* 1989;71(2):273-277.

24. Patel M, Paley D, Herzenberg JE: Limb-lengthening versus amputation for fibular hemimelia. *J Bone Joint Surg Am* 2002;84(2):317-319.

25. Naudie D, Hamdy RC, Fassier F, Morin B, Duhaime M: Management of fibular hemimelia: Amputation or limb lengthening. *J Bone Joint Surg Br* 1997;79(1):58-65.

26. McCarthy JJ, Glancy GL, Chnag FM, Eilert RE: Fibular hemimelia: Comparison of outcome measurements after amputation and lengthening. *J Bone Joint Surg Am* 2000;82(12):1732-1735.

27. Choi IH, Kumar SJ, Bowen JR: Amputation or limb-lengthening for partial or total absence of the fibula. *J Bone Joint Surg Am* 1990;72(9):1391-1399.

28. Herring JA: Symes amputation for fibular hemimelia: A second look in the Ilizarov era. *Instr Course Lect* 1992;41:435-436.

29. Walker JL, Knapp D, Minter C, et al: Adult outcomes following amputation or lengthening for fibular deficiency. *J Bone Joint Surg Am* 2009;91(4):797-804.

30. Birch JG, Walsh SJ, Small JM, et al: Syme amputation for the treatment of fibular deficiency. An evaluation of long-term physical and psychological functional status. *J Bone Joint Surg Am* 1999;81(11):1511-1518.

31. Osebold WR, Lester EL, Christenson DM: Problems with excessive residual lower leg length in pediatric amputees. *Iowa Orthop J* 2001;21:58-67.

32. Hantes ME, Malizos KN, Xenakis TA, Beris AE, Mavrodontidis AN, Soucacos PN: Complications in limb-lengthening procedures: A review of 49 cases. *Am J Orthop (Belle Mead NJ)* 2001;30(6):479-483.

33. Hamdy RC, Makhdom AM, Saran N, Birch J: Congenital fibular deficiency. *J Am Acad Orthop Surg* 2014;22(4):246-255.

34. Cummins D, Kapp S: Lower limb pediatric prosthetics: General considerations and philosophy. *J Prosthet Orthot* 1992;4:203.

35. Gibson D: Child and juvenile amputee, in Banjerjee S, Khan N, eds: *Rehabilitation Management of Amputees.* Baltimore, MD, William and Wilkins, 1982, pp 394-414.

Chapter 74

Congenital Longitudinal Deficiency of the Tibia

Jorge A. Fabregas, MD   Rebecca C. Whitesell, MD, MPH

Abstract

Congenital deficiency of the tibia or tibial hemimelia is characterized by partial or complete absence of the tibia. Many of these patients have other associated anomalies. Although the true incidence of this condition is unknown, it has a bilateral presentation in approximately 30% of patients. Treatment varies depending on the amount of tibia that is absent and the presence or absence of the extensor mechanism.

Keywords: Brown procedure; congenital limb deficiency; congenital longitudinal deficiency; Syme ankle disarticulation; tibial deficiency; tibial hemimelia

Introduction

Congenital longitudinal deficiency of the tibia is the term used to describe a longitudinal deficiency of the tibial (medial) side of the lower limb. The tibia and the medial aspect of the foot are involved to various degrees. This condition has been known by many names in the literature, including tibial hemimelia, tibial meromelia, tibial anomaly, congenital tibial absence, congenital aplasia/dysplasia of the tibia, and congenital preaxial deficiency of the lower extremity.[1-3] The two most frequent terms used in modern literature and practice are congenital longitudinal deficiency of the tibia and tibial hemimelia.

Congenital longitudinal deficiency of the tibia is defined as partial or complete absence of the tibia, with a relatively unaffected fibula. Associated limb anomalies that occur in conjunction with the tibial deficiency include varying degrees of limb shortening, an equinovarus foot, knee joint abnormalities, and longitudinal deficiencies of the foot.[4-7] Frequently, there is bilateral involvement (up to 30% in some case series), and patients may have other limb anomalies such as proximal femoral focal deficiency (PFFD), a lobster claw hand deformity, or radial longitudinal deficiency of the upper limbs. The incidence of longitudinal congenital deficiency of the tibia has historically been estimated as 1 in 1 million live births in the United States,[8] but the true current incidence of the disease has not been reported. The database of the National Center on Birth Defects and Developmental Disabilities of The Centers for Disease Control and Prevention groups all limb deficiencies into either upper or lower limb deficiencies. The annual incidence of reduction deformity in the lower limbs is approximately 2 in 12,000 births; however, further data identifying only tibial deficiencies are unavailable.[9]

Clinical Presentation

In some instances, congenital longitudinal deficiency of the tibia can be difficult to distinguish from the much more common fibular deficiency, especially because it is difficult to precisely palpate and differentiate the soft, cartilaginous tibia and fibula in a small infant. The best clinical clue is that patients with a fibular deficiency always have an equinovalgus foot deformity, whereas patients with tibial deficiency always have an equinovarus foot deformity[6,10] (**Figure 1**). If there are associated ray abnormalities in the foot, patients with fibular deficiencies will have lateral ray deformities or deficiencies, and patients with tibial deficiencies will have medial ray deformities or deficiencies. The knee should be evaluated for the presence of a palpable patella and quadriceps and a patella tendon. It should also be determined if there is active extension of the knee because this will guide surgical decision making.

History

Otto is widely accepted as the first person to report on a patient with tibial hemimelia in the English literature in 1841.[1] In 1877, Albert described the transference of the fibula to the distal aspect of the femur to create a fibulofemoral arthrodesis. In the early 1900s, Myers[1] described fibular transfer to re-create a knee joint. Helferich, Patrona, Motta, Busachi, and Joachimstal all individually reported single procedures in which they made slight modification to Albert's described procedure to achieve a fibulofemoral arthrodesis.[1] Brown[11] was the first to report on a series of three patients in which he performed a fibulofemoral transfer to re-create the knee joint.

Dr. Fabregas or an immediate family member serves as a paid consultant to Integra. Neither Dr. Whitesell nor any immediate family member has received anything of value from or has stock or stock options held in a commercial company or institution related directly or indirectly to the subject of this chapter.

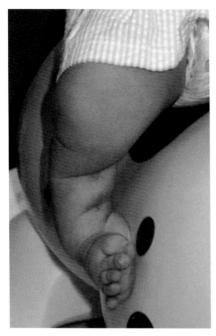

Figure 1 Clinical photograph of a 3-month-old infant with an absent tibia shows the typical equinovarus position of the foot. Note the dimpling along the medial border of the missing tibia.

In 1961, Frantz and O'Rahilly[12] were the first to attempt to define a unified language to describe all limb deficiencies. Jones et al[13] were the first to create a classification system designed specifically to distinguish types of tibial deficiencies (known as the Jones classification). In an effort to create a classification system that would help dictate potential surgical interventions, Kalamchi and Dawe[7] modified the Jones classification scheme.

After Brown[11] first described his fibular transfer technique in 1965, a substantial number of articles regarding tibial hemimelia were published until the early 1980s. By the early 1980s, some authors estimated there were up to 300 reported cases of the deficiency.[3] Since the 1980s, there have been relatively few articles published regarding this deficiency, and most of the current literature focuses on the genetic aspects of the disorder. Tibial hemimelia is unique among congenital limb deficiencies because it is genetically transmitted in a substantial number of patients.[3] For example, bilateral tibial deficiency associated with central cleft defect is inherited as an autosomal dominant condition.

Classification

The ideal classification system for congenital longitudinal deficiency of the tibia would incorporate treatment guidelines, help determine a prognosis, and aid in future research. The classification system would categorize the deficiency by the variables known to affect the patient's outcome and help identify potential interventions.

In tibial deficiencies, quadriceps function and strength, the length of the tibial remnant, the degree of ankle joint and foot involvement, and any associated musculoskeletal anomalies help determine potential interventions and can affect the patient's overall outcome.[6,14] The Jones classification system, which was published in 1978, remains the most widely used system to describe tibial deficiencies.[13] This system, however, is based on radiographic appearance and does not incorporate any of the variables known to influence patient outcomes. The classification system developed by Kalamchi and Dawe[7] attempts to incorporate some clinical factors in the classification scheme, but this system is less widely used by clinicians. Most recently, Weber[15] developed a classification and scoring system, but it is a rather detailed system and has not achieved wide popularity among clinicians.

Jones System

In the Jones classification system, groups are separated by radiographic appearance.[13] In type 1 deficiencies, the tibia is not visible on radiographs. In type 1a deficiencies, the proximal tibia is completely absent, and the distal femoral epiphysis is hypoplastic. In type 1b deficiencies, the proximal tibia is absent on radiographs, but unossified small tibial cartilaginous anlage can be viewed by ultrasound, arthrogram, and MRI or can be appreciated on surgical dissection. The most distinguishing radiographic characteristic between type 1a and type 1b deficiencies is the normal distal femoral epiphysis in a type 1b deficiency. Williams et al[4] performed surgical dissections on several patients classified as having a type 1b deficiency and found no tibial anlage despite that finding in the patient cohort used to create the Jones classification in which all type 1b patients had a tibial anlage on surgical exploration.[13] An additional distinguishing feature between Jones type 1a and type 1b deficiencies is a usual lack of quadriceps function (absent active knee extension) in the type 1a group.

In type 2 deficiencies, the proximal tibia is visible on radiographs, but the tibia is substantially shortened, with the distal part at least partially absent or substantially hypoplastic. In type 3 deficiencies, the distal tibial epiphysis is visible as either a fully ossified entity or as localized calcification with the proximal tibia poorly defined. Type 3 deficiencies are very rare. In type 4 deficiencies, the tibia is shortened, and there is tibiofibular diastasis. The Jones classification is very useful for defining various tibial deficiencies based on radiographic appearance, but outcome-based factors, such as quadriceps strength, foot anomalies, and overall limb length, are not used as a basis for classification.[13]

Kalamchi and Dawe System

The Kalamchi and Dawe[7] classification system is based on the type and degree of deformity, which the authors proposed would lead to defined treatments. Three groups are described based on clinical and radiographic findings. Type I is characterized by total absence of the tibia, proximal fibular migration, and distal femoral epiphysis hypoplasia on radiographs. Clinically, patients with type I deficiency have knee flexion contractures greater than 45°, no quadriceps function, marked equinovarus foot deformity, and, occasionally, medial ray deficiencies. Type II deficiency is defined as distal tibial aplasia. On radiographs, the proximal fibular migration is not as severe as in type I, and the distal femoral metaphyseal width and epiphyseal ossification are normal. Clinically, patients with type II deficiency have milder knee flexion contractures (25° to 45°), positive quadriceps function, and a relatively normal knee joint articulation. Type III deficiency is defined as dysplasia of the distal tibia, with diastasis of the tibiofibular syndesmosis. Radiographically, the distal tibia shows varying degrees of hypoplasia and shortening, the amount of syndesmotic diastasis can vary, the foot is in varus, and the talus may have a nearly vertical orientation. Clinically, patients with type III deficiency have normal knee joints and well-developed quadriceps function.

Weber System

In 2008, Weber[15] proposed a new classification and scoring system for tibial deformities. The classification system was developed to create a more modern system that incorporates correct anatomic terms, all types of deficiencies, and the inclusion of a scoring system to weight various associated anomalies in accordance with their effects on clinical decisions. The classification system identifies seven types of tibial deficiencies (I through VII), and five of the types have subgroups, depending on whether a cartilaginous tibial anlage is present or absent. The higher the number assigned to the classification, the more severe the tibial deficiency.

The scoring system assigns points for the presence or absence of a patella and the state of the hip, the femur, the fibula, the foot, and associated muscle function. The scoring system has a minimum score of 0 and maximum assigned value of 39; the higher the score, the less severe the impairment.

Type I is tibial hypoplasia, and type II is tibial fibular diastasis; these types

have no subgroups. Type III is distal aplasia, type IV is proximal aplasia, type V is biterminal aplasia, type VI is agenesis with double fibulae, and type VII is tibial agenesis with a single fibula. Types III through VII each include two subgroups: in subgroup a, cartilaginous anlage is present; in subgroup b, cartilaginous anlage is absent.

Comparisons

Despite the efforts of Kalamchi and Dawe[7] and, most recently, Weber,[15] the classification system most widely accepted and used by surgeons remains the Jones system.[13] Although the Kalamchi and Dawe[7] system more clearly defined the clinical correlates of each type of deformity, it did not add any new information regarding patient treatment. Weber's classification is more thorough, includes all variants (no matter how rare they may be), and attempts to provide a scoring system to indicate outcomes; however, it is rather difficult to understand, is cumbersome to use, and its reproducibility is questionable. All three classification systems (**Figure 2**) fail to incorporate the importance of associated foot anomalies in the decision-making process for amputation versus limb salvage.

Foot Abnormalities

Although Kalamchi and Dawe[7] addressed the knee and tibial deformity in their classification system, there is no scheme that has incorporated the degree of foot deformity. Radiographic and clinical examination may show duplication or absence of the medial rays (**Figure 3**). The degree of tibial deficiency does not correlate with the degree of foot abnormality.[5] Dissection studies[4,5,16] have further defined the various anomalies. The investigators found that nearly all of the patients had subtalar coalitions, as well as various other midfoot and hindfoot coalitions. The cuboid was larger than normal. The talus was elongated, and its joint surfaces were in abnormal sagittal

alignment. These dissection studies found abnormal muscle and tendon development. Vascular anomalies are common, and they have been defined as being similar to the embryonic vascular structure of the distal limb with a prominent two-vessel system.[17]

Although foot anomalies are not incorporated into the classification schemes for tibial deformities, they are important in clinical practice for prognosis and determination of appropriate surgery. The more deformed the foot, the more likely amputation is the appropriate surgical option. Nearly normal or normal feet are an indication for reconstruction surgery. Knowledge of abnormal vasculature may be beneficial in determining surgical flap or reconstruction options. Miller and Armstrong[16] advocate the use of arteriography to help in this process.

Other Associated Anomalies

In addition to foot abnormalities, tibial deficiencies are frequently associated with other skeletal anomalies. A review of several of the largest patient studies found that hip and hand abnormalities are the most common associated anomalies.[6,10,13,18] The most common hip abnormalities include developmental hip dysplasia, PFFD, coxa valga, and a congenitally shortened femur.[19,20] The most common hand anomalies include a lobster claw hand and thumb abnormalities.[7,21] Schoenecker et al[10] described a 21% incidence of spine abnormalities, including hypoplastic vertebra and hemivertebra, in their patient population. Visceral anomalies, including hypospadias, imperforate anus, cardiac abnormalities, hernia, cryptorchidism, and learning disabilities, also have been documented.[7,13]

There are two defined conditions involving tibial deficiency. Warner syndrome involves tibial dysplasia, triphalangeal thumbs, and prehallucal polydactyly. The second group of disorders involves tibial deficiency, split-hand

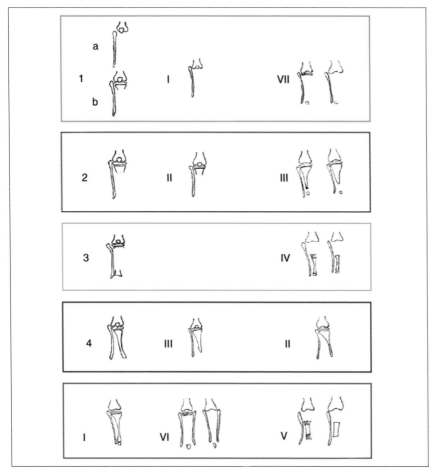

Figure 2   Illustration comparing the common characteristics of three classification systems (Jones, Kalamchi and Dawe, and Weber) for congenital longitudinal deficiencies of the tibia. Jones types 1a and 1b, Kalamchi and Dawe type I, and Weber type VII all demonstrate absence of the tibia (green box). Jones type 2, Kalamchi and Dawe type II, and Weber type III all demonstrate the presence of the proximal tibia with absence distally (red box). Jones type 3 and Weber type IV demonstrate the absence of the proximal tibia, with the distal tibia present (blue box). Jones type 4, Kalamchi and Dawe type III, and Weber type II demonstrate diastasis of the distal tibiofibular joint (purple box). Weber types I, VI, and V do not have any corresponding types in the other classification systems (pink box).

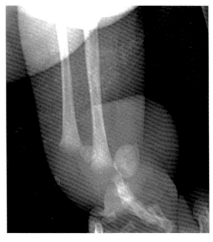

Figure 3   AP radiographs shows a tibial deficiency with an abnormal distal tibia and medial rays.

deformity, and femoral bifurcation or ulnar defects (also known as split hand/foot malformation with failure of long deficiency). Tibial deficiency has been identified as a rare component (not present in all patients) of various other syndromes, including Gollop-Wolfgang complex and Langer-Giedion syndrome.[22,23]

Etiology

The etiology of most tibial deficiencies is unknown, but several theories have been proposed in the literature. Given the skeletal and vascular anomalies found on dissection, some authors have suggested an embryologic incident in approximately the fifth gestational week.[2,12,17] In the early 20th century, tibial deficiency occurred in several patients who had been exposed to thalidomide in utero.[6]

Because of several case reports of similar congenital abnormalities in family members, some authors have suggested genetic transmission.[6,21,24,25] Clark[21] documented an autosomal dominant inheritance pattern with variable penetrance. Pashayan et al[25] documented a review of

several reports of family inheritance in a father and daughter, a father and son, and a father and daughter/daughter and daughter. McKay et al[24] documented an autosomal recessive inheritance pattern.

A single genetic mutation that leads specifically to tibial deficiency has yet to be identified. A *PITX1* gene mutation was implicated as being associated with various malformations of the lower limbs, including clubfoot, polydactyly, and tibial deficiency.[26] A genetic mutation at chromosome 17p13.3 has been implicated in split-hand/split-foot syndrome in patients with long bone deficiency syndrome. Cho et al[27] identified a 404 G>A mutation in the sonic hedgehog cis-regulator in patients with tibial hemimelia-polydactyly-triphalangeal thumb syndrome.

Surgical Planning

The goal of any surgical intervention for tibial deficiency is to obtain nearly normal knee function with as normal a gait as possible. Prior to proceeding with any surgical intervention, the patient must be thoroughly evaluated. The association of tibial deficiency with multiple syndromes has been well documented, and the involvement of any syndrome should be considered when planning surgery. Other limb anomalies, such as bilaterality, may play a role in the overall functional outcome of the patient. Tibial hemimelia can sometimes be associated with PFFD. In these patients, the treatment of PFFD takes precedence. In a patient who has a very short limb with no extensor mechanism associated with PFFD, consideration should be given to arthrodesis of the fibula to the femur in combination with a Syme ankle disarticulation to increase the lever arm of the femoral segment.

The foot must be considered in surgical planning. Anatomic variations in the foot may preclude limb salvage. Congenital anomalies, such as coalitions, instability, and missing rays, must all be considered. Universal recurrence of a deformed, rigid plantigrade foot and a substantial limb-length discrepancy at maturity can be problematic. Amputation and prosthetic fitting is usually the preferred treatment for substantial foot deformity.

The next management decision concerns the functionality of the knee. The most important deciding factor in the treatment of tibial deficiency is the presence of active knee extension,[5] which implies an adequate active quadriceps muscle. Quadriceps function is a prerequisite for a successful Brown procedure or any procedure other than a knee disarticulation. It may be possible to identify the extensor mechanism clinically, which is the preferred method. Other techniques, such as arthrography, direct surgical exploration, ultrasound, CT, or MRI (**Figure 4**), can be used but are rarely needed. The extensor mechanism should be considered inadequate or absent if a trained physical therapist and/or physician is unable to identify active knee extension after a careful examination.

Treatment Options

The classification system described by Jones et al[13] is used in the following discussion of treatment options for tibial deficiencies.

Jones Type 1a Deficiency

In a type 1a tibial deficiency, there is complete absence of the tibia seen on the radiograph taken at birth. In a type 1a deficiency, the infant's contracted limb is positioned proximal and lateral to the femoral condyles, with an absent patella but normally functioning hamstrings. The foot is in extreme varus and is nonfunctional. There is no extensor mechanism, which precludes the possibility for reconstruction.

Knee Disarticulation

Most patients with complete tibial hemimelia will require knee disarticulation. Loder and Herring[5] reported on functional outcomes in children treated with knee disarticulation and prosthetic fitting. Gait analysis showed nearly normal gait velocity (81%) and energy expenditure within normal range. Although their speed for a 50-yard dash was below the fifth percentile, an appropriate prosthesis allowed for both a stable knee and return to recreational sports.[5] In one study, approximately 17% of the patients returned to recreational skiing after a knee disarticulation.[14]

Knee disarticulation is usually indicated when the child begins to pull to stand. In some patients, surgery may be delayed past this milestone up to 1 year of age. This allows additional time for the parents to be convinced of the nonfunctionality of the limb and the need for amputation.

A knee disarticulation is performed using a long curved transverse incision, with the anterior flap larger than the posterior flap. The dressing, with or without a plaster shell, must be secured with suspension above the pelvis. Compression garments can be used to control swelling for 2 to 3 weeks postoperatively, followed by prosthetic fitting. Some patients may require epiphysiodesis later in life to accommodate prosthetic componentry and achieve symmetric knee levels.

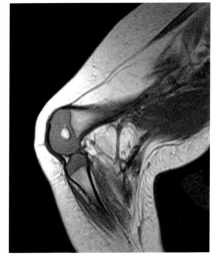

Figure 4 Sagittal MRI of the lower limb of a child with tibial deficiency shows absence of an extensor mechanism.

Brown Procedure

Centralization of the fibula (Brown procedure) combined with a Syme ankle disarticulation has been mentioned often in reference to type 1 tibial deficiencies. This procedure is likely successful only in patients with a type 1b deficiency because the complete lack of an extensor mechanism (as in a type 1a deficiency) is said to be a contraindication. This procedure is distinct from synostosis of the fibula to the tibia. Apparently, although not observed by Brown and Pohnert,[28] there are tibial deficiencies in which the extensor mechanism occasionally will insert into the fibula. This would make the Brown procedure a more viable option.

A lack of the proximal portion of the tibia is associated with a lack of an extension mechanism across the knee. Failure of the Brown procedure has resulted from the unopposed action of the hamstrings across the knee joint, which leads to flexion contracture and difficult (if not impossible) prosthetic fitting. In most patients, the Brown procedure results in less functionality because of recurrent knee flexion contractures.

The family of the patient should be fully counseled before a Brown procedure is performed because of the high failure rates and probability of an eventual knee disarticulation. Although early studies reported successful outcomes, many surgeons have been unable to be reproduce those outcomes.

The Brown procedure attempts to produce a limb with a useful knee segment.[11] The procedure entails transposing the fibula into the intercondylar notch. This allows the fibula to undergo hypertrophy and become a tibia-like structure, resulting in adequate knee function. A successful procedure can produce a proprioceptive knee with active knee extension and flexion. Although the procedure was described by Myers[1] and by Sulamaa and Ryoeppy,[29] it was popularized by Brown[11] after he published a case series of three patients with tibial deficiencies.

Key points in performing a Brown procedure include shortening the femur, remodeling the upper fibula, and creating a long posterior flap for the Syme ankle disarticulation to avoid wound closure problems if an attempt is made to preserve the foot. A longitudinal incision is made along the lateral border of the quadriceps. The absence of the tibial remnant, which should have been determined preoperatively with MRI, should be confirmed. If a tibial remnant is present, transfer should be delayed until the segment is ossified. If the tibial remnant is absent, the surgeon can proceed with the fibular transfer. The epiphysis is dissected and half of its attachment to the soft tissue is maintained to preserve the epiphyseal blood supply. The proximal fibula is cut with a knife to fit into the condylar notch area of the femur. Muscle balance is established and immobilizaton is provided in a reduced and extended position.

Based on outcomes, it is unclear if results of the Brown procedure justify its use. Loder and Herring[5] reported poor results in 53 of 55 patients who were treated with fibular transfer for congenital absence of the tibia. Although the Brown procedure invariably results in

varus and valgus instability, this does not usually pose a substantial problem because it can easily be corrected with a prosthesis. However, the progressive development of flexion contractures is a complication that cannot be accommodated with a prosthesis. Flexion contractures are unremitting because of the unopposed hamstrings, and they frequently lead to the need for knee disarticulation. Attempted preservation of the foot also is controversial. An unstable ankle results in the permanent use of a brace, unless an arthrodesis is performed. Despite the aforementioned controversies, Simmons et al[30] reported that patients were satisfied with the results of their Brown procedure based on the patients' own objective assessment of their daily functioning.

Jones Types 1b and 2 Deficiencies

In patients with type 1b and 2 tibial deficiencies, the proximal tibia is present but the distal portion is absent. Importantly, the hamstrings and quadriceps are both present and function normally. Unlike patients with a type 1a deficiency, these patients typically have instability and problems occur distally. The foot is in varus and is displaced medially. In infants, the proximal tibia may not be initially apparent at birth and may be cartilaginous.

Although fusion of the fibula to the tibia may result in excellent outcomes, if the proximal tibial segment has not ossified (is still cartilaginous), surgery should be delayed until ossification occurs. This will facilitate fusion between the fibula and the tibia. After fibular tibial synostosis is performed, a Syme ankle disarticulation can be done at 1 year of age, followed by prosthetic fitting (**Figure 5**). This primary reconstruction of the proximal tibial remnant via fusion to the fibula by translation to the more medial position is the favored procedure of the authors of this chapter. A Syme ankle disarticulation is typically needed because of ankle instability. Salvage of

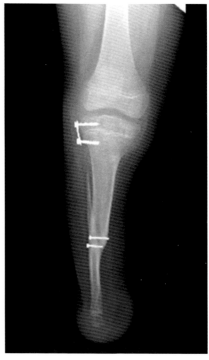

Figure 5 AP radiograph of child with a Jones type 2 tibial deficiency who was treated with synostosis of the fibula to the tibial remnant and a Syme ankle disarticulation.

the deformed foot will lead to a rigid nonfunctional foot, whereas ankle disarticulation will allow a prosthesis to be fitted so that patients can participate in normal activities.

The fibular centralization procedure can be performed by end-on-end fusion of the tibia to the fibula, followed by fixation with a medullary rod or by side-to-side fusion with screw fixation and cast immobilization to maintain alignment. In both techniques, removal of the proximal fibula should be considered to avoid prosthetic fitting difficulties and allow more mobility of the fibula. This will lead to more appropriate mechanical alignment under the tibial remnant.

Jones Type 3 Deficiency

In patients with a type 3 tibial deficiency, the knee is unstable and the tibial remnant is present distally. The patient typically has good quadriceps function and a very small proximal tibial remnant. A unique amorphous osseous structure develops characteristics of the distal tibial shaft. Distinction must be made between patients with a type 3 tibial deficiency and those with a short tibia and a varus foot.[17] In patients with a short tibia, the full tibia is present and clearly seen on radiographs. Depending on the anatomy of the ankle, some patients may be considered candidates for tibial lengthening. With tibial lengthening, however, there tends to be severe varus deformity of the limb. Type 3 tibial deficiency is rare, and few studies have been published. Based on the limited available data, patients achieve good function after a modified Syme ankle disarticulation or a Chopart amputation.[31]

Jones Type 4 Deficiency

In a type 4 tibial deficiency, diastasis of the distal tibia and fibula causes a severe rigid varus foot positioned between the fibula and tibia. Moderate limb shortening is present, and there is no articular surface of the tibiotalar joint. Care must be taken to differentiate this condition from clubfoot. The correct diagnosis of a type 4 deficiency may not be apparent until resistance to clubfoot correction is encountered. These patients are candidates for a Syme ankle disarticulation.

A functional articulation of the foot at the ankle joint is possible, but it is extremely rare. In some instances, an attempt to retain the foot is reasonable if the condition is less severe or if a contralateral deficiency is present. In either case, surgery should be delayed until the child has reached walking age. Some techniques of tibial lengthening and foot repositioning may permit a plantigrade foot to be retained;[32] however, this may be difficult because of talocalcaneal coalitions, deformities, and other congenital foot anomalies.

Reconstruction of the ankle may result in a limb-length discrepancy of greater than 8 cm. In a study of patients who had a type IV deficiency, 9 of 10 patients were treated with ankle reconstruction, and the foot was retained.[10] However, 5 of those 9 patients eventually elected conversion to a Syme ankle disarticulation because of concerns regarding the resultant limb-length discrepancy and the magnitude of the lengthening required.

Summary

Congenital longitudinal deficiencies of the tibia can have various clinical and radiographic presentations. Regardless of the type of tibial deficiency, the characteristics of the patient, the psychological and financial effects on the patient and family, the need for multiple surgeries, and the possibility of eventual knee disarticulation should all be considered in the decision-making process before treatment begins. It is imperative that the family be fully informed about treatment options and expected outcomes.

References

1. Myers H: Congenital absence of the tibia: Transplantation of the head of the fibula. Arthrodesis at the ankle joint. *Am J Orthop Surg (Phila PA)* 1905;23(1):72-85.

2. Epps CH Jr, Tooms RE, Edholm CD, Kruger LM, Bryant DD III: Failure of centralization of the fibula for congenital longitudinal deficiency of the tibia. *J Bone Joint Surg Am* 1991;73(6):858-867.

3. Wehbé MA, Weinstein SL, Ponseti IV: Tibial agenesis. *J Pediatr Orthop* 1981;1(4):395-399.

4. Williams L, Wientroub S, Getty CJ, Pincott JR, Gordon I, Fixsen JA: Tibial dysplasia: A study of the anatomy. *J Bone Joint Surg Br* 1983;65(2):157-159.

5. Loder RT, Herring JA: Fibular transfer for congenital absence of the tibia: A reassessment. *J Pediatr Orthop* 1987;7(1):8-13.

6. Epps CH Jr, Schneider PL: Treatment of hemimelias of the lower extremity: Long-term results. *J Bone Joint Surg Am* 1989;71(2):273-277.

7. Kalamchi A, Dawe RV: Congenital deficiency of the tibia. *J Bone Joint Surg Br* 1985;67(4):581-584.

8. Brown FW: The Brown operation for total tibial hemimelia, in Aitken GT, ed: *Selected Lower-Limb Anomalies: Surgical and Prosthetics Management.* Washington, DC, National Academy of Sciences, 1971, p 20.

9. Centers for Disease Control and Prevention: Birth defects: Data and statistics. Available at: http://www.cdc.gov/ncbddd/birthdefects/data.html. Accessed September 1, 2015.

10. Schoenecker PL, Capelli AM, Millar EA, et al: Congenital longitudinal deficiency of the tibia. *J Bone Joint Surg Am* 1989;71(2):278-287.

11. Brown FW: Construction of a knee joint in congenital total absence of the tibia (paraxial hemimelia tibia): A preliminary report. *J Bone Joint Surg Am* 1965;47(4):695-704.

12. Frantz CH, O'Rahilly R: Congenital skeletal limb deficiencies. *J Bone Joint Surg Am* 1961;43(8):1202-1224.

13. Jones D, Barnes J, Lloyd-Roberts GC: Congenital aplasia and dysplasia of the tibia with intact fibula: Classification and management. *J Bone Joint Surg Br* 1978;60(1):31-39.

14. Christini D, Levy EJ, Facanha FA, Kumar SJ: Fibular transfer for congenital absence of the tibia. *J Pediatr Orthop* 1993;13(3):378-381.

15. Weber M: New classification and score for tibial hemimelia. *J Child Orthop* 2008;2(3):169-175.

16. Miller LS, Armstrong PF: The morbid anatomy of congenital deficiency of the tibia and its relevance to treatment. *Foot Ankle* 1992;13(7):396-399.

17. Hootnick DR, Levinsohn EM, Randall PA, Packard DS Jr: Vascular dysgenesis associated with skeletal dysplasia of the lower limb. *J Bone Joint Surg Am* 1980;62(7):1123-1129.

18. Aitken GT: Amputation as a treatment for certain lower-extremity congenital abnormalities. *J Bone Joint Surg Am* 1959;41(7):1267-1285.

19. Sedgwick WG, Schoenecker PL: Congenital diastasis of the ankle joint: Case report of a patient treated and followed to maturity. *J Bone Joint Surg Am* 1982;64(3):450-453.

20. Wolfgang GL: Complex congenital anomalies of the lower extremities: Femoral bifurcation, tibial hemimelia, and diastasis of the ankle. Case report and review of the literature. *J Bone Joint Surg Am* 1984;66(3):453-458.

21. Clark MW: Autosomal dominant inheritance of tibial meromelia: Report of a kindred. *J Bone Joint Surg Am* 1975;57(2):262-264.

22. van de Kamp JM, van der Smagt JJ, Bos CF, van Haeringen A, Hogendoorn PC, Breuning MH: Bifurcation of the femur with tibial agenesis and additional anomalies. *Am J Med Genet A* 2005;138(1):45-50.

23. Stevens CA, Moore CA: Tibial hemimelia in Langer-Giedion syndrome: Possible gene location for tibial hemimelia at 8q. *Am J Med Genet* 1999;85(4):409-412.

24. McKay M, Clarren SK, Zorn R: Isolated tibial hemimelia in sibs: An autosomal-recessive disorder? *Am J Med Genet* 1984;17(3):603-607.

25. Pashayan H, Fraser FC, McIntyre JM, Dunbar JS: Bilateral aplasia of the tibia, polydactyly and absent thumb in father and daughter. *J Bone Joint Surg Br* 1971;53(3):495-499.

26. Klopocki E, Kähler C, Foulds N, et al: Deletions in PITX1 cause a spectrum of lower-limb malformations including mirror-image polydactyly. *Eur J Hum Genet* 2012;20(6):705-708.

27. Cho TJ, Baek GH, Lee HR, Moon HJ, Yoo WJ, Choi IH: Tibial hemimelia-polydactyly-five-fingered hand syndrome associated with a 404 G>A mutation in a distant sonic hedgehog cis-regulator (ZRS): A case report. *J Pediatr Orthop B* 2013;22(3):219-221.

28. Brown FW, Pohnert WH: Construction of a knee joint in meromelia tibia (congenital absence of the tibia): A fifteen-year follow-up study. *J Bone Joint Surg Am* 1972;54(6):1333.

29. Sulamaa M, Ryoeppy S: Congenital absence of tibia. *Acta Orthop Scand* 1963;33(1-4):262-270.

30. Simmons ED Jr, Ginsburg GM, Hall JE: Brown's procedure for congenital absence of the tibia revisited. *J Pediatr Orthop* 1996;16(1):85-89.

31. Fernandez-Palazzi F, Bendahan J, Rivas S: Congenital deficiency of the tibia: A report on 22 cases. *J Pediatr Orthop B* 1998;7(4):298-302.

32. Blauth W, Hippe P: The surgical treatment of partial tibial deficiency and ankle diastasis. *Prosthet Orthot Int* 1991;15(2):127-130.

Chapter 75

Amputations Distal to the Knee: Pediatric Prosthetic Considerations

Ramona M. Okumura, BS, CP

Abstract

Specific prosthetic principles and considerations are applicable in managing pediatric amputations distal to the knee. The etiology of the amputation can affect socket modifications, alignment, and prescription considerations. Frequently, skeletal asymmetries associated with pediatric amputation and limb deficiency cause alignment challenges affecting standard prosthetic fitting procedures. It is also helpful to be familiar with the transition between component sizes to optimize the useful life of a prosthesis.

Keywords: ankle disarticulation; fibular deficiency; partial foot amputation; rotationplasty; tibial deficiency

Introduction

This chapter discusses amputations distal to the knee in pediatric patients. In the past, partial foot, transtibial, and ankle disarticulation amputations were referred to as below-knee amputations. Although this classification terminology has since been replaced by the International Organization for Standardization (ISO),[1] the term below-knee is helpful when broadly referring to various amputation levels distal to the knee. Pediatric limb deficiencies distal to the knee can result from congenital, traumatic, and disease-related causes. It is helpful to be familiar with the most common presentations along with prosthetic options for treating these patients.

Before the age of 4 years, a child is rapidly developing and changing, thus requiring unique prosthetic alignments and only simple components. By the age of 7 years, the typical prosthesis should couple high performance with increased durability to meet elevated activity levels while accommodating rapid skeletal growth. Children wear out prosthetic components much faster than do adults. This may mean that at the same time they are outgrowing cracked, broken, or otherwise damaged prosthetic feet, pylons, and sockets, they also require fitting with a new and larger prosthesis. The replacement of outgrown components can sometimes benefit from prior planning in selecting the original componentry because the attachment mechanisms of differently sized components may or may not be compatible.

As in adults with unilateral and bilateral limb loss distal to the knee, children with amputations at these levels can achieve very high function. Unlike children with unilateral upper limb loss, those with below-knee prostheses are likely to use them, even when fit is compromised by growth changes. If the lower limb prosthesis looks brand new, it is likely that it is not being used. A thorough evaluation is then indicated to determine problems with the fit or function of the device.

Alignment and Foot Function

As the infant learns to ambulate, the alignment of the prosthesis should match that of normal infant ambulation. Infant gait begins with the hips and knees flexed, the ankles dorsiflexed, and a wide base of support similar to an athlete's "ready" body position. This positioning allows the infant's hips, knees, and ankle joints to react in many directions before his or her center of mass falls outside the base of support. Although it appears that the foot is "toed out," when the rotational axis of the knee is considered, it should be recognized that the foot position is a result of the external rotation of the hip. The vertical reference line through the anteroposterior bisection of the socket at the knee falls closer to the midfoot of the prosthetic foot than in adult alignment because the knee is flexed and the ankle is dorsiflexed. Because the infant walks with more of a flatfoot loading response and rolls over the medial border of the foot in terminal stance, the foot itself, lacking heel-off, does not require dynamic response characteristics. Because the foot placement at loading response is variable, a simple soft foam foot will conform to the ground, aiding the child's balance and ambulation.

The preschool-age child adopts a more adult-like ambulation pattern, with a heel strike at loading response and a heel rise at terminal stance and preswing.[2] The alignment of both the

Neither Ms. Okumura nor any immediate family member has received anything of value from or has stock or stock options held in a commercial company or institution related directly or indirectly to the subject of this chapter.

anteroposterior and the mediolateral vertical reference lines is similar to adult alignment. The preschool-age child typically does not have a sophisticated, high-performance running gait, but a cushioned heel is still a necessary part of the prosthetic foot design.

After school-age children develop the ability to run and jump, they can benefit from a variety of available high-performance prosthetic foot designs. Such feet and ankles become available when the foot size reaches 15 cm (approximating a US size 8 shoe).

Despite their small mass, reduced moment arms, and the decreased associated forces, children place greater demands on components than the average adult. Accordingly, split-toed carbon feet are not typically available in pediatric sizes because they would not be durable enough to last for the projected lifespan of the component. However, because of decreased loading forces, the residual limbs of children have better tolerance of ground reaction forces than those of adults, and children can run and jump with less optimally designed components.

Gait Deviations and Skeletal Asymmetry

Pediatric limb absences from etiologies such as congenital limb deficiencies and traumatic or disease-related amputation frequently result in skeletal asymmetries in the length, rotation, and angulation of bony segments. Even if the original proportions of the bony segments maintain the same relationships during growth, the actual measured differences increase. For example, a 20% limb-length discrepancy in an infant's tibia translates to a small length differential during early childhood; however, assuming proportional growth, the measured difference in length becomes substantially larger when the child reaches full skeletal maturity. In these patients, some gait deviations found in adulthood can be traced back to pediatric skeletal origins.

In such patients, the normal skeletal reference points used in the prosthetic management of adult-onset amputation can cause incorrect length, alignment, and anatomic prosthesis loading. For example, when the ipsilateral lower limb segments are deficient, the hemipelvis may also become hypoplastic over the course of skeletal maturation. This may cause the iliac crest, the posterior superior iliac spine, or the trochanter to be a poor observational reference point for the overall length of the prosthesis. As in children with scoliosis, having good vertical compensation with a centered trunk and the head at midline during gait might be a more functional reference for determining the appropriate length for the prosthesis.

For the same reasons, when managing limb deficiencies distal to the knee, the length of the femur should be assessed to determine the extent to which any surgically guided growth procedures intended to correct for angulation deformities or other developmental anomalies may have shortened its overall length.

A common gait deviation in the transverse plane occurs when the lateral femoral condyle is hypoplastic. This is common in patients with fibular deficiencies. Because the knee joint axis is higher on the lateral side, increasing knee flexion causes the tibia to externally rotate. The foot can be seen traveling in an arc, with the heel migrating medially with increased swing flexion. As the knee maintains flexion during swing, the heel remains medial and may even strike the contralateral limb during midswing. In extension, the opposite occurs, causing the shin to rotate externally during preswing. In such patients, the toe-out of the prosthesis should be aligned to the least problematic orientation. Some children learn to modify their gait by adding compensatory internal or external rotation during the swing phase for more consistent foot tracking in the line of progression.

Because the transverse cross section of a pediatric, Syme-style ankle disarticulation–type socket is round, it tends to rotate about the limb. Patellar tendon–bearing brims are often added in these sockets to reduce the socket rotation caused by ground reaction forces. In contrast, because Boyd amputations provide bony shapes for transverse plane rotational control, patellar tendon–bearing brims may not be necessary for rotational control, but they may still be prescribed for proximal weight bearing or for management of the coronal plane ground reaction force moments.

In cases in which the knee axis is not parallel to the floor, such as in the presence of a hypoplastic femoral condyle as previously described, the patellar tendon–bearing brim will rotate in the transverse plane and can shear against the medial patella and lateral femoral condyle. The height and trim lines of the Boyd, Syme, and transtibial patellar tendon–bearing socket brims must be evaluated throughout the range of motion of the functional swing phase to ensure a comfortable fit.

A common transverse plane skeletal aberration occurs during skeletal growth of a limb with a fibular deficiency because the tibia tends to internally rotate so that the anterior distal tibia is rotated as much as 45° at skeletal maturity when referenced to the axis of knee rotation. The anterior bow of the proximal tibia is also somewhat internally rotated, although not as much as the distal end. For the adult with an ankle disarticulation caused by a congenital fibular deficiency, the socket modifications made to offload this anterior bow will most likely be more lateral to its apex.

Coronal plane gait deviations can result from limb-length discrepancies that accompany growth spurts. When the prosthesis becomes short, for the sake of efficiency, children with below-knee prostheses learn to shift their trunk laterally over the prosthesis. This reduces the socket stresses needed for the normal excursion of the center of mass through the prosthetic foot. For different reasons, children with longitudinal femoral deficiencies also often ambulate using this method. They have a compensated Trendelenburg gait arising from the inefficiency of the hip abductor mechanism in ipsilateral midstance. For these children, shifting the trunk shortens the acting moment arm of the hip abductors to keep the pelvis level. When fitting a prosthesis in patients with longitudinal femoral deficiencies, leveling the pelvis by increasing the overall length of the prosthesis may unroof the femoral head if the acetabulum has not fully developed. Lengthening the prosthesis adducts the femur relative to the pelvis and changes the vector loading in the acetabulum to femoral areas that may not have been loaded with an asymmetric pelvis. The change in hip joint loading that accompanies changes in the length of the prosthesis is more obvious in children with Aitken type A or B presentations[3] with a more acute femoral neck angle.

In contrast, for patients with knee valgus, which is common in longitudinal fibular deficiencies, lengthening the prosthesis increases the valgus load at the knee. In this instance, the foot inset needs to be evaluated to transfer the ground reaction force through the knee and try to equalize the mediolateral loads through the socket at the knee joint.

In the knee of a limb with a fibular deficiency, valgus increases during the last few degrees of extension. By increasing the socket flexion (or ankle dorsiflexion) from the adult standard of 5° to 10° while maintaining the sagittal orientation of the socket over the foot, the abducted orientation of the socket over the foot is reduced. Because gait deviations accompany excessive dorsiflexion, the patient must also learn to ambulate with more knee flexion at loading response. This results in a slightly shorter step length, but the trade-off for more

normal loads through the knee over a lifetime is beneficial.

Over time, because of the repetitive hip abduction loading of the limb, the residual limb below the knee can drift into substantial varus. This is best seen during a lateral varus thrust during single-limb support. Fortunately, clinical observations suggest that when a patient stabilizes his or her knee by contracting the thigh muscles, much of the lateral thrust is eliminated, and the adduction alignment is minimized. This method is preferable to alignment accommodations because the resultant progressive increases in the relative outset of the foot to reduce these varus moments become increasingly unsightly.

Traumatic Amputation Considerations

New prosthetic prescriptions for children with traumatic amputations distal to the knee are generally similar to adult treatment options. However, variations may occur during the process of skeletal maturation from normally expected growth as a consequence of trauma to the growth plates or because of overloading of the growth plates secondary to alignment.

Partial Foot Amputation

For the pediatric patient with a partial foot amputation, the ipsilateral limb may not grow as much over time as the contralateral limb; therefore, with skeletal maturation there may be an increasing limb-length discrepancy. This discrepancy should be accommodated at each prosthetic fitting. In patients with partial foot amputation resulting from pediatric etiologies, the overall length of the residual limb should be measured at each prosthetic fitting.

The plantar surface of the partial foot amputation is generally pressure tolerant in early childhood because of the minimal loading mass of the child's body. However, these pressures increase

exponentially with maturity because of increasing mass and biomechanical moments, without comparative increases in the plantar surface area for pressure distribution. In addition, during growth of the child, complications often arise that are similar to adult pathologies. For example, bone spurs may form on transected metatarsals or affected tarsals.

Boyd and Syme Procedures

In children fitted with a Boyd-level prosthesis, low-profile feet are generally available so that the overall length of the prosthesis is not too long compared with that of the contralateral limb. However, the use of extremely low-profile feet greatly reduces dynamic response and durability. Prosthetic advantages and disadvantages of the Boyd amputation level in children are similar to those experienced by adults. Fortunately, in children, surgically guided growth can shorten the limb during skeletal maturation to accommodate the use of higher-performance, more durable feet as the child grows taller. With a Boyd amputation, it is somewhat difficult to cosmetically hide the bulk and shape of the socket in the prosthesis.

Considerations for a Syme ankle disarticulation prosthesis are similar to those of a Boyd amputation prosthesis, except that the reduced bulk of the distal residual limb can be more easily hidden in the shape of the prosthesis and there is less required shortening of the limb with skeletal maturity and surgically guided growth. However, as with adult prescriptions, there is often a lack of good transverse plane rotational control in the socket, which necessitates a higher socket profile containing a patellar tendon–bearing brim.

Because many children with ankle disarticulations and Boyd amputations also have some knee valgus, the foot should be inset to preserve even weight bearing through the knee joint. However, in doing so, it is also biomechanically optimal to transfer the weight bearing proximally through the knee of the prosthesis rather than maintaining distal end bearing with an inset foot. End bearing over an inset foot will introduce a varus moment through the knee, more so than a more axial load through the knee with proximal weight bearing.

Transtibial Amputation

Because the transtibial level of amputation is commonly affected by appositional overgrowth, provisions should be made for distal socket lengthening in the event that this occurs early in the lifespan of the socket. Additional pads of varying hardnesses can be applied distal to the gel liner or inside the socket liner using molded distal end pads. During the rapid growing years of the child, overgrowth can occur more than once a year, so pads can substantially reduce the lifetime cost of socket replacements. In addition, current techniques of distal soft-tissue suspension using pin-locking gel liners can apply traction on the distal soft tissue that can elongate the soft-tissue envelope and prolong the time before bony overgrowth penetrates through the skin. This strategy also increases the time before revision surgery is needed.

Although total surface bearing sockets have increased distal end pressure compared with proximal weight-bearing designs such as patellar tendon–bearing brims, the ability to lengthen the socket by removing pads allows the bone to fit in the longer soft-tissue envelope and extends the useful life of the socket. Alternatively, high socket brims, such as supracondylar designs, can accommodate longitudinal growth by allowing the limb to grow out of the socket. Padding can be added to the tibial flares for proximal weight bearing and rotational control and to allow space for distal growth or overgrowth. Other socket configurations that do not cause hammocking of the distal soft tissues can also increase the time between

revision surgeries necessitated by skin penetration of the bony overgrowth. For example, socket interfaces that reduce shear forces that cause skin traction, such as thin Surlyn (DuPont) linings in a traditional pelite insert, are helpful for reducing distal skin traction and hammocking leading to skin breakdown.

When the proximal tibial physis is unaffected by a traumatic injury, the limb continues to grow enough to provide an adequate functional limb length at skeletal maturity. Guided growth can be helpful when the limbs are exceptionally long and high-performance components will require additional clearance at skeletal maturity.

Traumatic injuries requiring transtibial amputations can often cause asymmetric injury to the proximal tibial physis. This can lead to angular growth of the tibial segment because the proximal tibia provides an average of 60% of the tibial growth or approximately 6 mm of the 1 cm in average overall growth per year. If one side of the tibial physis is fused in the original injury, the opposite side will contribute approximately 6 mm of annual growth at the angle of deformity. The associated socket loads at the distal end of the tibial deformity will progressively increase, and eventual socket accommodations will be needed. Additional adjustments may also be needed to the proximal brim opposite the fusion site to maintain limb comfort and prevent skin breakdown. If the socket is on an endoskeletal system, the socket alignment can also be adjusted to accommodate changes in the tibial femoral angle, along with translation of the foot to keep the weight line of the socket located through the foot both anteroposteriorly and mediolaterally.

If the angulation is severe and the anteroposterior and mediolateral alignment over the foot exacerbates compression on the side of the growth plate that needs expansion, the physis contribution of the compressed growth plate may be reduced because excessive compression

on the growth plate will hinder growth. When possible, alignment of the ground reaction force through the socket should be positioned to reduce this pressure by shifting the tilt of the foot or the socket.

If the tibia and fibula are connected by a bone bridge early in growth, the increased differential contribution of the proximal femoral growth plate causes the limb to drift into varus at skeletal maturity,[4] which often makes it difficult to achieve weight bearing against the medial tibial flare. When this occurs, it can be cosmetically difficult to hide the distal tibia in the limb shaping. It can also affect the ability to align the pins into the locking mechanism holes and may affect traction loads on the distal limb when using pin-locking liner suspensions.

Although the fibula does not provide critical function for the knee, it provides transverse plane rotational stability for a transtibial socket, especially for patellar tendon–bearing designs. When the fibula is absent because of traumatic injury, socket rotational control is problematic for the higher performance loading typically needed in children. Although the head of the fibula is intolerant to high axial, sagittal, and coronal plane loads, it has enough tolerance for the reduced torsion loads. However, children with complete fibular deficiency often have adequate tibial contours to assist with rotation stability in a socket.

Congenital Limb Presentations
Partial Foot Prostheses

Some syndromes such as Möbius syndrome are associated with transverse partial foot deficiencies. Longitudinal partial foot deficiencies are more commonly associated with fibular deficiency or ectrodactyly. Because fibular deficiencies also have associated hindfoot and tarsal anomalies that cause ankle instability, greater attention must be given to holding the hindfoot in a more neutral position with respect to inversion and eversion while accommodating the absent anatomy. The feet of children with ectrodactyly are often very wide, which makes it difficult to fit into ready-to-wear shoes. Because the tarsals are often coalesced and more stable in those with transverse deficiencies, adult-like prostheses can be prescribed.

Boyd and Ankle Disarticulation Prostheses

In children with congenital limb deficiencies, Boyd amputations and ankle disarticulations are usually performed to revise longitudinal fibular or tibial deficiencies. In infants and preschool-age children there is little space for prostheses, and low-profile feet, which have very limited dynamic response, are usually prescribed. By the time children require higher performance feet, there is generally enough clearance to the floor to fit some form of dynamic response foot to the socket.

Fibular Deficiency Prostheses

The residual limb of a child with a congenital fibular deficiency who is treated with an elective Boyd amputation or ankle disarticulation may have a tibial bow that provides some rotational socket stability; therefore, the proximal socket modifications that are often needed for those with traumatic etiologies are usually unnecessary. If a high socket brim is used for coronal plane stability and proximal weight bearing, care must be taken to evaluate the transverse rotation of the brim about the femoral condyles during swing flexion because of the tilted knee axis. Until guided growth alters the higher lateral knee flexion axis, both the socket and the foot will rotate beneath the femur during the swing phase into increased toe-out during flexion and will return to toe-in at full extension. Increasing the knee flexion or the foot dorsiflexion at the bench alignment should be considered to reduce knee valgus from the tilted knee axis. This technique maintains the distal end of the residual limb in more of an axial position and achieves improved cosmetic foot alignment when paired with good gait training. Dorsiflexion of the foot is associated with a shortened step length, but this is less disadvantageous than uneven loading to the knee joint if the foot is outset relative to the ground reaction force through the knee.

During skeletal growth, the tibia corkscrews internally so that the distal "anterior" tibia is often oriented 45° internally at skeletal maturity. When modifying areas of relief in the socket, attention should be given to the orientation of the bony prominences relative to the line of progression of the socket.

The distal insertions of the hamstrings can present as two separate medial and lateral insertions or can be one coalesced insertion at the middle of the posterior tibia. Relief modifications to the posterior socket should reflect these anatomic variations to optimize the height of the posterior proximal force couple for sagittal plane stability of the limb in the socket, ultimately protecting the anterior distal limb.

Because older children often need increased knee stability when the knee is flexed for running or jumping, they learn to contract their gastrocnemius muscle in the closed kinetic chain. This action can cause migration of the heel pad, which uncovers the anterior distal tibia and makes it very susceptible to high sagittal plane forces in loading response. Running is usually powered by the hamstrings and the gastrocnemius, which keep the knee in slight flexion and power gait from hip extension. This helps to pull the distal tibia away from the anterior socket. During limb evaluations, the clinician should palpate both the distal insertions of the hamstrings and the proximal insertion of the gastrocnemius when they are contracted to ensure appropriate reliefs for these tendons within the socket.

Tibial Deficiency Prostheses

The proximal fibula is positioned lateral to the tibia. If the proximal fibula is fused at the level of the distal tibia at the time of amputation for the purpose of fashioning the tibia into a longer Syme-type limb, the longitudinal growth of the fibula will occur proximally and laterally to the femoral condyle. Surgically guided growth management of the proximal fibular physis can be performed to prevent this aberrant proximal growth of the fibula and any associated socket modifications. In children with Boyd amputations or Syme ankle disarticulations, guided growth to shorten the residual limb will allow for fitting high-performance feet and achieving better cosmesis at skeletal maturity.

Longitudinal Femoral Deficiency Prostheses

Some children with longitudinal femoral deficiencies are treated with Boyd amputations or Syme ankle disarticulations. In those with Aitken type A and B deficiencies,[3] the femoral segment is often short. The relatively proximal location of the anatomic knee makes the below-knee prosthesis very long compared with the contralateral normal limb. Because of the femoral length discrepancy, there is ample space for dynamic feet. Because the sagittal moment arm over the foot when running is substantially longer than the normal moment arm for a child of a matching height and weight, the selected functional dynamic category of the foot should be higher than normal to obtain the expected spring loading. If the dynamics of the foot are properly selected, running and walking should not be problematic.

Sitting can be problematic because chair depth is symmetric and, because of the short thigh segment, the proximal location of the knee prevents the ipsilateral pelvis from touching the back of the chair. Thus, the child's trunk is always rotated in the chair. If the child's knee must flex past 90° for the foot to lay flat on the floor, the posterior trim line of the socket may need to be lowered to accommodate this flexion, without forcing the limb to migrate out of the socket when using typical distal suspension. Because the knee is much higher off the floor than the sound-side knee, the distal loading of the leg during sitting is mainly concentrated on the child's ipsilateral buttock.

Rotationplasty Prostheses

Children with Aitken type C and D longitudinal femoral deficiencies are challenging to fit with a prosthesis. By surgically rotating the lower limb segment with the ankle at the height of the contralateral knee, rotationplasty can fashion an anatomic segment that functions as a knee joint, with the foot acting as the "transtibial" limb segment. However, there is still no direct bony connection between the foot and the pelvis. Because the individual's body weight ultimately needs to be transferred through the pelvis and the prosthesis to the ground, the proximal prosthesis should be shaped similar to an ischial weight-bearing transfemoral socket brim. The prosthesis should be similar to a transtibial socket, with side joints and a molded thigh corset. Management of the proximal brim is the same as that used for a transfemoral prosthesis, except that the thigh segment is not a closed volume, so an ischial seat is necessary to transfer the ground reaction force through the prosthesis to the pelvis. Contact along the hip extensor muscles is necessary to transfer hip extension power to the socket. In particular, the hamstrings muscles are traveling horizontally and laterally to the anatomic knee, and their path should be reflected in the socket shape.

It is commonly believed that it is appropriate to place 50% of the weight-bearing forces in the distal socket and 50% at the brim. However, this strategy is biomechanically inefficient. If the ground reaction force of the prosthesis is partially end bearing, the prosthesis will shorten in stance as weight is transferred through the foot, tibia, and residual femur until the soft tissue connecting the femur to the pelvis is compressed and the socket contacts the pelvis. During the swing phase of gait, the weight of the prosthesis will stretch the soft tissues of the hip, and the length of the affected limb/prosthesis will increase, making it difficult to clear the floor in swing. Because this strategy has been used to manage weight bearing, patients typically are fitted with an intentionally shortened prosthesis, which results in poor prosthetic gait. To correct this problem, one solution is to have the patient's weight borne at the proximal brim at the pelvis, allowing the rotated anatomic foot and ankle complex to be used for cadence control and the replication of flexion and extension of knee function with minimal weight bearing. Although this type of prosthesis is designated as a transtibial prosthesis for billing purposes, the alignment of the hip, knee, and foot is the same as used for transfemoral function, with consideration of the trochanter-knee-ankle line to ensure that the knee axis is stable and the foot is appropriately under the center of mass.

The rotated foot is molded with the residual limb in maximum plantar flexion to match the ankle angle in the stance phase. Ankle stability after rotationplasty can be a concern. For example, when a femoral deficiency is accompanied by a fibular deficiency, the ankle mortise will have limited stability. In addition, a plantarflexed ankle is much less stable than an ankle in a dorsiflexed, close-packed position where the joint surfaces have their greatest congruency. However, even in a close-packed position, the ankle of a limb with a fibular deficiency is unstable in the coronal plane and poorly suited for weight bearing.

Management of the prosthetic knee axis can be problematic because, during growth, the surgically rotated foot segment often derotates, causing the knee flexion axis to lose its perpendicular orientation to the line of progression. In such cases, knee flexion at heel-off will introduce aberrant rotation into the swing phase. When the anatomic axis of the ankle is excessively externally rotated, the heel can catch on the sound-side limb during midswing.

Because the orientation of the residual hip musculature causes the thigh segment to internally rotate with hip flexion, the proximal socket will also rotate unless rotational control is designed into the socket shape using transfemoral socket techniques. Having good rotational control built into the proximal pelvic socket brim and using an auxiliary nonelastic Silesian belt will assist in maintaining the alignment of the knee axis. This will minimize unwanted transverse plane rotation through the unstable ankle joint.

The range of motion necessary to have a fully functioning knee joint for both ambulation and sitting is larger than the typical ankle range of motion. Although most of the necessary motion can come from the ankle joint, some additional motion comes from the forefoot. Also, the normal ankle hindfoot axis moves in a conical track. There are not many prosthetic sidebar knee joints that can track with the foot through this large range of motion. Fortunately, extreme flexion of the rotationplasty prosthesis primarily occurs in the non–weight-bearing conditions of the swing phase around a hypermobile, fibular-deficient ball-and-socket ankle joint. However, if the foot is used for power transference when ascending stairs in a step-over-step manner, the foot will migrate in the socket as the anatomic axis shifts to the axis of the mechanical knee joint. This can cause skin problems or possible internal bony wear and tear over time.

The foot and ankle must fit through the narrow ankle shape of the prosthesis. The prosthetist may be tempted to make the posterior socket section with soft material to protect the tibial crest and dorsum of the foot from the loads of the prosthesis; however, the three-point pressure system that controls knee extension must transfer forces to these areas, and this transfer must not be affected by compliance of the socket.

Suspension of the prosthesis can be accomplished with a heel strap. Frequently, using a nonelastic Silesian belt for secondary suspension can aid in achieving coronal and transverse plane stability of the prosthesis because of the lack of a hip abduction mechanism.

When growth adjustments are made to the prosthesis to accommodate the increasing length of the tibial segment, the ischial seat must be raised so that pelvic weight bearing on the prosthesis can be maintained. This can be achieved by moving the thigh section more proximally on the side joints or padding the ischial seat. After ischial weight bearing is corrected, the balance of the overall prosthesis length can be increased in the shin segment.

Moseley Prosthesis

The Moseley prosthesis, which is more commonly used in the Netherlands than in the United States, places the foot and ankle at the height of the knee without surgically rotating the foot. It is constructed in a similar manner to the rotationplasty prosthesis. Cosmesis is the major problem with this prosthesis because the foot is in neutral or slightly dorsiflexed position when the prosthetic knee is in full extension. Because the foot is in dorsiflexion during stance phase, it has a more stable hindfoot than that observed in the plantarflexed rotationplasty limb. If the femoral deficiency is accompanied by a fibular deficiency, additional care should be taken in molding the foot socket for ankle support because a domed talus is often present. Because active dorsiflexion powers prosthetic knee extension, it may not be possible to actively ascend stairs as can be done a with rotationplasty prosthesis. In other respects, the fit and function of the Moseley prosthesis is similar to a rotationplasty prosthesis. Suspension of the prosthesis can be achieved with an instep strap. The addition of a non-elastic Silesian belt will assist in coronal and transverse plane control as well as provide auxiliary suspension.

There are only two sidebar knee joints that track well with the foot and ankle motion through the entire range of knee flexion necessary for good prosthetic function. The knee joints of the Townsend Rebel series (Townsend Design) are fabricated with stainless steel and, although rather large, can track well with ankle and forefoot motion. In addition, the polycentric Hyperextension Knee Orthosis joint (SureStep) is also available, but is suitable only for patients weighing less than 100 lb (45.36 kg).

Limb Salvage Rotationplasty Prostheses

In children with cancer, limb salvage using Van Nes rotationplasty is usually performed in the first two decades of life before skeletal maturity. The prostheses for patients undergoing these procedures resemble transtibial prostheses with side joints and a thigh corset.

Unlike children with longitudinal femoral deficiency, these children have good hip joints and can fully bear weight through their foot segment. They can also use their active muscle power to ascend stairs in a step-over-step fashion and can function at a much higher level than children with congenital femoral anomalies. To have the necessary range of motion for knee function and cosmesis, the ankle is positioned in maximum plantar flexion when the prosthesis is in full extension. Usually, the outside hinges on these prostheses do not track well with the motion of the foot and ankle through the necessary range of motion because they are subjected to heavy loads. As a result, the foot either migrates in the socket or the tarsals are loaded in ways that the foot is not normally used, potentially leading to joint degeneration over time. Because these children have good hip joints, a simple corset on the thigh can provide some weight bearing and coronal plane stability for the ankle joint.

Good cosmesis is a major challenge with this type of prosthesis because the primary growth plates of the femur and tibia are at the knee, with the distal femur and proximal tibia contributing an average of 70% and 60%, respectively, of segmental growth. The thigh length should be substantially longer after surgery to allow the sound-side femur to catch up with the newly made ipsilateral thigh segment. The short shin will have a faster swing time than the longer sound-side shin because of the short length of the pendulum. However, because the ankle can actively control the timing of the foot, the problems associated with the shorter shins of knee disarticulation prostheses are not observed in this population. As these children grow and cancer treatment is completed, the distance between the residual foot and the floor typically allows for the use of high performance feet. Other than these considerations, these prostheses can be fitted as previously described for other rotationplasty prostheses.

Considerations for Component Choice

As with components for adults, attention needs to be paid to height and weight tolerances when selecting components. The main complications occur when prostheses must be adjusted for the child's growth.

Below-knee prostheses for children have an average useable life of 9 to 18 months, and they sometimes can be used for much longer periods.

The socket materials should be locally adjustable over bony prominences for growth. Acrylic resins have thermoplastic properties. If the reinforcing materials (such as knits) used over bony areas can be stretched, the sockets can be heated and stretched to accommodate growth.

Because children often play in water or other wet environments, the aluminum used in their prosthetic components can corrode, causing stress risers in the form of tiny cracks. When carbon materials are used adjacent to unanodized aluminum, an electrolytic process occurs when wet, which further corrodes connections. Titanium is less corrosive, but it is brittle and notch sensitive. Tube clamps made of titanium should not be overtightened because they are especially prone to cracking. Stainless steel components, although much heavier, are more durable and less likely to sustain catastrophic failure than titanium components. Similarly, if wood exoskeletal ankle blocks are needed, hard oak or maple is more water tolerant than traditional, softer poplar blocks. Durable materials should be used in prosthetic devices for children, and the prostheses should be monitored for damage at the child's regular checkups.

When smaller components, such as feet and pylons, require replacement because of the child's growth, attention must be given to the prosthesis connectors. Endoskeleton foot adapters are available, as well as different size pylons, depending on the weight of the child.

Prosthetic feet do not all have the same heel height built into the sole. Most pediatric feet have a 6 mm heel height, which is common to children's athletic shoes. However, when the child's shoe size transitions to more adult sizes at 22 cm, the heel height changes to 1 cm. The commonly used Seattle LightFoot (Trulife) offers several other heel height options depending on the shoe size.

When moving from a pediatric-sized prosthetic foot to an adult-sized foot for a heavier child without making a new prosthesis, the initial pediatric foot can be fitted with an adult-sized pyramid and a 30-mm pylon system by using an 8-mm bolt solid ankle cushion heel foot adapter and later switching to a 10-mm pyramid. If the child is quite small in stature, an adult-sized pyramid receiver on a 22-mm pylon can be fitted on the adult foot and pyramid until an adult pylon system is appropriate.

In special instances, manufacturers may be willing to customize pediatric components for special uses, such as custom-made feet that can function well for running but also can be used for normal ambulation.

Summary

A child with amputation or congenital limb loss distal to the knee can function well with prostheses designed according to principles appropriate for the child's age and activity level. When possible, prostheses for children should be designed with options that allow for their rapid growth to extend the life of the prosthesis before a replacement is needed. The prosthesis should be durable. Sockets should be designed to transfer the high ground reaction loads in all three planes through the prosthesis. When a child is very small, pediatric-sized socket interfaces are available and have some options that are similar to those available for adults. As the child's growth stabilizes in his or her later teen years, adult component options can be used to allow comfortable participation a wide range of chosen activities.

References

1. International Organization for Standardization: *IS 8548-1: Prosthetics and Orthotics. Limb Deficiencies: Part 1. Method of Describing Limb Deficiencies Present at Birth.* Geneva, Switzerland, International Organization for Standardization, 1989, pp 1-6.

2. Sutherland D: The development of mature gait. *Gait Posture* 1997;6:163-170.

3. Aitken GT: Proximal femoral focal deficiency: Definition, classification, and management, in Aitken GT, ed: *Proximal Femoral Focal Deficiency: A Congenital Anomaly.* Washington, DC, National Academy of Sciences, 1969, pp 1-22.

4. Blount WP: *Fractures in Children.* Baltimore, MD, Williams & Wilkins, 1955.

Chapter 76

Congenital Deficiencies of the Femur

Ian P. Torode, MD, FRACS

Abstract

To appropriately manage a child with a limb deficiency, it is first necessary to understand the natural history of the condition and the associated functional implications. It also is important to be able to adequately communicate important findings to the child's parents and family members. Some children can be managed with a simple procedure, whereas others will require a number of major reconstructive surgeries to achieve optimal function. Because treatment may extend over many of the childhood years, the support of the family is essential to achieve the best outcome for the child.

Keywords: amputation; femur; femur absence; deficiency; deformity; reconstruction; rotationplasty.

Introduction

Although the femur is the largest skeletal component in the lower limb, congenital deficiencies of the femur must be considered along with the associated anomalies that frequently coexist in the lower segments of the limb. The functional compromise that can arise from a more distal deficiency may play an important role in the plan for managing a femoral deficiency. The relationship between deficiencies of the fibula and tibia are briefly discussed in this chapter as they relate to femoral deficiencies. The diagnosis, management, and treatment of femoral deficiencies from the antenatal period to maturity also are addressed. The terms congenital short femur and proximal femoral focal deficiency (PFFD) are used because they adequately differentiate the extremes of longitudinal deficiencies, particularly regarding management.

Etiology

Congenital deficiencies of the femur differ from other typical skeletal anomalies in the extent of the variations and the lack of a definite inheritance pattern. For example, although tibial hemimelia varies in the degree of the deficiency, an autosomal dominant inheritance is common. In contrast, in congenital below-elbow deficiencies, the degree of the clinical presentation has little variation, and most of these deficiencies have a similar appearance to each other, although there is no inheritance pattern.

Thalidomide can produce lower limb deficiencies, but the deficiencies typically have a phocomelic pattern. A causative teratogenic agent for the typical deficiency has not been identified. Femoral facial syndrome is an exception to the sporadic inheritance pattern.[1] Femoral hypoplasia is also seen in the rare Goltz syndrome, which is associated with a gene mutation on the X chromosome[2] (**Figure 1**).

Presentations

Congenital deficiencies of the femur have essentially three modes of presentation for orthopaedic management. These modes are a prenatal presentation, which is detected by an ultrasound

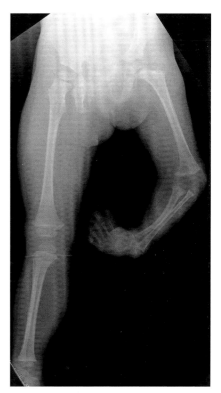

Figure 1   Radiograph of the lower limbs of a female infant with Goltz syndrome demonstrates the hypoplastic left lower limb.

examination; initial detection at the time of birth; and later referral of an older child who had not been evaluated earlier because of some extenuating circumstance, such as residence in a remote area without access to a surgeon with expertise in managing limb deficiencies.

Prenatal Presentation

In developed countries, many pregnant women have an ultrasound examination during pregnancy. Because the first ultrasound examination performed at approximately 12 weeks' gestation may be cursory and done only for pregnancy confirmation, a substantial number of

---

Dr. Torode is deceased. At the time this chapter was written, Dr. Torode or an immediate family member served as an unpaid consultant to Medtronic Sofamor Danek.

skeletal limb deficiencies may be overlooked. Limb deficiencies may not be detected until the 20-week ultrasound examination, which may present an issue if pregnancy termination is a consideration.[3] The orthopaedic surgeon may be asked to provide advice on the likely extent and natural history of a detected limb deficiency (**Figure 2**).

The surgeon should be able to reasonably differentiate between a congenitally short femur and a true PFFD. In cases in which the available information does not allow a definite opinion, some reassurance of a favorable outcome may still be possible and will help to decrease the parents' distress and guilt during the remainder of the pregnancy.

Postnatal Presentation

Ideally, the newborn will be treated by the same surgeon who provided prenatal advice. This continuity of care prevents the dissemination of well-intentioned but often erroneous information given by family members and the nursing staff, most of whom are unfamiliar with such an abnormality. If a diagnosis has not been made before birth, the pediatrician will refer the infant to a surgeon for care; the treating surgeon should address any misinformation received by the infant's family and offer reassurance. The family will want to know if the child will walk. In infants with a true PFFD, the surgeon can often offer reassurance that the child will walk, even if a prosthesis may be needed (**Figure 3**).

Delayed Presentation

In some instances, there may be a delay in the child being seen for treatment. If an older child is referred for treatment, the surgeon may need to allocate considerable time to explain the child's condition and review treatment options with the parents.

Classification Systems

The numerous classification systems for congenital femoral deficiencies suggest

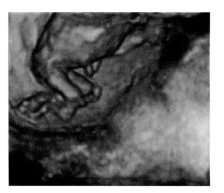

Figure 2   Prenatal ultrasound image shows a bowed and short tibia, a foot in valgus, and a slightly short but intact femur. After birth, the child will be best managed with foot ablation (usually in the second year of life when the child wants to walk to explore his or her world) and prosthetic fitting.

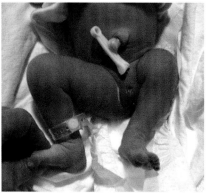

Figure 3   Photograph of a newborn female with a very short left femur, with a good foot and normal-appearing leg.

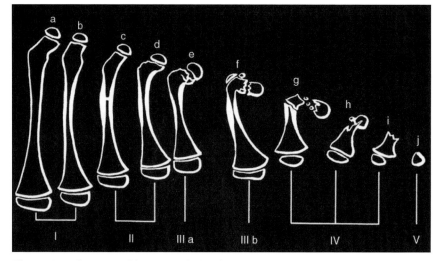

Figure 4   Illustration of the Hamanishi classification system for femoral deficiency. This system demonstrates the large number of variations that may be present, ranging from a virtually normal femur (a) to a vestigial bone (j).

that no single system is satisfactory for all patients. The Hamanishi[4] classification system demonstrates that there are many radiologic appearances and degrees of severity in congenital femoral deficiencies (**Figure 4**). Gillespie and Torode[5] categorized congenital longitudinal femoral abnormalities into two major groups. At the moderate end of the severity scale is the congenital short femur, and at the more extreme end is the true PFFD. Later, Gillespie revised the classification system by adding a third group that consisted of children

with a very short femoral residual limb, which is often fused to the tibia.[6] In this group, no intervention around the knee is necessary (**Figure 5**). The revised Gillespie classification system is useful in formulating a treatment plan and is readily understood by parents. In most instances, the classification system helps the surgeon determine if reconstruction or prosthetic assistance would be the most appropriate course of treatment. It is important that the distal components of the limb also be considered when formulating a treatment plan.

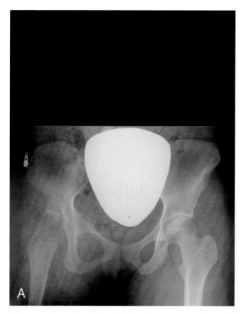
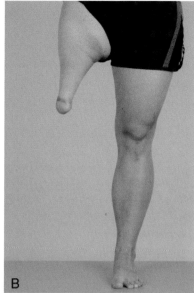
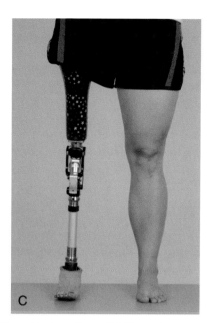

Figure 5   Images of a female patient with a Gillespie type 3 femoral deficiency. **A,** Radiograph of the pelvis shows the vestigial femoral component. Clinical photographs of the deficient limb (**B**) and the patient wearing a prosthesis (**C**).

In children with an intermediate level of femoral abnormality, the Fixsen and Lloyd-Roberts[7] classification system is useful in making treatment decisions. If the proximal end of the femoral fragment is bulbous (the stable sign), the femoral head and neck will later ossify. In some patients, this later ossification will allow an apparent PFFD to be managed as a congenital short femur, with reconstruction rather than ablation (**Figure 6**).

The Aitken classification divides PFFDs into four types. Type A includes children with a radiographically abnormal proximal femur, with a pseudarthrosis that will ossify progressively with time and a varus femoral neck. These femora can be reconstructed. A type B deficiency is more severe, with a persistent defect between the femoral head in the acetabulum and the femoral shaft. These femora may be reconstructible. In type C deficiencies, just a small ossicle is present as the femoral head, and the femur has a spindle shape; however, there is no stability between the pelvis and limb. Attempts to reconstruct the proximal femur in these children are unlikely to be warranted. In type D

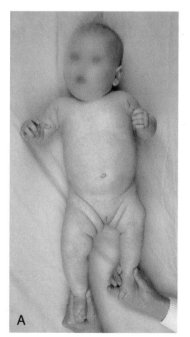
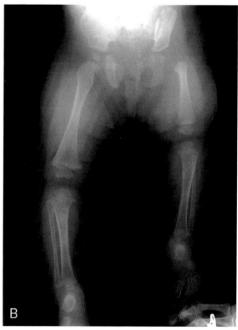

Figure 6   **A,** Photograph of a baby girl with a congenital short femur. Note the foot of the affected limb is at the midtibial level of the unaffected limb. **B,** Radiograph of the patient's lower limbs taken at 9 months of age.

deficiencies, the femur is rudimentary, and no proximal reconstruction should be attempted[8] (**Figure 7**).

The classification by Paley and Stannard[9] is useful for guiding surgical intervention and reconstruction, particularly

in patients with more severe proximal femoral and diaphyseal deficiencies. On one end of the severity spectrum, congenital femoral deficiency management involves treatment of a modest limb-length difference, and at the other

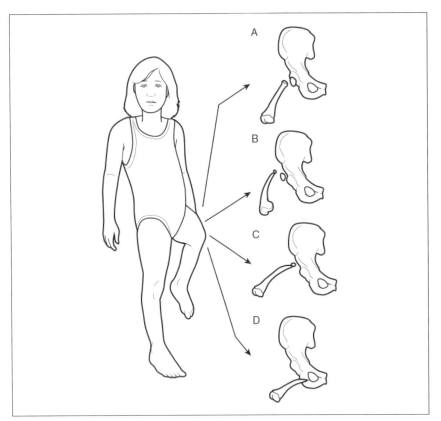

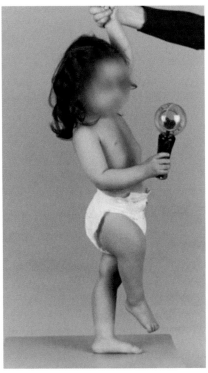

Figure 8   Standing lateral photograph of a girl with a congenital short right femur.

Figure 7   Illustration of the Aitken classification of femoral deficiency. **A,** In a type A deficiency, there is stability, with a bulbous proximal femur and a femoral head in the acetabulum. **B,** In a type B deficiency, the femur is more spindle shaped proximally, which implies a lack of connection between the ossified bone in the acetabulum and the femur. The lack of stability is accompanied by failure of ossification and the continued existence of motion between the femur and pelvis. **C,** In a type C deficiency, the femoral head is lacking, and the femur is less well developed. A tuft of ossification is seen at the proximal femur, but there is no articular relationship between the femur and acetabulum. The acetabular development is poor. **D,** In a type D deficiency, the femoral deficiency is severe, and there is no proximal tufting. The acetabular development is poor, the hip is unstable, and there is a marked limb-length discrepancy.

end is a gross limb discrepancy and the need for prosthetic assistance. Within this spectrum is a dividing line between patients who can be treated with limb reconstruction and those who are best treated with limb ablation and prosthetic fitting. Treatment decisions are influenced by the mores of the society in which the patient resides, the skill and experience of the surgeon, and the wishes of the family.

Clinical Examination
The patient will typically lie or stand with the affected limb in a position of flexion and external rotation. Examination of the hip may reveal telescoping,

which is a sign of a true PFFD and indicates a likely lack of integrity between the femoral shaft and the head and neck. In infants, the hip flexion deformity is often relatively fixed. It becomes less fixed in patients with a congenital short femur, whereas it remains fixed in patients with true PFFD. The affected knee will often demonstrate laxity in the AP plane of the joint. Paradoxically, the laxity is more obvious in patients with lesser degrees of limb shortening, because the contractures around the knee with the PFFD will often disguise the instability (**Figure 8**).

Below the knee, it is important to assess the degree of tibial and fibular

involvement. In milder cases, the degree of shortening may be minimal, but in more severe cases the tibia may be bowed, with a linear dimple over the midtibia. In the foot, the integrity of the ankle joint, the extent of tarsal coalitions, and the number of rays in the foot must be considered. Although the number of rays is readily apparent, it is often less important than the integrity of the ankle joint.

Radiographic Features
Plain radiographs will complement and clarify clinical findings. In an infant, a radiograph of the lower half of the patient's body will provide useful information. At the pelvic level, the acetabulum of the unaffected limb should be noted. Although most lower limb deficiencies are unilateral, some patients have bilateral involvement that is expressed as acetabular dysplasia, whereas others may have more marked bilateral involvement. On the involved side, acetabular dysplasia is common

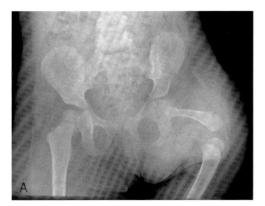 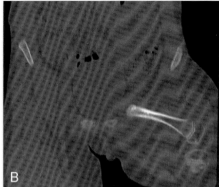 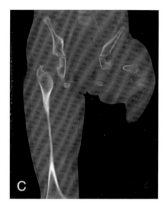

Figure 9   **A,** AP radiograph of the pelvis of a 3-year-old girl with marked femoral deficiency. Note the bulbous proximal femur. CT scans of the pelvis of the child at 8 years of age shows the femur lying anterior to the superior pubic ramus, with the proximal end adjacent to the bladder (**B**) and the ossified femoral head fused to the ischium (**C**).

and requires treatment.

In a patient with a milder level of congenital short femur, the femur will be short with a degree of midshaft sclerosis and an anterolateral bow. The proximal femur will be ossified, and there may be a varus deformity. The external rotational deformity and valgus of the distal femur will become more obvious over time. In patients with a higher level of congenital short femur, the femur will be shorter than in those with a milder deformity, will lack ossification proximally, and the proximal femur will be bulbous. The bulbous femur implies the presence of an unossified femoral head, which is supported by the presence of a reasonably well-formed acetabulum. Radiographic findings can be confirmed with ultrasound, but it is important to note that the varus of the femoral neck will make the unossified greater trochanter proud, and this can be interpreted as a congenital dislocation. The findings also can be confirmed with MRI. Although sedation may be required in infants, MRI may be performed if there is doubt about the diagnosis or confirmation is needed.

In children with a true PFFD, the femur is very short, the proximal end is poorly developed, and there is substantial involvement of the diaphysis. The acetabulum is shallow, and no ossification is seen in the acetabulum. The foot lies at the level of the contralateral knee.

Below the knee, the tibia and fibula can be variably involved. At the milder end of the severity spectrum, the tibia and fibula may appear equal in length or minimally shorter than each other, whereas at the more severe end of the spectrum, the fibula is absent and the tibia is short and bowed anteriorly. In these patients, the foot is in equinus and the talus is subluxated posterolaterally to the tibia.

As time passes, ossification continues and the outcome for an individual patient becomes clearer. Clinical findings and radiographic features will usually allow the surgeon to develop a working plan for the child so the family can understand the likely course of the disorder; however, accurate classification of a deficiency is difficult to determine in some children. For example, clinical findings suggested a true PFFD in a 3-year-old girl (**Figure 9**). Radiographic findings showed a bulbous proximal femur and a femoral head that was present but completely ossified to the ischium. The proximal femur was located anterior to the superior pubic ramus and posterior to the femoral neurovascular bundle.

Abnormality of the hip joint is a hallmark characteristic in these children, but true dislocation of a developed femoral head from the acetabulum is rare. For example, **Figure 10** shows a three-dimensional reconstruction of the hip of a child who appeared to have a dislocated femoral head, but the femoral head and neck were actually markedly underdeveloped. During an attempted open reduction of the femur, a complete lack of development of the pubic segment of the acetabulum was found; the proximal femur was returned to the presurgical articulation.

Treatment Planning

If the infant is examined by the surgeon in the first few weeks after birth, the parents should be reassured that the deficiency is not the mother's fault, there is no specific treatment necessary for the deficiency, no surgery will be necessary in the child's first year of life; and the deficiency will not prevent the child from crawling or pulling to a standing position. No special physiotherapy is required. The family should be reassured that the child will be able to walk. Parents should be informed if their child is a candidate for surgical reconstruction, with the goal of the child walking on his or her own feet, or whether the femoral or foot and ankle deficiency will necessitate a prosthesis for ambulation. A management plan should be formulated and discussed with the family early in the child's life. It is expected that these children will undergo several surgical procedures over their growing years, which can be a source of anxiety for the family. However, if the family is informed of the treatment plan and is aware of the serial steps, they will likely be involved in the process and experience less anxiety.

In patients with lesser degrees of femoral deficiency and a good foot and ankle, judicious use of epiphysiodesis and/or femoral lengthening should lead to satisfactory outcomes. In a child with a more severe deficiency, such as a typical congenital short femur with the foot at the midshaft level of the contralateral tibia, the expected limb-length discrepancy at maturity requiring accommodation is approximately 20 cm. Resolving such a discrepancy in a series of small surgical steps is less daunting and more readily achievable.

In a child with a good foot and ankle and a minor degree of tibial involvement, the management plan should include tibial lengthening (expected gain of 4 to 5 cm) in the preschool years, pelvic lengthening and correction of acetabular dysplasia using a modification of the Hall technique (expected gain of 2 cm),[10] and correction of the coxa vara (expected gain of 2 cm). Instead of lengthening the femur with a frame, an alternative plan is to wait and lengthen the femur with intramedullary nails using a pertrochanteric approach when the child is approximately 10 years of age (expected gain of 5 cm), coupled with a judicious contralateral epiphysiodesis (expected gain of approximately 3 cm), followed by a final femoral lengthening using a nail when the patient is a teenager. A guided-growth system can be used to correct valgus malalignment of the distal femur, and the rotational malalignment can be addressed at the time of femoral lengthening (**Figure 11**).

If the condition of the foot and ankle is poor and the tibia is bowed, a foot ablation (Syme amputation) and prosthetic fitting are indicated.[11,12] Knee valgus in later childhood can be managed with a transphyseal screw[13] (**Figure 12**). A guided-growth system using a plate can readily correct the valgus, but the presence of a plate and screws under the prosthesis may be problematic. Although children can generally tolerate a difference in knee heights and a prosthesis can readily cope with leg-length issues, a contralateral epiphysiodesis or a femoral lengthening should be

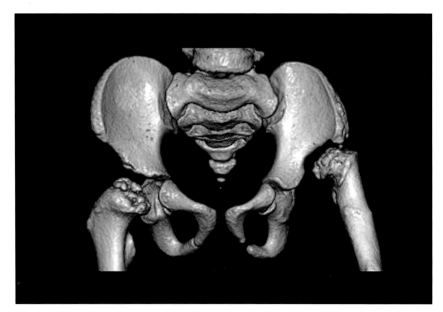

Figure 10   Three-dimensional CT scan of the pelvis of a child showing a deficient left femur articulating with a pseudoacetabulum that had been stable for 3 years.

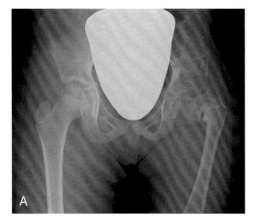
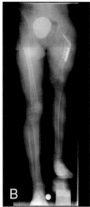
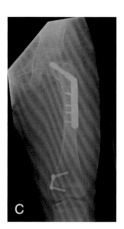
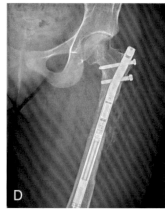

Figure 11   Radiographs of the patient shown in Figure 6. **A,** AP radiograph of the pelvis taken when the child was 9 years old. The shadow of the carbon fiber block used to lengthen the left hemipelvis can be seen. The femoral head and neck have ossified in varus. **B,** Standing radiograph of the legs and pelvis after correction of the coxa vara. **C,** Radiograph of the femur after correction of coxa vara. A guided-growth system using a plate is in place to treat the genu valgum. **D,** Radiograph of the left femur after lengthening using a PRECICE nail (Ellipse Technologies).

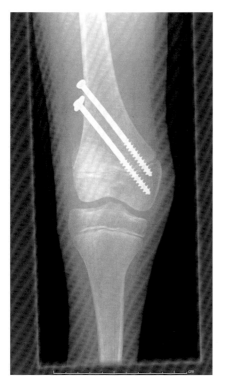

Figure 12 AP radiograph of the right knee of a boy with a congenital short femur who was treated with a foot ablation. Two screws were used to correct the genu valgum, although one screw will suffice.

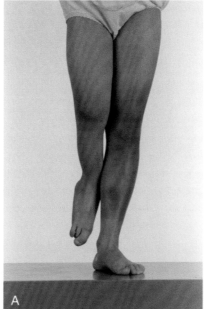

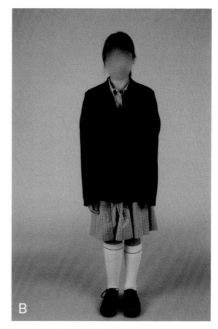

Figure 13 **A,** Photograph of the lower limbs of an 8-year-old girl after multiple surgical procedures had been performed on her hypoplastic right leg. The patient requested foot ablation rather than undergoing further attempts at limb reconstruction. **B,** Photograph of the patient after foot ablation and fitting with a prosthesis. The patient was very satisfied with the outcome.

considered for some patients.

In more severe cases, the femoral deficiency is the most obvious abnormality; however, the integrity of the foot and ankle requires early assessment. Experience has shown that attempts to salvage a marginally functioning foot will compromise long-term function. If the foot is saved, there is often great reluctance to undergo foot amputation until the child reaches his or her teenage years and becomes aware of the functional limitations of the saved foot (**Figure 13**).

Children with a poor foot and ankle and a femur that is not reconstructible may be best treated with foot ablation and knee fusion. This surgery can be done as soon as ossification around the knee is adequate. Patients with a tiny femur that is often already fused to the tibia (Gillespie group C) are included in this group. In this group, no knee fusion is needed.

Children with a good foot and ankle and a poor femur are candidates for rotationplasty. This procedure is done through the knee and combined with a knee fusion. If the child's parents do not want the child to be treated with a rotationplasty, the child should be treated with methods used for a patient with a poor foot.

In a child with a stable femur (albeit short) and a femoral head in the acetabulum, there is a role for delayed treatment and further investigation before committing the child and family to several surgical procedures, including at least two femoral lengthening procedures. In the child with a poor foot, the need for below-knee reconstruction and tibial lengthening can be avoided, and length can be attained by a prosthesis after foot ablation.[9]

Surgical Techniques
Foot Ablation

In patients requiring foot ablation, this chapter's author prefers to use a Syme amputation approach or ankle disarticulation. A Boyd amputation can be used, but the talus and os calcis are often fused and difficult to deliver distally. The Boyd procedure provides no functional gain in these patients. A useful adjunct is to divide the Achilles tendon through a small incision at approximately the junction of the middle and distal thirds of the leg. This allows a simpler delivery of the talus and calcaneus for the posterior capsular resection and removal of those bones for either a Syme or Boyd procedure. It should be noted that the tibial kyphosis commonly seen in children with more severe deficiencies should be corrected by a tibial osteotomy with internal fixation at the time of the foot ablation. Failure to do so may compromise long-term prosthetic fitting and comfort (**Figure 14**).

Knee Valgus

Knee valgus in a femoral deficiency is often overlooked. Previously, a distal femoral opening osteotomy with a fibular graft was advocated to gain some

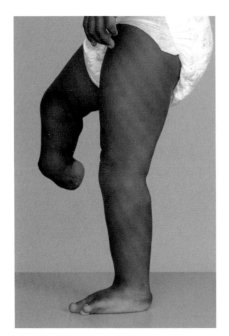

Figure 14 Clinical photograph of a young boy who was treated with a foot ablation but did not undergo correction of the tibial kyphosis. This deformity substantially compromises prosthetic fit and comfort.

length and stimulate growth. Although the outcome was usually satisfactory, correction with a staple, a plate, or a transphyseal screw is a much simpler procedure and can be done with same-day release from the hospital.[13,14] Use of a transphyseal screw in patients using a prosthesis avoids metal under the skin adjacent to the prosthesis. Correction of the genu valgum also needs to be done when a foot ablation has been performed. If correction is not done, the leg will often be aligned to the tibia, which will magnify knee valgus or, alternatively, the fitting should allow for a bulge in the lateral aspect of the prosthesis so that the prosthetic limb is correctly aligned to the patient. It is also necessary to appreciate that the genu valgum may disguise the external rotation deformity of the femur, which may require correction by osteotomy or derotation at the time of femoral lengthening.

Correction of Coxa Vara

In a patient with a completely ossified intact femur, the procedure to correct coxa vara is straightforward. In more complicated instances, particularly if there is an ossification defect (pseudarthrosis), coxa vara correction is more difficult and requires either a soft-tissue release or femoral shortening. Rather than compromise the soft-tissue integrity of muscle units, the author of this chapter prefers femoral shortening. It is necessary to adequately correct the coxa vara so the healing of the compromised bone of the proximal femur is not impaired because of poor biomechanics. In these patients, the use of bone morphogenetic protein has been advocated to stimulate ossification.[9]

Correction of Acetabular Dysplasia

Acetabular dysplasia is common in children with a congenital deficiency of the femur, but it may be overlooked on radiographic studies because the shorter limb may be abducted. If the hip subluxates during lengthening, it is very difficult to resolve the problem. It is better to overtreat children with acetabular dysplasia. A modification of the Hall innominate osteotomy has been used with consistent results.[10] This modified procedure uses iliac crest bone grafts and a carbon fiber insert to provide immediate stability because these grafts tend to collapse when used alone in small children with dysplasia and require protection in the spica cast. In the experience of this chapter's author, none of the children treated with this modified procedure had hip subluxation during subsequent femoral lengthening procedures.

Tibial Lengthening

A minor degree of tibial shortening is often present in children with femoral deficiency. Tibial lengthening of approximately 4 to 5 cm is readily achievable in these children during the preschool years. If there is any doubt about the stability of the foot and ankle, a calcaneal wire should be used. If a knee flexion contracture develops, a simple orthotic extension from the frame will suffice during the lengthening phase.

Knee Fusion

A knee fusion can be performed as soon as the ossification centers around the knee are present. The need to retain or remove the growth plates around the knee will depend on the degree of deficiency of the femur and tibia and the expected desired length at maturity. The distal aspect of the "new" thigh should be slightly shorter than the contralateral side at maturity to accommodate the prosthetic knee. If the fusion is held by a smooth pin or nail, growth will continue if a growth plate has been retained for that purpose (**Figure 15**).

Femoral Lengthening

Many femora have been lengthened using a frame; however, the advent of lengthening nails has provided a method that is more acceptable because it avoids the considerable scarring and muscle entrapment that accompanies the use of a frame. Excellent results have been obtained with various nails, including the Albizzia nail (DePuy), the Phenix nail (Phenix Medical), the Intramedullary Skeletal Kinetic Distractor (Orthofix), and the PRECICE nail (Ellipse Technologies). The femur must be large enough to accommodate the nail. In addition, although a lateral bow can be accommodated with an osteotomy, an anterior bow is often more distal and a second osteotomy or a shorter nail may be required. These issues should be addressed when planning the procedure. For a teenager, a two-stage correction using a corrective osteotomy and nail followed by lengthening with a nail is preferable to the use of a frame around the thigh for an extended period of time (**Figure 11, D**).

Rotationplasty

The major advance in rotationplasty was changing the site of rotation from the tibia[15,16] to the knee, as described by Torode and Gillespie.[17] With experience, the safety net provided by using a tibial osteotomy can be avoided to completely rotate the leg through the knee.[18] It is much easier to adjust limb length through the knee. Children treated with rotationplasty generally achieve excellent mobility, but they have a Trendelenburg gait. An alternative approach is stabilization of the limb by fusing the femur to the pelvis.[19] The knee is retained in a rotated position to provide flexion and extension close to the hip. The distal femoral growth plate should be ablated to prevent excessive growth, which will locate the weight-bearing axis anterior to the trunk. Further studies are needed to determine if it is better to preserve motion at the expense of energy and joints or provide stability by fusing the femur to the pelvis (**Figure 16**).

Rotationplasty Prosthesis

Initially, the limb may appear too long in a younger child but, with growth of the unaffected limb, the rotated limb will become relatively shorter and the knee will come to lie at a more appropriate level. It is important to consider the future growth of the retained growth plates and the need for additional procedures to prevent compromise of future function that could result from leaving the limb too long.

The early rotationplasty prosthesis was relatively heavy with a thigh structure incorporating long hinge arms and a "thigh lacer" component. In recent years, the prosthesis has been substantially modified and, although external hinges are still used at the "knee" level, the thigh segment is self-suspending (**Figure 17**). Care should be taken to place the hinges at the axis of rotation of the talus. Radiographic determination of optimal positioning of the hinges will be aided by placing markers on the skin.

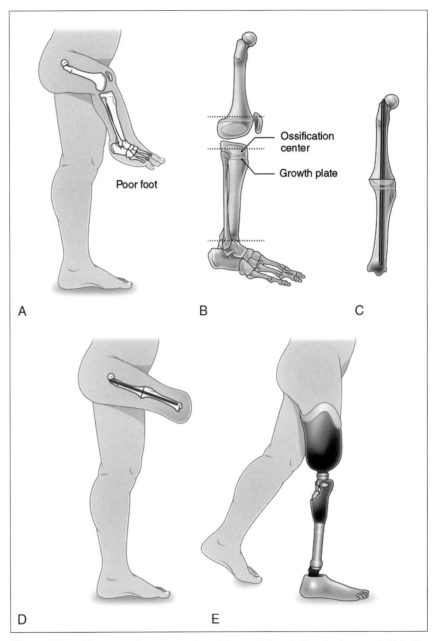

Figure 15 Diagrammatic representation of the procedure to fuse the knee and ablate the foot. **A,** The deficient limb is not suitable for a rotationplasty; a foot ablation and knee fusion is planned. **B,** The skeleton of the limb is shown, with possible resection levels at the knee marked by the dotted lines. In this example, the proximal tibial growth plate is retained and the distal femoral growth plate is removed. The decision regarding these levels depends on the desired overall limb length at maturity as indicated by the distal dotted line incorporating the combination of existing segmental lengths and the available growth potential. **C,** The final position of the femur and tibia, with fixation using an intramedullary nail. Rotational control is superfluous because the foot has been amputated. **D,** The limb after foot ablation and knee fusion. **E,** The patient fitted with a prosthesis.

As children grow and make use of their new "knee," the range of plantar flexion may increase. However, the temptation to make the prosthesis as cosmetically pleasing as possible by casting the foot in maximal plantar flexion should be

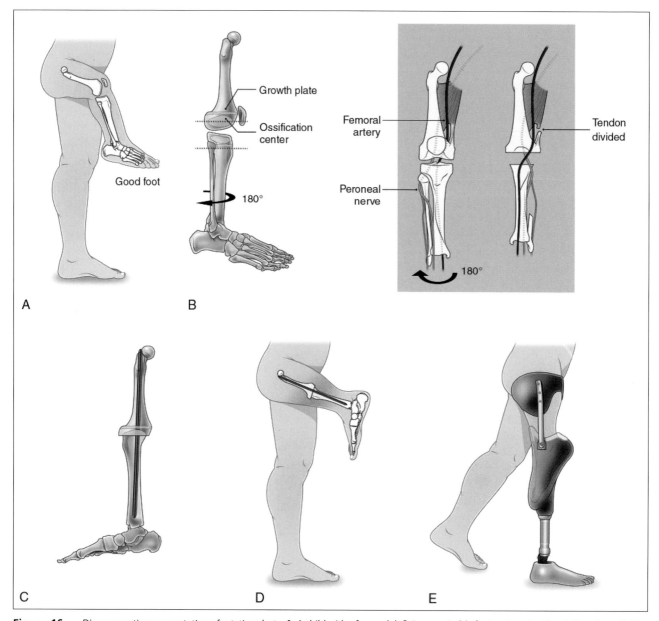

Figure 16 Diagrammatic representation of rotationplasty. **A,** A child with a femoral deficiency suitable for treatment with rotationplasty. **B,** The ossific nuclei around the knee are shown. The possible resection levels are indicated by the dotted lines. If there is adequate femoral length, the femoral resection line moves more proximally to remove the distal growth plate and a portion of the femoral metaphysis; the amount is dictated by the assessment of the expected limb lengths at maturity. **C,** The rotated leg with an intramedullary rod in situ. The cross bolts may be omitted and control obtained with a hip spica. This technique allows rotation to be adjusted in the postoperative period. **D,** The final limb position with the foot rotated. **E,** The rotated limb fitted with a rotationplasty prosthesis.

avoided because the joint will become inflamed as it operates at its limit, reducing the load-bearing capacity of the calcaneus and allowing for more pistoning in the prosthesis so that the joints are no longer optimally aligned.

Distal Femoral Focal Deficiency

Distal femoral focal deficiency is discussed as a separate entity for several reasons. First, in terms of occurrence, it is quite rare. There are isolated case reports in the English-language literature but no patient studies.[20-23] Second, the ossification of the proximal femur is

intact and the function of the hip joint itself appears normal, although Taylor et al[22] reported a case of distal deficiency associated with a hip dislocation.

The clinical appearance of a distal femoral focal deficiency is similar to that of a severe PFFD, with the foot of the affected limb at the level of the

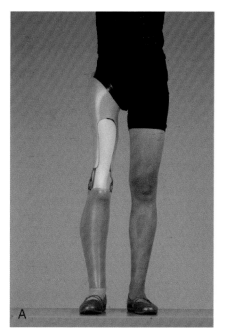 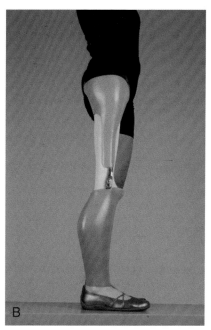

Figure 17   **A,** AP (**A**) and lateral (**B**) photographic views of a rotationplasty prosthesis.

contralateral knee. However, instability occurs through the diaphyseal defect of the distal femur. The knee joint may be nonexistent because the distal femoral condylar component may be fused to the proximal tibia.

In this setting, the child will require a prosthesis for ambulation. Alignment of the limb through fusion of the proximal femoral segment to the tibia will restore stability to the limb and allow better prosthetic function. Rotationplasty is another option to improve stability and function. This procedure should achieve a better gait than seen in patients after rotationplasty for PFFD.

Summary

Although congenital deficiencies of the femur are uncommon, the diagnosis can be demystified by knowledge of the natural history of the condition and an understanding of the expected development of the limb. At the milder end of the severity spectrum, management is essentially the same as that provided for a limb-length discrepancy, unless the distal segments of the limb are substantially involved. At the severe end of the spectrum, most children will be best managed by prosthetic fitting. Within these extremes, there will be children in whom the potential exists for essentially normal function; reconstructive procedures and femoral lengthening are justified in these patients. In some instances, the desire for reconstruction and normalization needs to be tempered by an appreciation of the number of surgical procedures and years of a child's life that will be involved in the attempt to achieve those goals. A close collaboration between the treating surgeon and the prosthetic team is essential for optimal care of children with a congenital deficiency of the femur.

References

1. Jones KL: Femoral hypoplasia: Unusual facies syndrome, in Jones KL, ed: *Smith's Recognizable Patterns of Human Malformations*, ed 4. Philadelphia, PA, WB Saunders, 1988, pp 268-269.

2. Goltz RW, Peterson WC, Gorlin RJ, Ravits HG: Focal dermal hypoplasia. *Arch Dermatol* 1962;86:708-717.

3. Filly AL, Robnet-Filly B, Filly RA: Syndromes with focal femoral deficiency. *J Ultrasound Med* 2004;23(11):1511-1516.

4. Hamanishi C: Congenital short femur: Clinical, genetic and epidemiological comparison of the naturally occurring condition with that caused by thalidomide. *J Bone Joint Surg Br* 1980;62(3):307-320.

5. Gillespie R, Torode IP: Classification and management of congenital abnormalities of the femur. *J Bone Joint Surg Br* 1983;65(5):557-568.

6. Gillespie R: Classification of congenital abnormalities of the femur, in Herring JA, Birch JB, eds: *The Child With a Limb Deficiency*. Rosemont, IL, American Academy of Orthopaedic Surgeons, 1998, pp 63-72.

7. Fixsen JA, Lloyd-Roberts GC: The natural history and early treatment of proximal femoral dysplasia. *J Bone Joint Surg Br* 1974;56(1):86-95.

8. Aitken GT: Proximal femoral focal deficiency: Definition, classification and management, in Aitken GT, ed: *Proximal Femoral Focal Deficiency: A Congenital Anomaly*. Washington, DC, National Academy of Sciences, 1968, pp 1-22.

9. Paley D, Stannard SC: Lengthening reconstruction surgery for congenital femoral deficiency. Available at: http://limblengtheningdoc.org/lengthening_reconstruction_surgery_congenital_femoral_deficiency_29.pdf. Accessed May 26, 2015.

10. Millis MB, Hall JE: Transiliac lengthening of the lower extremity: A modified innominate osteotomy for the treatment of postural imbalance. *J Bone Joint Surg Am* 1979;61(8):1182-1194.

11. Syme J: Amputation at the ankle joint. *London and Edinburgh Monthly J Med Sci* 1843;3:93.

12. Birch JG, Walsh SJ, Small JM, et al: Syme amputation for the treatment

of fibular deficiency: An evaluation of long-term physical and psychological functional status. *J Bone Joint Surg Am* 1999;81(11):1511-1518.

13. Métaizeau JP, Wong-Chung J, Bertrand H, Pasquier P: Percutaneous epiphysiodesis using transphyseal screws (PETS). *J Pediatr Orthop* 1998;18(3):363-369.

14. Blount WP, Clarke GR: Control of bone growth by epiphyseal stapling: A preliminary report. *J Bone Joint Surg Am* 1949;31(3):464-478.

15. Kritter AE: Tibial rotation-plasty for proximal femoral focal deficiency. *J Bone Joint Surg Am* 1977;59(7):927-934.

16. King R: Providing a single lever in proximal femoral focal deficiency: A preliminary report. *J Assoc Child Prosthet-Orthot Clin* 1966;6:23.

17. Torode IP, Gillespie R: Rotationplasty of the lower limb for congenital defects of the femur. *J Bone Joint Surg Br* 1983;65(5):569-573.

18. Krajbich I: Proximal femoral focal deficiency, in Kalamchi A, ed: *Congenital Lower Limb Deficiencies*. New York, NY, Springer-Verlag, 1989, pp 108-127.

19. Brown KL: Resection, rotationplasty, and femoropelvic arthrodesis in severe congenital femoral deficiency: A report of the surgical technique and three cases. *J Bone Joint Surg Am* 2001;83(1):78-85.

20. Tsou PM: Congenital distal femoral focal deficiency: Report of a unique case. *Clin Orthop Relat Res* 1982;162:99-102.

21. Gilsanz V: Distal focal femoral deficiency. *Radiology* 1983;147(1):105-107.

22. Taylor BC, Kean J, Paloski M: Distal focal femoral deficiency. *J Pediatr Orthop* 2009;29(6):576-580.

23. Joseph B: Distal focal femoral deficiency, in Loder RT, Torode I, Joseph B, Nayagam S, eds: *Paediatric Orthopaedics: A System of Decision-Making*. London, England, Hodder Arnold, 2009, pp 269-271.

Chapter 77

Knee Disarticulation and Transfemoral Amputation: Pediatric Prosthetic Considerations

David B. Rotter, CPO

Abstract

When fitting a growing child with a prosthesis at the knee disarticulation or transfemoral amputation level, the treating prosthetist should be aware of the special concerns regarding suspension and component options. As the child grows from infancy to adolescence, the main factor influencing component selection is the space available distal to the prosthetic socket. Congenital anomalies, such as proximal femoral focal deficiency, present unique challenges and require a separate fitting protocol.

Keywords: acquired amputation; congenital limb deficiency; mechanical locking and suction suspension; pediatric articulating knee; proximal femoral focal deficiency (PFFD); rotationplasty; Syme ankle disarticulation

Introduction

Several factors distinguish the care of pediatric limb deficiencies versus adult amputations. Data suggest that 70% of the children seen in pediatric clinics have a congenital limb deficiency, and the remaining 30% have acquired amputations resulting from causes such as trauma and sarcomas.[1] For the child who has a congenital limb deficiency, both advantages and challenges need to be addressed. Children who are born with a limb deficiency are incredibly adaptable because they know no other existence. The use of a prosthesis often becomes second nature if it is incorporated during the child's growth and development. When not wearing their prostheses, children also learn locomotion strategies, such as hopping, scooting, and crawling, which allows for the development of greater balance and strength in their sound limb. Patients with bilateral lower limb deficiency

use their upper limbs and torso to propel themselves forward on the ground when not using prostheses, thus affording greater muscle development and dexterity.

Challenges in care relate to the appearance of the affected limb. Congenital limb deficiencies can be associated with other anomalies, such as irregular bone and muscle development, joint instability, and joint malrotation.[2] Data further suggest that 40% of patients have multiple limb involvement, potentially increasing prosthetic fitting challenges.[3] Bony overgrowth is a challenge specific to an acquired amputation. The growth of the long bone overtakes the soft-tissue envelope, potentially resulting in bone piercing through the skin.[4]

When given the opportunity, it is always preferable for the surgeon to perform a knee disarticulation that preserves the end-bearing surfaces and avoids longitudinal bony overgrowth. In

the pediatric population, knee disarticulation is considered preferable to transfemoral amputation for many reasons. The primary concern in a growing child is that the development of the affected limb will keep pace with the sound-side limb. Knee disarticulation preserves the femoral epiphysis, allowing the growth mechanism in the femur to be unaffected. An end-bearing limb with primarily intact thigh musculature makes a knee disarticulation functionally superior to a transfemoral amputation.[5,6]

When to Begin Prosthetic Care

The literature suggests that it is appropriate to begin prosthetic fitting when a child reaches the developmental milestone of independently pulling to a stand.[7-9] However, varying opinions exist in the literature on when to provide a child with an articulated knee. Earlier studies suggested waiting until age 3 years,[10] but the more contemporary approach suggests that a child should be provided with an articulating knee early in development, in line with the pull-to-stand milestone.[11,12] The benefits of early fitting with an articulating knee include permitting a child to crawl and kneel even before standing is achieved.

Early Suspension and Knee Systems

If a summary statement can be made about suspension systems and knee components for the pediatric patient, it is that one can influence the other. This fact is most apparent when a child with a congenital limb deficiency is fit with

Mr. Rotter or an immediate family member serves as a board member, owner, officer, or committee member of the Association of Children's Prosthetic and Orthotic Clinics.

his or her first prosthesis. Component selection often is predicated on space allowance.

Just as liner technology has become ubiquitous for adult suspension systems, liners have steadily become an ideal suspension choice for the pediatric population. Liners are easy for parents to don on very young children. In addition, the elastic nature of the material allows for expansion as the child grows. Liners provide secure suspension, generally eliminating the need for a suspension belt. If the residual limb is short and lacks sufficient leverage, a belt can be used to augment suspension and stability. The disadvantage of using liners is that length is added to the end of the residual limb. If a liner system is chosen for suspension, the remaining overall length must be measured, and a decision must be made to determine which knee articulation system can be used.

An example of some liner and suspension considerations in the first prosthetic fitting for a child are demonstrated in **Figure 1**. It is important that parents be instructed on how to apply the liner and chosen suspension system. The prosthetist may use a temporary socket to determine the overall height of the prosthesis. In fitting the child shown in **Figure 1**, outside hinges were selected because there was insufficient space for an articulating knee below the socket, and the knee center would be impractically low. This would impede the child from crawling. A common strategy used with outside hinges is to couple them with an anterior elastic strap attached proximally to the socket and distally to the shin section. The elastic strap allows the child to crawl with a bent knee and is snug enough to ensure immediate knee extension on standing. This strap can be tightened or loosened depending on the child's ability to control the articulation throughout his or her maturation and development.

In patients with bilateral transfemoral amputations or knee disarticulations,

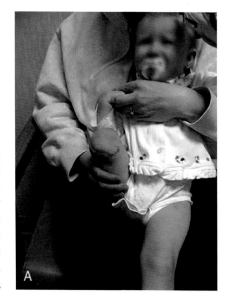
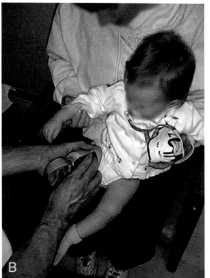
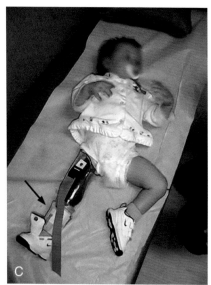
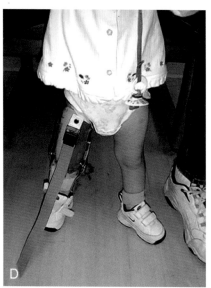

Figure 1 Clinical photographs demonstrate some steps and considerations in the first prosthesis fitting of 6-month-old child. **A,** The right limb was revised to a knee disarticulation because the child was born with an absent tibia and a nonfunctioning limb distal to the knee. **B,** The parent is instructed on the application of the gel liner. **C,** The donned liner is shown within the clear socket of the prosthesis. A distal lanyard was fed through the bottom of the socket to create a lanyard-style suspension system that is secured with a plastic clip. Also pictured is an exoskeletal wood block (arrow) attached to the temporary socket that is used to determine the overall height. After the appropriate height is determined, articulation can be added to the knee. **D,** Outside hinges were used because of insufficient space for an articulating knee below the socket. (Courtesy of David B. Rotter, CPO, Scheck and Siress, Chicago, IL.)

matching the anatomic knee center is no longer a primary consideration. The prosthetist may choose to use bilateral endoskeletal knee joints (**Figure 2**). Initially, such prostheses may be intentionally shortened to minimize the risk of injury from falls. However, as these children grow and become more stable, length is added to the shin sections to create better overall symmetry.

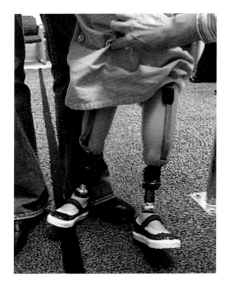

Figure 2 Clinical photograph of endoskeletal components being fit. (Courtesy of David B. Rotter, CPO, Scheck and Siress, Chicago, IL.)

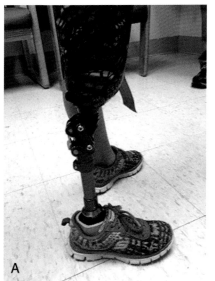

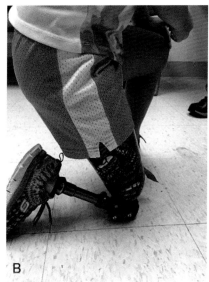

Figure 3 **A,** Clinical photograph of a pediatric four-bar knee. **B,** Clinical photograph of the advantages of using a four-bar knee system, which include greater range of flexion to allow kneeling. (Courtesy of David B. Rotter, CPO, Scheck and Siress, Chicago, IL.)

The Growing Child

The main factor influencing component selection is the space available distal to the socket. As a child grows and the relative distance between the distal end of the socket and the ground increases, a greater range of component choices becomes available. As more distance is gained, suspension options become less of a fitting consideration.

Despite a steady increase in component offerings for the pediatric population, selection is still limited, which is especially true for pediatric knee systems. As a child grows and gains sufficient clearance, various four-bar mechanical knee systems can be used (**Figure 3, A**). Polycentric knee mechanisms offer several advantages, specifically for pediatric fittings. The greater range of motion present when kneeling is both practical and helpful for an infant who is crawling and an older child who kneels on the ground during play (**Figure 3, B**).

As greater clearance is achieved with a child's continued growth, a polycentric five-bar mechanism can be fit (**Figure 4**). The advantage of this system is the increased stability present with a

mechanical locking feature at heel strike or when pressure is exerted on the heel of the foot. This feature allows for greater inherent stability as the child becomes more active and traverses uneven terrain during play and sport activities.

The Active Child

Nearly all children will eventually want to use their prostheses to run. This process might start with a double hop on the sound-side limb to a single hop on the prosthesis and will eventually progress to running leg over leg. Most pediatric knees have a manual friction setting that is good for level, steady speed walking but does not provide sufficient resistance to heel rise when running. The child will compensate by using an abducted circumduction motion, swinging through a stiff leg, or having the leg shank fully flexed and rebounding off the posterior aspect of the socket back into extension. Being highly adaptable, children will use their ingenuity to resolve any design shortcomings of the prosthetic knee. As the shank length gets longer, the effective pendulum length of the prosthesis elongates, increasing its swing-phase duration, thus

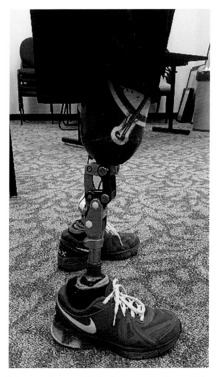

Figure 4 Clinical photograph of a pediatric polycentric five-bar knee. (Courtesy of David B. Rotter, CPO, Scheck and Siress, Chicago, IL.)

making it increasingly difficult to run with knees with only friction resistance.

A few fluid-controlled knees have been designed to address this deficit within the pediatric population (**Figure 5, A**). At present, further development of fluid-controlled knee systems is needed to better accommodate the growing and increasingly more active child.

Polycentric knees can be coupled with highly responsive pediatric carbon fiber feet (**Figure 5, B**); however, such dynamic feet will subject the knee mechanism to greater torques in swing as the child goes from walking to running. This further supports the need for mechanisms that will provide greater swing phase control for pediatric patients.

Transitioning to Adult Components

As a child becomes an adolescent, the prosthetist is encouraged to consider adult components as soon as a child's limb length and body weight allow. Adult components offer a far greater array of choices for fluid-controlled knees and dynamic feet to accommodate the active adolescent. Endoskeletal components can adapt the standard pediatric 22-mm diameter pylon to an adult 30-mm pylon, which allows for mixing and matching of adult and pediatric components.

As previously mentioned, liner technology is used extensively in pediatric fittings. When a child is young and the bony anatomy is difficult to palpate, an elastomeric liner will provide good soft-tissue load bearing in addition to a secure form of suspension (**Figure 6, A**). As the child with a knee disarticulation grows older and his or her anatomy becomes more defined, more traditional means of suspension, such as suspension system with a supracondylar door, can be used (**Figure 6, B and C**). This type of suspension will reduce the distal build height of the prosthesis and allow a more symmetric knee center.

A modern variant to true suction suspension is a seal-in liner (**Figure 6, D**), which can be used after a child develops sufficient dexterity and strength to don and doff the liner independently. Given the rapid growth considerations that must be accounted for, true suction suspension is challenging in pediatric prosthetic management.[13] The seal-in liner system offers a better alternative because it does not have to

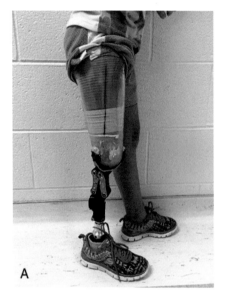
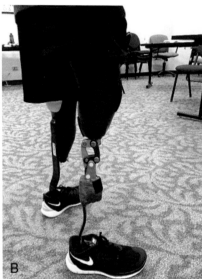

Figure 5 **A,** Clinical photograph of a fluid-controlled pediatric knee. **B,** Clinical photograph of responsive carbon fiber feet. (Courtesy of David B. Rotter, CPO, Scheck and Siress, Chicago, IL.)

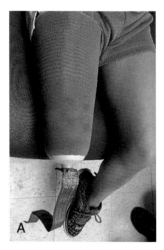
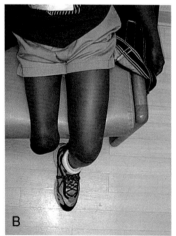
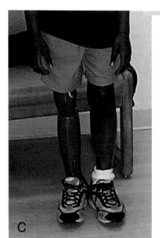
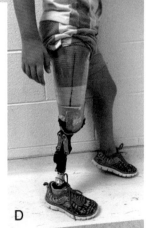

Figure 6 Clinical photographs of suspension prostheses. **A,** Locking liner with lanyard strap. **B,** Knee disarticulation with palpable prominent condyles. **C,** Supracondylar medial door suspension. **D,** Seal-in liner. (Courtesy of David B. Rotter, CPO, Scheck and Siress, Chicago, IL.)

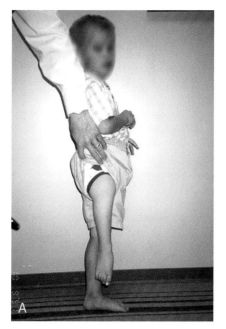 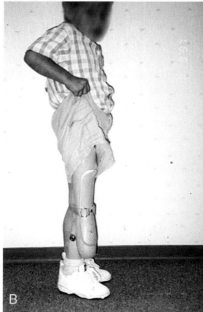

Figure 7 Clinical photographs of a child with a proximal femoral focal deficiency. **A,** Untreated. **B,** The child wearing an extension prosthesis. (Courtesy of David B. Rotter, CPO, Scheck and Siress, Chicago, IL.)

fit as snugly as a true suction socket. The initial fit can be intentionally loose, requiring the use of fitting socks. As the limb grows, removal of the interface socks will accommodate growth and maintain a reasonable socket fit. Importantly, a positive suction suspension is preserved throughout the initial socket fitting and subsequent growth accommodations.

Congenital Anomalies

Children born with congenital anomalies may have unique fitting challenges. A prosthetist may encounter uniquely formed limbs and must think creatively to accommodate the anatomy into a functional prosthesis. The most commonly seen congenital deformity treated with a transfemoral prosthesis is a proximal femoral focal deficiency (PFFD), which is also known as longitudinal deficiency of the femur, partial. PFFD results in a shortened anatomic femoral length, which raises the ipsilateral ankle and foot closer to the height of the contralateral (sound-side) knee.

Three potential courses of action exist for pediatric patients with congenital anomalies at or distal to the knee. The first option is to fit the limb as is with a modified extension prosthesis (**Figure 7**). The foot is placed in full equinus to accommodate the donning of pants. The articulation is placed as proximally as possible to gain ground clearance during swing and should be as compact as possible to allow comfortable sitting. This option accommodates the anatomy the child was born with and allows the child's input into future decision making if rotationplasty or ankle disarticulation is considered at a later date.

The second option is for the surgeon to perform rotationplasty of the foot (also known as Van Nes rotationplasty). In this procedure, the surgeon rotates the affected foot 180° to allow the foot to function as a quasi-knee joint (**Figure 8, A and B**). The dorsiflexors act as knee flexors, and the plantar flexors act as knee extensors.[14] Outside hinges should be used on the prosthesis to contour around the malleoli and create

a mechanical joint center that is congruent with the anatomic joint center to create a smooth reaction at the joint (**Figure 8, C**). As the child grows older and larger, stronger outside hinges are required to accommodate the forces generated in gait. The foot is positioned in full equinus to generate maximum power for each movement. The shape of the foot in equinus allows for good suspension over the heel as it becomes prominent enough for self-suspension. Suspension can be achieved using an anterior door, a strap over the heel, or a stovepipe-style cushion insert in the distal foot portion.

After rotationplasty, it is common for the foot to start to derotate back to its original position with the passage of time. As this occurs, the prosthetist must creatively fashion the articulations to maintain a semblance of fluid ankle articulation. If the joint incongruity becomes too severe, surgery is required to reset the limb at an appropriate angle.

The third option for patients with congenital anomalies at or distal to the knee is surgical ablation of the foot with a Syme ankle disarticulation. The advantage of this procedure is that it allows the fitting of traditional prosthetic knee components. The disadvantages include the loss of a functional joint under physiologic control. In some instances, the decision to perform a Syme ankle disarticulation can be delayed until the child is old enough to make his or her own decision regarding the procedure (**Figure 9**).

Summary

Children who require transfemoral prostheses may have a wide range of limb shapes and fitting challenges. Children who have a congenital limb deficiency are likely to have atypical bone shapes, muscle placements, and joint irregularities and may have multiple limb involvement. When surgery is the appropriate course of action to remove

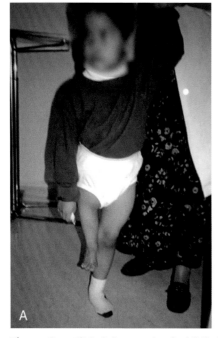
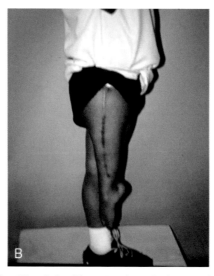
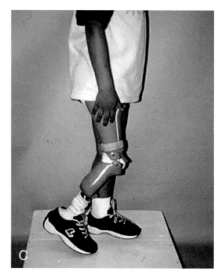

Figure 8   Clinical photographs of a child before (**A**) and after (**B**) rotationplasty. **C,** Photograph of a pediatric rotationplasty prosthesis. (Courtesy of David B. Rotter, CPO, Scheck and Siress, Chicago, IL.)

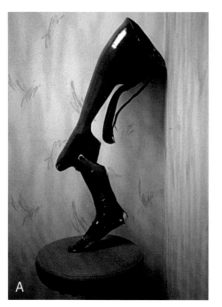
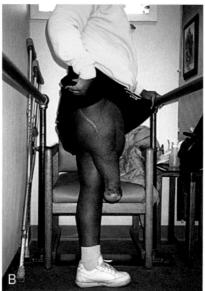
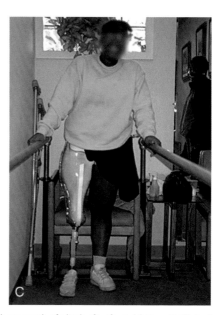

Figure 9   **A,** Clinical photograph of a prosthesis worn prior to elective foot ablation. **B,** Clinical photograph of a limb after foot ablation. **C,** Clinical photograph of the fitting of traditional prosthetic knee components in an adolescent. (Courtesy of David B. Rotter, CPO, Scheck and Siress, Chicago, IL.)

a nonfunctioning residual limb distal to the knee, a disarticulation procedure is preferred. Children with acquired transtibial amputations are more susceptible to bony overgrowth. A prosthetic fitting that can accommodate bony overgrowth may delay the need for revision surgery.

The prosthetist must be mindful of the limitation in the available components to construct a prosthesis for the child with a limb deficiency caused by a transfemoral amputation or a knee disarticulation. This is especially true for the youngest patients being fit for the

first time. Congenital anomalies such as PFFD offer unique challenges and have a separate fitting protocol.

The pediatric patient with a transfemoral amputation, a knee disarticulation, or a lower limb congenital anomaly is faced with unique challenges. Those challenges should be viewed by the prosthetist as unique opportunities to fashion a well-functioning device that will improve the quality of life for the growing child.

References

1. Challenor YB: Limb deficiencies and amputation surgery in children, in Molnary GE, ed: *Pediatric Rehabilitation*. Baltimore, MD, Williams and Wilkins, 1985.

2. Aitken GT, Pellicore RJ: Introduction to the child amputee, in *Atlas of Limb Prosthetics: Surgical and Prosthetic Principles*. St. Louis, MO, CV Mosby, 1981, pp 493-500.

3. Gibson D: Child and juvenile amputees, in Banjerjee S, Khan N, eds: *Rehabilitation Management of Amputees*. Baltimore, MD, Williams and Wilkins, 1982, pp 394-414.

4. Aitken GT: Overgrowth of the amputation stump. *Interclin Info Bull* 1962;1:1-8.

5. Loder RT, Herring JA: Disarticulation of the knee in children: A functional assessment. *J Bone Joint Surg Am* 1987;69(8):1155-1160.

6. Hughes J: Biomechanics of the through-knee prosthesis. *Prosthet Orthot Int* 1983;7(2):96-99.

7. Morrissy RT, Giavedoni BJ, Coulter-O'Berry C: The limb-deficient child, in Morrissy RT, Weinstein SL, eds: *Lovell and Winter's Pediatric Orthopaedics*, ed 5. Philadelphia, PA, Lippincott Williams & Wilkins, 2001, vol 2, pp 1217-1272.

8. Coulter-O'Berry C: Physical therapy management in children with lower extremity limb deficiencies, in Herring JA, Birch JS, eds: *The Child With a Limb Deficiency*. Rosemont, IL, American Academy of Orthopaedic Surgeons, 1998, pp 319-330.

9. Krebs DE, Edelstein JE, Thornby MA: Prosthetic management of children with limb deficiencies. *Phys Ther* 1991;71(12):920-934.

10. Stanger M: Limb deficiencies and amputations, in Campbell SK, Palisano RJ, Vander Linden DW, eds: *Physical Therapy for Children*. Philadelphia, PA, WB Saunders, 1994, pp 325-351.

11. Wilk B, Karol L, Halliday S: Characterizing gait in young children with a prosthetic knee joint. *Phys Ther Prod* 1999;10:20.

12. Giavedoni BJ, Coulter-O'Berry C, Geil M: Movement masters. *Adv Direct Rehab* 2002;11:43-44.

13. Thompson GH, Leimkuehler JP: Prosthetic management, in Kalamchi A, ed: *Congenital Lower Limb Deficiencies*. New York, NY, Springer-Verlag, 1989, pp 211-235

14. Van Nes C: Rotation-plasty for congenital defects of the femur: Making use of the ankle of the shortened limb to control the knee joint of a prosthesis. *J Bone Joint Surg Br* 1950;32:12-16.

Chapter 78

Hip Disarticulation and Hemipelvectomy in Children: Surgical and Prosthetic Management

Joseph Ivan Krajbich, MD, FRCS(C)   Todd DeWees, BS, CPO

Abstract

Hip disarticulation and hemipelvectomy (transpelvic amputation) are uncommon in pediatric patients. However, in acute situations, it is helpful to be familiar with the surgical approaches and prosthetic options for children undergoing high-level lower limb amputations. Classification based on etiology may affect overall patient management. The components available for prosthetic fitting may be limited based on the age of the patient.

Keywords: hemipelvectomy; high-level pediatric amputee; hindquarter amputation; hip disarticulation; prosthetic management; surgical management

Introduction

Pediatric amputees represent between 10.3% and 11.7% of the overall amputee population.[1,2] Patients with hip disarticulations and hemipelvectomies (transpelvic amputations) represent approximately 2% of the amputee population.[1] Therefore, pediatric patients with high-level lower limb amputations represent only 0.2% of the overall amputee population. Because of the very small number of children with hip disarticulation or hemipelvectomy, surgeons and prosthetists often have limited experience in managing these patients, who have special needs and require special considerations. It is likely that only tertiary referral centers for pediatric limb deficiency treat enough of these children to collect adequate objective data to establish both surgical and prosthetic treatment principles. However, virtually any practicing orthopaedic surgeon can be faced with an acute situation where hip disarticulation or hemipelvectomy is necessary to save the life of a child. Traumatic injury and sepsis are among the main etiologic causes of these high-level amputations. It is important to be familiar with the basic management principles that guide treatment and prosthetic fitting to provide these children with optimal care.

Surgical Management: Anatomic Considerations

In most instances of acquired high-level amputation, the surgical treatment is likely to be dictated by the type of injury or the condition leading to the amputation. Therefore, the surgeon should be well versed in the anatomy and the surgical exposures around the hip and pelvis and able to adapt the approach to the individual circumstances.

Children usually have a healthy proximal blood supply, resilient tissues, and good healing potential. All three main blood supplies to the proximal part of the limb can be used as dictated by the circumstance. A posterior gluteal flap based on gluteal vessels, an anterior flap based on external iliac/femoral vessels, and a medial flap based on the obturator vessels can all be used. It is important to be aware that the bony pelvis and the proximal femur serve as attachments to a host of central skeleton muscles; their loss or loss of their anchorage can lead to secondary issues related to pelvic floor support, abdominal wall integrity, and spinal balance (JI Krajbich, MD, unpublished data presented at the Association of Children's Prosthetic-Orthotic Clinics annual meeting, Springfield, MA, 1988).

The pelvis is also the site of several internal organs whose preservation or removal will depend on the existing pathology and surgeon's skill. Because a procedure of this magnitude will have a substantial effect on the patient's quality of life and future health, an intimate knowledge of the underlying pathology and pelvic anatomy is imperative.

Terminology and Classification
Hip Disarticulation

In general, in hip disarticulation it is assumed that there is loss of the bony structures distal to the hip joint. That is, all of the femur is absent, but the pelvis, including the acetabulum, is intact and present. The integrity of the soft tissues can vary with etiology. A special case is the presence of a very short femoral

Dr. Krajbich or an immediate family member serves as a board member, owner, officer, or committee member of the Association of Children's Prosthetic and Orthotic Clinics and the Scoliosis Research Society and is a member of a speakers' bureau or has made paid presentations on behalf of K2m. Neither Mr. DeWees nor any immediate family member has received anything of value from or has stock or stock options held in a commercial company or institution related directly or indirectly to the subject of this chapter.

segment that cannot serve as a functional proximal femur for the purpose of prosthetic fitting. In such instances, the child will likely require a hip disarticulation–like prosthetic fitting. This is relatively important in a very young child facing transfemoral amputation because loss of the distal femoral growth plate may preclude a functional transfemoral fitting; therefore, the patient eventually may require a hip disarticulation–like prosthesis. In some congenital deficiencies, such as phocomelia, a hip disarticulation–like prosthesis may be required if the vestigial limb cannot provide transfemoral-like function.

Hemipelvectomy

Partial or complete hemipelvectomy is also called transpelvic or hindquarter amputation. The limb loss involves not only the whole limb but also a portion of the central skeleton (the pelvis). Clearly, the complexity of the surgical approach, if needed, and prosthetic fitting depends on the presence and integrity of the remaining bony pelvis, the soft-tissue structures, and the underlying pathologic process.

Classification According to Etiology

Similar to other limb deficiencies in children, high-level lower limb loss can be either acquired (trauma, neoplasm, or sepsis) or congenital (amelia), phocomelia (intercalary deficiency), or another type of loss (conjoined twins).

Trauma

Trauma likely accounts for most high-level amputations in the lower limbs. Motor vehicle crashes (the child is usually a pedestrian), lawnmower injuries, and injuries sustained in a war zone are high-energy injuries that devastate the proximal soft tissues. Frequently, these injuries are complicated by massive wound contamination and loss of bony integrity. Because these are serious, life-threatening injuries,

resuscitation of the child by establishing cardiopulmonary stability is the first priority. Stopping major blood loss is an integral part of this effort. Initially, simple manual pressure and packing is all that can be done. After the patient's condition has stabilized and adequate ventilatory support and fluid resuscitation has been accomplished, careful assessment of the extent of the injuries is necessary for a rational approach.

Surgical control of major bleeding and débridement of contaminated tissue is the next mandatory step. At this point, the treatment team must decide if any emergent limb salvage procedure can be used. Revascularization is an important consideration because a relatively short window of a few hours exists in which an avascular limb can be saved. Attempts also should be made to preserve and use any relatively intact and viable tissue to increase the length of the limb and diminish functional loss. As already mentioned, the ability to preserve the distal femoral physis can be of major importance in the functional outcomes of very young children. A major impediment of instituting such reconstructive procedures in the setting of acute trauma is the absence of an onsite specialized surgical team. Transfer of the child to an institution with these capabilities should be considered if feasible.

Additional interventions can be instituted after the patient is stabilized. Treatment by experienced surgeons in an operating room setting may lead to more judicial débridement and may optimize the survival of remaining tissues. A number of débridements with the wound remaining temporarily open or treated with vacuum suction dressing may be necessary before final wound closure. Any needed bone or soft-tissue reconstruction can be part of this process.[3-5]

Additional techniques can be used to obtain optimal functional results for each patient. Bone transport, free flaps, rotational flaps, and composite vascularized graft can all be used.[6-9]

Neoplasms

In children, Ewing sarcoma is the most common neoplasm found in the proximal femur or pelvis; however, osteogenic sarcoma and some soft-tissue sarcomas also occur at these sites. Among the soft-tissue sarcomas in children with neurofibromatosis type I (von Recklinghausen disease), peripheral nerve sheath sarcoma is the most frequently encountered neoplasm.

Because modern treatment of these tumors has shifted toward chemotherapy and limb salvage, a primary amputation is performed only in a situation in which limb salvage is not possible because of the involvement of vital structures and inability to obtain clear resection margins.[10-15] Primary amputation is a relatively rare treatment in a modern pediatric oncology surgical practice. In the experience of one of this chapter's authors (JIK), primary amputation is most likely in a patient with pelvic neurofibrosarcoma. This neoplasm is resistant to chemotherapy and radiation therapy and frequently involves several vital structures in the pelvis; a complete hemipelvectomy is often the only chance for a cure. Failure of a primary limb salvage procedure, such as endoprosthetic or allograft replacement in the femur or internal hemipelvectomy is another situation in which hip disarticulation or formal hemipelvectomy may be required. Substantial postoperative complications are possible.[15-17]

Sepsis

Purpura fulminant septicemia, necrotizing fasciitis, and other causes of infected gangrenous limbs may necessitate proximal limb amputation as a lifesaving measure.[18] The surgical principles used to treat septic shock will apply. Cardiopulmonary resuscitation, fluid resuscitation, the administration of massive doses of antibiotics, and débridement of any obvious necrotic contaminated tissue are also critical to the patient's survival. However, the need for a proximal amputation usually does not apply in patients with purpura fulminans because systemic sepsis generally leads to ischemia of various body parts, which quite commonly includes the limbs. In this situation, limbs or parts of a limb can become ischemic but are not contaminated by infection (dry gangrene). In such a situation, it is necessary to wait until the final demarcation of necrotic and viable tissue occurs before deciding on the level of amputations. This final demarcation may take several days or even weeks; a very proximal amputation is rarely necessary.

In any of these situations, the usual course of treatment involves multiple débridements and delayed wound closure until a healthy, uninfected wound is obtained. Modern, complex wound care techniques, such as vacuum-assisted dressings, flaps, and skin grafts, are usually used to achieve wound closure.[4]

Congenital Defects
Unilateral Congenital Absence of the Whole Limb
Unilateral congenital absence of the whole limb, also known as amelia, is a rare condition. The treatment mainstay is prosthetic fitting determined by the extent of the pelvic involvement. Surgical intervention is limited to the treatment of secondary effects of such a limb deficiency.

Phocomelia
Lower limb phocomelia is not technically a hip disarticulation. Quite frequently, however, a small deficient, minimally functional foot contributes little to limb function other than perhaps acting as an improved anchor for a prosthetic socket. Children with lower limb phocomelia frequently require hip disarticulation–like prostheses. Surgical intervention is rarely indicated unless the position or alignment of the affected limb at the pelvis interferes with prosthetic fitting. In such patients, a realignment procedure may be indicated. Many of these

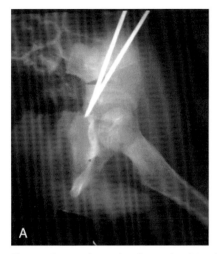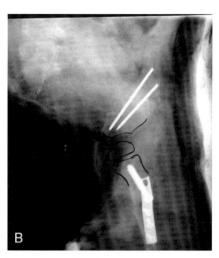

Figure 1   Radiographs of secondary hip subluxation treated by Salter innominate osteotomy (**A**) and innominate osteotomy and proximal femoral varus osteotomy (**B**).

children have other limb deficiencies and warrant an individualized approach to maximize their function.

Separated Conjoined Twins
Pygopagus conjoined twins (Siamese twins) may be candidates for a separation procedure. After separation, either one or usually both children will have a hemipelvectomy-like situation. Separation is a very complex surgical procedure performed by a multidisciplinary surgical team, and it usually requires double teams of general pediatric surgeons, pediatric urologists, pediatric orthopaedic surgeons, and pediatric plastic surgeons. The soft-tissue defects can be quite large and may require prolonged treatment before the child is ready for prosthetic fitting.

Hemipelvectomy in Very Young Children
The absence of a hemipelvis has a substantial influence on the development of a child's spine and contralateral hip. The loss of abdominal wall integrity, paraspinal muscle integrity, and iliopsoas integrity all lead to early paralytic-like lumbar scoliosis convex to the side of the absent hemipelvis. The remaining hemipelvis is at the caudal end of the scoliotic curve and tilts into

abduction. Consequently, the remaining hip is forced into an adducted position with respect to its acetabulum. This leads to uncovering of the femoral head and, in a young child, the development of further hip dysplasia and eventually hip subluxation. Both surgical and prosthetic techniques are needed to treat these patients.

Initially, prosthetic treatment incorporates a spinal brace into the prosthetic design. However, a progressive worsening of the deformity may require surgical treatment. Surgical treatment of scoliosis and/or osteotomies around the hip, on the femoral as well as the pelvic side, may be required (**Figure 1**). In some of these children, other organ deficiencies and their treatment (for example, colostomies and other enterostomies) can make treatment even more challenging. A child with a colostomy or enterostomy on the prosthetic side may be more functional without a prosthesis; a walker or crutches and a swing-through gait may provide more effective locomotion.

Prosthetic Management
As previously stated, pediatric patients with hip disarticulation or hemipelvectomy are a small and specialized population. Studies of adults with hip disarticulations or transpelvic

amputations have traditionally shown high prosthetic rejection rates[19,20] because of the combination of socket discomfort and the high-energy cost of ambulation. Although these factors exist in the pediatric population, prosthesis rejection rates have been found to be as low as 10%.[21]

It should be noted that there are important differences between pediatric patients with high-level lower limb loss and their adult counterparts. The first major physiologic distinction is the rate of energy consumption. For pediatric patients with hip disarticulation and transpelvic amputation, the oxygen consumption cost has been reported at 151% and 161% of normal, respectively.[22] Their adult counterparts have energy consumptions levels reported as high as 200% of normal.[23] A second difference between pediatric and adult amputees is the most common causes of amputation. In adults older than 60 years, the most common causes are vascular disease or trauma. In pediatric patients, the primary causes of amputation are tumor or congenital amputation.[1] In addition, the smaller body mass of a pediatric patient, particularly at younger ages, decreases the force on weight-bearing areas of the body. This in turn decreases the need for additional padding or thermoplastic material to create a comfortable socket and reduces the overall weight of the socket without compromising structure.

Prosthetic fitting in pediatric patients is complicated by their constantly changing body size, changes in functional levels, the limited availability of appropriately sized prosthetic components, and conflict between the weight of the prosthesis and its durability. These challenges can be mitigated by following the sound prosthetic fitting principles of good communication, regular patient follow-up, appropriate component selection, and flexibility in prosthetic design.

Biomechanics and Prosthetic Alignment

No studies are available that show differences in the biomechanics of gait between pediatric and adult patients treated with hip disarticulation or transpelvic amputation; therefore, the descriptions of the gait biomechanics of hip disarticulation and transpelvic amputation will follow the descriptions of Radcliffe,[24] Raiford and Epps,[25] and Solomonidis et al.[26] At initial contact, the ground reaction line runs posterior to the ankle, anterior to the knee, and anterior to the hip. Solomonidis et al[26] subdivided and described hip disarticulation gait in terms of axial force, anterior-posterior knee moment, anterior-posterior hip moment, medial-lateral hip moment, and torque. The axial force follows a double-bump pattern, which reaches a maximum force at approximately 20% of the gait cycle, maintaining a force approximately equal to body weight until approximately 50% of the gait cycle, and then it diminishing to zero at toe-off. The anterior-posterior knee moment begins with a small extension force until 30% of the gait cycle; at that point, it increases to its maximum force, which is maintained to 55% of the gait cycle. At that point it starts its decrease to zero at toe-off. The anterior-posterior hip moment is described as a flexion moment caused by contact of the hip joint with the flexion limiter. There is a brief reversal of this force between 10% and 20% of the gait cycle, then the force returns to an extension moment, which reaches its maximum just before toe-off. The medial-lateral hip moment follows that of an able-bodied individual, with the moment adducting the hip with a maximum force at 35% of the gait cycle. Torque was also shown to be very similar to that of able-bodied individuals, with maximum force occurring at approximately 50% of the gait cycle in the internal direction.[24-26] This brief description of the biomechanics highlights both the similarities and differences between hip disarticulation and normal gait.

Prosthetic alignment in a pediatric patient with a high-level lower limb amputation should follow similar biomechanical principles to that of an adult. The primary goals are to allow maximum stability in stance and necessary mobility in the swing phase of gait. However, the alignment of the prosthesis should not be overly stabilized. The adult standard of placing the weight line 1.0 to 1.5 inches anterior to the knee joint at midstance[27] should be scaled appropriately for the size of the pediatric patient. For example, the aforementioned offset may be appropriate for an adult with a hip-to-floor length of 91 cm but a pediatric patient with a hip-to-floor length of 45 cm would require a midstance offset of approximately 0.5 to 0.75 inch.

Hip Disarticulation Versus Transpelvic Amputation

Throughout the remainder of this chapter, the prosthetic care of pediatric patients with hip disarticulation or transpelvic amputation will often be treated synonymously. It is necessary at this point to delineate important and specific differences in the treatment of these two high-level amputations. These differences are primarily centered on the pelvic anatomy and socket designs.

For the patient with a hip disarticulation and a fully intact hemipelvis, weight-bearing forces are distributed over both bony and soft-tissue surfaces (**Figure 2**). This distribution allows the prosthetist to maintain maximum control over the prosthetic device by taking advantage of the ischial tuberosity, high anterior and posterior socket walls, and containment of the iliac crest. It should be noted that patients with very short femurs or those with phocomelia with a deficient foot attached at the hip are fitted with a prosthesis as though they had a hip disarticulation. Although they technically do not have a hip disarticulation, these nonfunctional distal elements necessitate prosthetic treatment with a hip disarticulation prosthesis.

Conversely, because the patient with a transpelvic amputation may have few, if any, of these bony structures, weight bearing will be necessary through hydrostatic forces applied to the soft tissues of the amputated side. Suspension of the prosthesis for a patient with a transpelvic amputation may be further enhanced by the use of a suction socket to help maintain intimate contact with the soft tissues.[28] Both of the sockets will likely require iliac crest containment of the contralateral side to improve coronal plane stability, which is typically done through the use of a single-piece socket with a flexible posterior element. The transpelvic socket design often includes the addition of a lumbar or thoracic extension on the amputated side. This extension is integral to the socket and designed to address the likely development of scoliosis, which is almost universal in this patient population (**Figure 3**). This design allows easy donning of the prosthesis while maintaining enhanced rotational control. The transpelvic socket typically has a taller proximal trim line in an attempt to reduce the risk of induced scoliosis. The patient with a hip disarticulation may be able to obtain contralateral iliac crest containment using a two-piece prosthetic design with the segments connected with nylon or polyethylene terephthalate straps. The advantages of this design over a one-piece socket are reduction in overall socket weight and increased comfort.

In the patient with bilateral high-level amputation, the use of prostheses is rare except for therapeutic standing. For this population, the primary purpose of a prosthetic socket is to provide a balanced pelvis for sitting, spinal support, and containing abdominal viscera.

Pediatric Considerations

Pediatric patients tend to be more active and have a higher functional level,

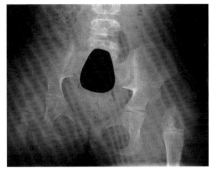

Figure 2 AP radiograph of the pelvis of a child with right-sided phocomelia. The patient will be fitted with a functional hip disarticulation prosthesis.

decreased oxygen consumption, and more pressure-tolerant soft tissues, and they may be more motivated than adults with the same level of amputation.[29] These advantages, however, are offset by the disadvantages of limited choice in prosthetic components, high relative prosthetic weight, and the limited experience of clinicians in treating children with high-level lower limb amputation.

Limitations in prosthetic components specifically designed for pediatric patients represent a substantial barrier to producing a prosthesis that is functional, durable, and sufficiently lightweight. Weight is extremely important considering that the typical adult prosthesis for a high-level lower limb amputation weighs between 5.75 and 6.20 kg.[23] This means that for the typical 6-year-old child weighing approximately 21 kg,[30] a prosthesis built with adult components and based on adult principles would represent greater than 25% of the child's body mass.

Current options for pediatric hip joints include the Child's Play Littig Hip Disarticulation System (Trulife), the 7E8 hip joint (Ottobock), and 3K51 Modular Hip Joint (Euro International). Knees produced for pediatric amputees provide a larger variety of options, but not as many as available to adult patients. When choosing a knee, mechanical or pneumatic options should be considered because they tend to be lighter in

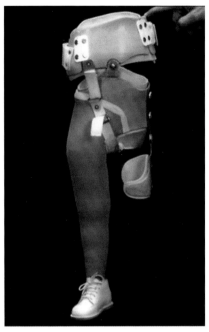

Figure 3 Photograph of a hemipelvectomy prosthesis with a thoracic extension to control 2° of scoliosis.

weight than hydraulic options. When the knee is to be used in functional gait, the selection of a polycentric option is encouraged. A polycentric knee will provide an effective shortening of the prosthetic limb in the swing phase of gait. The knee is the only pediatric prosthetic component that provides this benefit because polycentric hip joints are currently available only in adult sizes. The foot component of the prosthesis provides the greatest variety of pediatric options, nearly equaling those available to the adult amputee. When selecting components for a child's prosthesis, the goals of minimal weight and high durability are often at odds, but both must be a priority to achieve a successful outcome.

The anatomy of a pediatric patient with a high-level lower limb amputation should be taken into special consideration when attempting to produce a good fitting and high-functioning prosthetic device because of a combination of factors, including body size and the cause of amputation. The small body size, particularly of a preteen, often

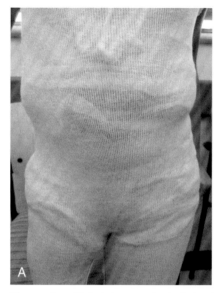
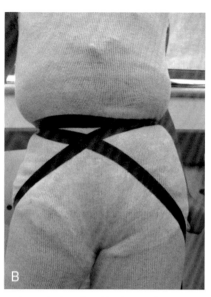

Figure 4 Clinical photographs depicting the casting technique for a hip disarticulation prosthesis. **A,** The patient with casting garment applied, providing little definition to the waist groove. **B,** Tape is applied to define and accentuate the waist groove.

provides only minimal surface area for weight bearing and control of the prosthesis. Structures such as the ischial tuberosity may be too small to provide sufficient surface area for a classic socket design. In some children, the anatomy may also create additional fitting complications, such as a child with a congenital hip disarticulation who has a nonfunctional proximal femoral segment or a child with a congenital transpelvic amputation with a partial but atrophic hemipelvis.

Casting and Modification

Although casting methods for hip disarticulation and transpelvic amputees are substantially different, both procedures start with a thorough physical examination. Whenever possible, this should include the examination of pelvic radiographs to provide a full understanding of the remaining bony structure. An interview with the patient and family is also indispensable in determining functional level and realistic goals, as well as providing appropriate education to patients and their families. Only after establishing this knowledge base should the casting process begin.

Hip Disarticulation

Prosthetic casting for the patient with a hip disarticulation should follow the principles applicable to an anatomic hip disarticulation socket.[31,32] This casting method relies primarily on containment of the hemipelvis, including the ischial tuberosity and pubic ramus. To obtain an intimate socket fit with this design, the patient is placed in a snug fitting casting sock suspended over the shoulders to maintain suspension. Electrical tape is then applied from the sound-side greater trochanter anteriorly around to lay superior to the iliac crest on the amputated side. The tape is then continued across the lumbar region and over the top of the sound-side iliac crest. Finally, the tape is continued across the midline, thus well defining the waistline above the iliac crest (**Figure 4**). This is an excellent method of defining the waist without distorting the shape of the impression through the use of tubing. Following this step, bony landmarks and areas of notable anatomy should be marked on the casting garment with an indelible marker and appropriate measurements taken.

Casting is now ready to begin. At the Shriners Hospital for Children in Portland, Oregon, a flexible fiberglass casting tape is used over plaster. This is a quick and clean method that provides excellent tissue compression while sacrificing very little in shape capture. When applying the casting medium, complete coverage of the amputated side, including the ischial tuberosity and the pubic ramus, is necessary. The cast should be extended completely around the waist to provide two distinct advantages: (1) It suspends and compresses the mold and (2) it will provide a mold for the pelvic support for the sound side. After the casting tape is applied, a casting stand may be used to provide weight bearing and stability while the clinician uses his or her hands to mold the contours of the socket. At this point in the casting procedure, anterior and posterior casting wedges should be used to achieve a snug anterior-posterior dimension.[33] For younger children, it may be more practical for a clinician to provide support and stability because the support surface of a casting stand may be too large for a child. The mold should be removed at the anterior midline. After removal, it should be examined to ensure that the appropriate shape has been captured. If the resulting cast does not have easily identifiable relief for all bony structures, recasting is necessary. This may appear to be an unnecessary step; however, when modifying an unfamiliar socket shape it is better to smooth than to sculpt.

Transpelvic Amputation

Casting of the child with a transpelvic amputation should be done using the suspension casting technique. This method of casting gives an excellent approximation of the hydrostatic pressures that the patient will experience in the prosthetic socket.[34,35] It has the added advantage of freeing the practitioner's hands to mold around any residual pelvic anatomy and give the cast the desired shape.

The process of casting the child with a transpelvic amputation begins with the application of a casting garment of sufficient strength to provide support for at least 50% of the patient's body weight because 50% or more of his or her weight will be supported by the sound-side lower limb. Any residual pelvic anatomy as well as the sound-side bony structures should then be marked with an indelible pen. The patient is then wrapped in casting media; fiberglass is recommended rather than plaster because fiberglass provides superior compression of the soft tissues. This mold should wrap around the sound side at the waist groove in the same manner as described for the hip disarticulation casting procedure. The medial border of the cast should be extended well past the midline of the body. This is important because the medial trim line of the socket will extend as far across the midline as possible to prevent herniation of the viscera.[36] After the casting material is applied, anterior and posterior casting blocks may be used to give the socket the appropriate shape. This increases control for the patient and creates the proper anterior shape for placement of the hip joint lamination plate.

Prior to filling and modification of the model, it should be checked against measurements taken at the time of molding. This is particularly important of the anterior-posterior dimension because this provides the basis for control of the prosthetic limb. If the anterior-posterior dimension of the cast is greater than the measurement, it can be decreased by cutting through the floor of the cast and overlapping the cut. This should allow sufficient adjustment to the anterior-posterior dimension. The cast should be then filled and modified as appropriate for the type of socket being fabricated.

Prosthetic Design
Ages 9 to 18 Months
At the time a child starts to demonstrate the desire to pull to stand, it is

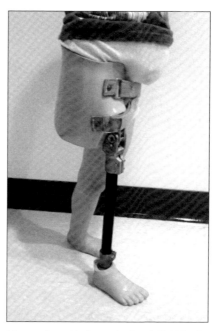

Figure 5 Photograph of an initial hip disarticulation prosthesis with a hip joint, no knee, and a basic foot. Note the anterior bulge of an ostomy bag, which further complicated this fitting.

appropriate to begin prosthetic treatment of a child with a high-level lower limb amputation. The child with amputation at this level may be delayed in reaching the pull-to-stand milestone, depending on the cause of amputation. For example, the child who has undergone amputation for tumor removal will likely be delayed because of extensive medical interventions and hospitalizations. It is also beneficial to begin educating the child's family as early as possible because this relationship will be extremely important in the ultimate success of prosthetic intervention. A simple lightweight design consisting of a laminated socket, hip joint, pylon, and foot is suggested (**Figure 5**). Examples of appropriate prosthetic hips would include the 7E8 hip joint and 3K51 Modular Hip Joint. Foot options include offerings by various manufacturers, such as Trulife, Kingsley MFG Company, and TRS. These foot prostheses are lightweight, simple, and stable, and they meet the needs of weight-bearing support appropriate for early locomotion.

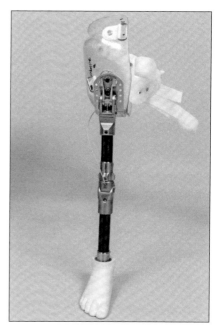

Figure 6 Anterior photographic view of a hip disarticulation prosthesis in the dynamic alignment phase. Components include a hip joint, a locking knee, and a basic foot.

Early gait often requires additional support in the form of furniture cruising, an appropriate push toy, or a walker. Children in this age group also greatly benefit from the intervention of a physical therapist, preferably with pediatric prosthetic experience.

Ages 18 to 48 Months
As the child grows, the first substantial change in prosthetic design is the addition of a monocentric manual locking knee (**Figure 6**), which provides the child with continued stability as well as allowing the knee to bend for sitting activities and eliminating the protrusion of the foot while sitting (a substantial drawback in a monolithic pylon system). Examples of this type of knee include the 3K41 knee (Euro International) or 3R30 knee (Ottobock). These and similar knees have the additional advantage of being very lightweight, thereby reducing the energy cost of gait. In contrast, patients in this age range with a transfemoral amputation would be fitted with an articulated knee.[37] Patients with

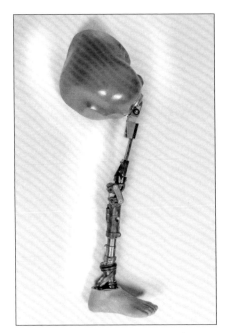

Figure 7 Lateral photograph of a hip disarticulation prosthesis with the Littig hip, a pneumatic knee, and a carbon fiber foot.

transfemoral amputations and knee disarticulations have better control of their prosthetic devices because of the longer lever arm of the prosthesis.

Ages 4 to 8 Years

As the child grows and matures, the transition to functional knees and more dynamic feet are appropriate next steps. The transition to a knee that flexes and extends as the prosthesis moves through the swing phase of gait allows a more natural and rapid gait.[38] An additional benefit can be gained by using a polycentric knee, which, when flexed, creates a functional shortening of the distal segment of the prosthesis. This in turn reduces the need for gait compensations such as vaulting and circumduction. Examples of this type of knee are the Total Knee Junior (Össur) and the PK-400 (TiMed). When selecting a knee for children in this age group, it is important to keep in mind the weight and durability of the component as well as the clearance above the foot because an overly long knee could result in uneven knee centers.

After the required prosthetic foot size exceeds approximately 13 cm, foot options expand. It is important to remember the balance between a dynamic foot and the stability necessary to control the hip and knee in stance. Examples of feet that provide this balance include the Truper Foot (College Park) or the Childs Play Foot (Trulife). These feet as well as other prosthetic feet provide the function necessary for a stable and efficient gait.

When a patient is transitioning from a locked knee to a functional prosthetic knee, it is highly beneficial for the patient to be treated by a physical therapist with experience in pediatric prosthetic gait training. The therapist can be a valuable resource and will greatly improve the likelihood of a successful prosthetic outcome.[39]

Ages 8 to 12 Years

For a child with a hip disarticulation or transpelvic amputation who is 8 to 12 years of age, a full spectrum of pediatric prosthetic components are available because body size is generally sufficiently large. These options include the pediatric Child's Play Littig Hip Disarticulation System, which allows for greater alignment adjustability and has a carbon fiber femoral pylon (**Figure 7**). This carbon strut functions to capture energy during stance, which is released during swing, resulting in a more energy efficient gait as well as a more natural path for the center of mass throughout the gait cycle.[40]

For children in this age range, prosthetic knee choices are similar to those available for children 4 to 8 years of age. Exceptions include four-bar pneumatic knees such as the TK-4P0C (DAW Industries). This type of knee is slightly longer than those previously mentioned and requires a greater body height for adequate clearance above the foot. These knees are advantageous because they functionally decrease in length when flexed and pneumatic control

allows greater control of the knee motion through the swing phase. The swing phase control is achieved with a smaller weight penalty compared with hydraulic-controlled knees, which is important in maintaining efficient gait. A few more prosthetic foot options are available, and more dynamic carbon fiber options are appropriate. Children of this age usually have adequate muscular strength and body awareness necessary to control a prosthetic hip and knee over a more dynamic foot. When selecting components for a specific patient, it is important to keep in mind not only the patient's needs and desires but the interplay of the components and their increasing complexity.

Ages 13 to 21 Years

The principles applicable to patients aged 13 to 21 years also applies to very active patients of all ages with high-level lower limb amputations. As pediatric patients enter this age group, they approach adult stature, but their body mass is usually less than that of adults. This is especially true for female patients, who physically mature approximately 2 years ahead of males.[41] For a pediatric patient with a nearly adult-sized body, the full spectrum of adult components is available for use in creating the appropriate prosthesis.

The socket can now be altered to include the use of soft thermoplastics or gel to provide increased comfort and improved pressure distribution. In this older pediatric population, the objections to using such materials are negated because the prosthesis represents a smaller percentage of total body mass and therefore has a smaller relative drag on walking efficiency. The use of many types of materials may be appropriate if the goals of comfort and prosthetic control are maintained. Alterations can range from the simple addition of gel in the area of the ischial tuberosity and ramus to a full flexible inner socket with a rigid frame to a complete custom gel interface. The needs of the patient should be paramount in making decisions, keeping in mind that socket discomfort is the primary reason for rejection of hip disarticulation or transpelvic prostheses.[20]

The selection of a hip joint for these patients is limited to the few hip joints on the market, which have changed little from the first hip joints used in the early 1950s. This is true with the notable exceptions of the Child's Play Littig Hip Disarticulation System and the Helix 3D hip (Ottobock). The former device, which was described earlier, is a single-axis hip that incorporates a carbon fiber strut to capture and return energy to increase the efficiency of gait. The Helix 3D hip is a polycentric joint with hydraulic control of both the swing and stance phases of gait. In addition, this joint is designed to link hip flexion and extension with transverse plane hip rotation.[42] These design advantages allow for the functional shortening of the prosthesis during swing through the use of a polycentric mechanism and a gait pattern that very closely simulates that of able-bodied peers.[26,42] Drawbacks to the Helix 3D hip include cost and the necessity to use the C-leg knee (Ottobock) and a compatible foot (also from Ottobock). Another potential drawback is the incompatibility of a microprocessor-controlled knee with the lifestyle of many pediatric patients, which can potentially expose the device to water and dirt. The patient must also be responsible enough to routinely charge the device. Although these knees have proven beneficial in some patients, the use of microprocessor components in lower limb prostheses is not recommended until the later teenage years when growth is complete.

Multiaxial knees with either pneumatic or hydraulic control of the swing phase of gait may also be appropriate for patients in this age group. Although hydraulic knees can be an excellent choice, they are slightly heavier than pneumatic knees, which may be a consideration particularly in a patient with a low body mass. Knees in this category include the 1325A knee (ST&G Corporation) and the Total Knee 2000/2100 (Össur). An additional knee choice is a knee similar to the KX06 knee (Endolite), which provides hydraulic control of both the swing and stance phases while maintaining a polycentric design that is important to toe clearance.

Patients in this age group may also benefit from the addition of a rotation adaptor such as the 4R57 (Ottobock). This component, which is typically installed directly above the prosthetic knee, allows the patient to rotate the prosthetic leg a full 360° at that point. This allows a patient to more easily enter the front seat of a car or to cross his or her legs. This device also allows the patient to move the prosthetic foot away from the gas and brake pedals when driving an automobile.

The choice of a prosthetic foot should be dictated by the activity level of the patient and his or her need for more stability or more mobility. Because it is important to carefully consider how the function of the foot will affect the other components in the prosthesis, the foot should be the last of the major components selected when formulating a prosthetic prescription. For example, the use of a carbon fiber foot with a long spring, such as the Silhouette (Freedom Innovations), may induce a greater knee flexion moment at heel strike while creating enhanced energy return as the patient transitions from terminal stance into swing. This provides a more dynamic but less stable prosthesis, which may be entirely appropriate for a highly active patient. However, the selection of a Trustep foot (College Park), which has greater heel compliance, decreases the knee flexion moment at heel strike and produces a more biomechanically stable prosthesis that may be more appropriate for a patient who requires more stability because of activity level or environment.

Summary

Both the surgical approach and subsequent prosthetic fitting can be quite challenging in a pediatric patient with a hip disarticulation or a transpelvic amputation. These children require an individualized approach depending on the integrity of their remaining tissue. The initial amputation procedure should concentrate on preserving as much bony skeleton as possible and, in young children, preserving the critical growth plates to enhance functional benefits as the child ages. Most of these children require a multidisciplinary team approach, both in the initial acute phase of treatment and until skeletal maturity and beyond.

The successful fitting of hip disarticulation or transpelvic prosthetic devices in pediatric patients is a complex task. Successful prosthesis use can be confounded by limitations in available componentry, extreme levels of activity, and the ever-changing body of the growing child. The constantly changing pediatric patient will require closer follow-up than an adult patient as well as the establishment of a positive, trusting relationship with both the patient and his or her family. Success is determined by careful attention to the needs of the specific pediatric patient and his or her family as well as socket fit, component selection, alignment, and the expertise of the members of the medical team.

References

1. Shurr D, Coot T, Buckwalter J, Cooper R: Hip disarticulation: A prosthetic follow-up. *Orthot Prosthet* 1983;37(3):50-57. Available at: http://www.oandplibrary.org/op/1983_03_050.asp. Accessed November 24, 2015.

2. Jeans KA, Browne RH, Karol LA: Effect of amputation level on energy expenditure during overground walking by children with an

amputation. *J Bone Joint Surg Am* 2011;93(1):49-56.

3. Bramer JA, Taminiau AH: Reconstruction of the pelvic ring with an autograft after hindquarter amputation: Improvement of sitting stability and prosthesis support. *Acta Orthop* 2005;76(3):453-454.

4. Canavese F, Krajbich JI, LaFleur BJ: Orthopaedic sequelae of childhood meningococcemia: Management considerations and outcome. *J Bone Joint Surg Am* 2010;92(12):2196-2203.

5. Labler L, Trentz O: The use of vacuum assisted closure (VAC) in soft tissue injuries after high energy pelvic trauma. *Langenbecks Arch Surg* 2007;392(5):601-609.

6. Boehmler JH, Francis SH, Grawe RK, Mayerson JL: Reconstruction of an external hemipelvectomy defect with a two-stage fillet of leg-free flap. *J Reconstr Microsurg* 2010;26(4):271-276.

7. Eldridge JC, Armstrong PF, Krajbich JI: Amputation stump lengthening with the Ilizarov technique: A case report. *Clin Orthop Relat Res* 1990;256:76-79.

8. Park HW, Jahng JS, Hahn SB, Shin DE: Lengthening of an amputation stump by the Ilizarov technique: A case report. *Int Orthop* 1997;21(4):274-276.

9. Sara T, Kour AK, Das De S, Rauff A, Pho RW: Wound cover in a hindquarter amputation with a free flap from the amputated limb: A case report. *Clin Orthop Relat Res* 1994;304:248-251.

10. Carter SR, Eastwood DM, Grimer RJ, Sneath RS: Hindquarter amputation for tumours of the musculoskeletal system. *J Bone Joint Surg Br* 1990;72(3):490-493.

11. Gebert C, Gosheger G, Winkelmann W: Hip transposition as a universal surgical procedure for periacetabular tumors of the pelvis. *J Surg Oncol* 2009;99(3):169-172.

12. Griesser MJ, Gillette B, Crist M, et al: Internal and external hemipelvectomy or flail hip in patients with sarcomas: Quality-of-life and functional outcomes. *Am J Phys Med Rehabil* 2012;91(1):24-32.

13. Grimer RJ, Chandrasekar CR, Carter SR, Abudu A, Tillman RM, Jeys L: Hindquarter amputation: Is it still needed and what are the outcomes? *Bone Joint J* 2013;95-B(1):127-131.

14. Han I, Lee YM, Cho HS, Oh JH, Lee SH, Kim HS: Outcome after surgical treatment of pelvic sarcomas. *Clin Orthop Surg* 2010;2(3):160-166.

15. Wirbel RJ, Schulte M, Mutschler WE: Surgical treatment of pelvic sarcomas: Oncologic and functional outcome. *Clin Orthop Relat Res* 2001;390:190-205.

16. Apffelstaedt JP, Driscoll DL, Spellman JE, Velez AF, Gibbs JF, Karakousis CP: Complications and outcome of external hemipelvectomy in the management of pelvic tumors. *Ann Surg Oncol* 1996;3(3):304-309.

17. Hillmann A, Hoffmann C, Gosheger G, Rödl R, Winkelmann W, Ozaki T: Tumors of the pelvis: Complications after reconstruction. *Arch Orthop Trauma Surg* 2003;123(7):340-344.

18. Brandt MM, Corpron CA, Wahl WL: Necrotizing soft tissue infections: A surgical disease. *Am Surg* 2000;66(10):967-970, discussion 970-971.

19. Nowroozi F, Salvanelli ML, Gerber LH: Energy expenditure in hip disarticulation and hemipelvectomy amputees. *Arch Phys Med Rehabil* 1983;64(7):300-303.

20. New York University: *Lower-Extremity Prosthetics*, New York, NY, New York University, 1973.

21. Schnall BL, Baum BS, Andrews AM: Gait characteristics of a soldier with a traumatic hip disarticulation. *Phys Ther* 2008;88(12):1568-1577.

22. Hector WK, Newman JD: Relative incidences of new amputations: Statistical comparisons of 6,000 new amputees. *Orthot Prosthet* 1975;29(2):3-16. Available at: http://www.oandplibrary.org/op/1975_02_003.asp. Accessed November 24, 2015.

23. Glattly HW: A statistical study of 12,000 new amputees. *South Med J* 1964;57(11):1373-1378.

24. Radcliffe CW: The biomechanics of the Canadian-type hip-disarticulation prosthesis. *Artif Limbs* 1957;4(2):29-38.

25. Raiford RL, Epps CH Jr: Experiences with the Canadian hip disarticulation prosthesis in the juvenile. *J Natl Med Assoc* 1974;66(1):71-75.

26. Solomonidis SE, Loughran AJ, Taylor J, Paul JP: Biomechanics of the hip disarticulation prosthesis. *Prosthet Orthot Int* 1977;1(1):13-18.

27. Zaffer SM, Braddom RL, Conti A, Goff J, Bokma D: Total hip disarticulation prosthesis with suction socket: Report of two cases. *Am J Phys Med Rehabil* 1999;78(2):160-162.

28. Sabolicn J, Guth T: The CAT-CAM-H.D.(tm): A new design for hip disarticulation patients. *Clin Orthot Prosthet* 1988;12(3):119-122.

29. Littig D, Lundt J: The UCLA Anatomical Hip Disarticulation Prosthesis. *Clin Orthot Prosthet* 1988;12(3):114-118.

30. Houdek MT, Kralovec ME, Andrews KL: Hemipelvectomy: High-level amputation surgery and prosthetic rehabilitation. *Am J Phys Med Rehabil* 2014;93(7):600-608.

31. Pasquina P, Cooper R: *Care of the Combat Amputee*, Washington, DC, Office of the Surgeon General, 2009

32. van der Waarde T, Michael JW: Hip disarticulation and transpelvic amputation: Prosthetic management, in Bowker J, Michael J, eds: *Atlas of Limb Prosthetics: Surgical, Prosthetic,*

and Rehabilitation Principles, ed 2. St. Louis, MO, Mosby-Year Book, 2002.

33. Stark G: Overview of hip disarticulation prostheses. J Prosthet Orthot 2001;13:50-53.

34. Fernández A, Formigo J: Are Canadian prostheses used? A long-term experience. Prosthet Orthot Int 2005;29(2):177-181.

35. Wilk B, Karol L, Halliday S, Cummings D, Haideri N, Stephenson J: Transition to an articulating knee prosthesis in pediatric amputees. J Prosthet Orthot 1999;11:69-74.

36. Average Weight for Children by Age. Available at: http://www.buzzle.com/articles/average-weight-for-children-by-age.html. Accessed October 7, 2015.

37. Isakov E, Susak Z, Becker E: Energy expenditure and cardiac response in above-knee amputees while using prostheses with open and locked knee mechanisms. Scand J Rehabil Med Suppl 1985;12:108-111.

38. Lundt J, Littig D, Choi G: The Littig Strut Hip Disarticulation System: An improvement in energy cost for the unilateral hip disarticulation prosthesis user. Orthopaedie Technik 1995.

39. Tanner JM: Foetus Into Man: Physical Growth From Conception to Maturity. London, UK, Castelmead Publications, 1989, pp 6-23.

40. Blumentritt S, Ludwigs E, Bellman M, Boiten H: The new Helix 3D hip joint. Orthopadie Technik 2008 2-5.

41. Ludwigs E, Bellmann M, Schmalz T, Blumentritt S: Biomechanical differences between two exoprosthetic hip joint systems during level walking. Prosthet Orthot Int 2010;34(4):449-460.

42. Rommers GM, Vos LD, Groothoff JW, Eisma WH: Clinical rehabilitation of the amputee: A retrospective study. Prosthet Orthot Int 1996;20(2):72-78.

Chapter 79

Rotationplasty: Surgical Techniques and Prosthetic Considerations

Joseph Ivan Krajbich, MD, FRCS(C)   *Sabrina Jakobson Huston, CPO*

Abstract

Rotationplasty is a surgical technique that maximizes the functional potential of children and young adults who have a high-level terminal amputation or were born with a significant intercalary lower limb deficiency, such as proximal femoral focal deficiency. It is helpful to be familiar with the surgical techniques for acquired and congenital deficiencies and prosthetic management of the residual limb.

Keywords: Aitken types A through D; limb salvage; osteosarcoma; proximal femoral focal deficiency; rotationplasty

Introduction

Rotationplasty, which is also referred to in the literature as a Borggreve procedure, a Van Nes rotationplasty, or a tibial or femoral turnaround procedure, has undergone several modifications since its original description. The principle of rotationplasty, however, remains the same: A healthy, functional joint (usually the ankle) is used as a substitute for the loss of a more proximal joint (usually the knee). For the ankle to function as a biologic knee substitute, it must be brought up to the level of the contralateral knee and turned 180° to function in the plane and range of a normal knee (**Figure 1**). The foot distal to the ankle joint is then a below-knee component of the limb and is fitted with a transtibial-like prosthesis (**Figure 2**). Ideally, the child's function then resembles that of a patient who has undergone a transtibial amputation.

Borggreve[1] first described the procedure in 1930 for a patient with tuberculosis of the knee. In the 1950s, Van Nes[2] published his variation of the procedure, which was used for congenital limb deficiency. Rotationplasty and its subsequent modification gained some popularity for the treatment of congenital femoral deficiencies,[3-5] most frequently proximal femoral focal deficiency (PFFD), and are used in several pediatric orthopaedic centers, primarily in North America and Europe. In the late 1970s in Vienna, Austria, Salzer et al[6] modified the procedure for limb salvage in patients with osteosarcoma of the distal femur. The procedure was further adapted for use in limb salvage of limbs with tumor in the proximal tibia and also in lesions involving the proximal femur, where the rotated knee can be used as a substitute for a hip joint. Since then, rotationplasty has been applied in a variety of conditions where the distal part of the limb with the functional distal joint can be salvaged, but a proximal joint cannot be salvaged. The greatest barrier to the wider acceptance of this technique appears to be unfamiliarity with the procedure.[7-9]

In addition to a cooperative patient, an optimal functional outcome in these procedures requires a successful surgical outcome, a diligent rehabilitation regimen, and expert prosthetic fitting. The rotationplasty prosthesis, albeit relatively inexpensive in terms of the prosthetic components, requires significant expertise on the part of the prosthetist to achieve a functionally optimal outcome.

Surgical Considerations
Indications

The primary reason for rotationplasty, compared with a transfemoral amputation, is to provide a patient with a biologic knee substitute that would improve gait efficiency, energy consumption of ambulation, and the ability to walk on uneven surfaces. Ideally, the resulting function is very similar to that of a transtibial amputation.

The indications for rotationplasty or its various modifications can be classified into two main categories: (1) congenital lower limb deficiency (usually but not always PFFD) and (2) acquired deficiency with rotationplasty as a form of limb salvage. The underlying condition is most frequently a malignant tumor in a child or a young adult, but it also is used for other etiologies, such as trauma, infection, and the failure of previous limb salvage or reconstruction procedures.

Dr. Krajbich or an immediate family member is a member of a speakers' bureau or has made paid presentations on behalf of K2m and serves as a board member, owner, officer, or committee member of the Association of Children's Prosthetic and Orthotic Clinics and the Scoliosis Research Society. Neither Ms. Jakobson Huston nor any immediate family member has received anything of value from or has stock or stock options held in a commercial company or institution related directly or indirectly to the subject of this chapter.

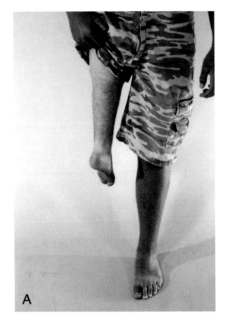 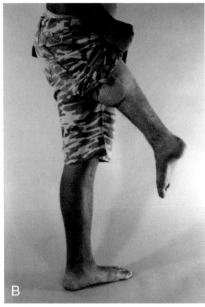

Figure 1 AP (**A**) and lateral (**B**) clinical photographs of a male patient treated with rotationplasty.

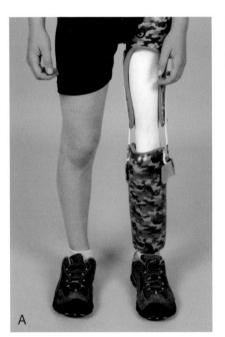 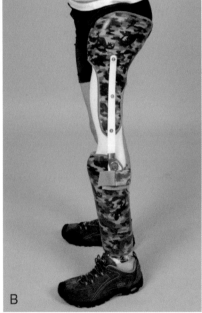

Figure 2 Clinical photographs of front (**A**) and side (**B**) views of a child with a rotationplasty prosthesis.

The surgical technique differs for each category, so each has a separate description in this chapter. However, some general principles apply to both categories.

Prerequisites

The joint to be transferred or rotated must have functional range of motion, and its nerve supply must be intact. Vascular supply to the distal part of the limb must be preservable or reconstructible. Motor supply to the newly reconstructed joint must be present and functional.

Absolute Contraindications

The absolute contraindications are a failure to satisfy the prerequisites. A poorly perfused or insensate foot with restricted range of motion is a poor substitute for other reconstructive methods or a modern transfemoral prosthesis. The procedure is contraindicated in patients with malignant tumors where adequate oncological resection margins do not allow for major nerve preservation.

Relative Contraindications

The relative contraindications are primarily subjective. In the opinion of one this chapter's authors (JIK), the primary reason that this procedure is not more widely performed, particularly in patients with PFFD and young (first and second decade) patients with cancer, is the treating surgeon's unfamiliarity with the procedure. The somewhat odd appearance of the reconstructed limb can occasionally be a deterrent. Functional expectations, particularly in patients with a tumor, also play an important role.[10] An active lifestyle versus a relatively sedentary lifestyle with potential multiple reoperations in the future may weigh on the child and any parental decision regarding the procedure chosen. The patient and the family must be comfortable with the decision to proceed with the proposed surgical approach. A lack of appropriate prosthetic services also is a relative contraindication; however, this criterion should be limited only to very underserved areas or countries. The prosthetic componentry is relatively simple, and the skill for making the prosthesis is acquirable and learnable. Having a well-functioning rotationplasty limb and prosthesis allows excellent function resembling that of a transtibial amputation. Having a functioning biologic knee-like joint provides for improved energy consumption in gait and improved agility and ability to walk on uneven surfaces.[11-15]

Rotationplasty for Children With PFFD

PFFD is a congenital abnormality of the femur that varies in severity from a deficit primarily in the subtrochanteric region of the femur to virtual complete absence of the femur[16-20] (**Figure 3**). For the purpose of this discussion, only true PFFD versus congenital short femur as described by Gillespie and Torode[21] will be considered. The most frequently used PFFD classification was developed by Aitken,[22] and all four types (A through D) are potentially suitable for rotationplasty if the child has a relatively normal foot and ankle complex. The presence or absence (or various degrees of dysplasia) of the hip is not a contraindication to the procedure. In patients with a reconstructible hip (Aitken types A and B), hip reconstruction is usually performed as a second procedure 1 or 2 years later. In addition, in normalizing the hip joint, the procedure allows for fine-tuning of the rotationplasty as to the length and rotation of the new thigh.[23]

The rotationplasty procedure has been modified several times since first being introduced by Van Nes.[2] Initially, the rotation was performed through the diaphysis of the tibia and the fibula, either alone or combined with knee fusion.[4,5,24] The addition of knee fusion has been a major contribution to the surgical treatment of PFFD, with or without rotationplasty. It was first described by King and Marks[25] and has become a standard part of PFFD treatment.[25-27] A single-bone thigh is aligned under the hip joint, thus allowing for restoration of the biomechanical axis of the limb in the sagittal plane.[25-27] Taking advantage of knee fusion, Gillespie and Torode[28,29] incorporated a substantial portion of the rotation through the knee fusion and the remainder through

the tibial diaphysis.[30] Still, the relatively common phenomena of derotation led one of this chapter's authors (JIK) to modify the procedure even further. In most patients, the entire rotation is carried through the knee fusion, which necessitates detachment of all vascular and tendon structures crossing the knee joint and careful mobilization of the neurovascular bundles to ensure a viable functional limb.[23]

Surgical Technique

The child is placed on a radiotranslucent table in a supine position, with the affected limb draped free. The posterior tibial and anterior tibial arterial pulses are marked on the skin for easy location and later monitoring. A "lazy S" incision is made over the knee area starting proximally and laterally, crossing the knee anteriorly at the level of the joint and curving medially and distally. The practice of one of this chapter's authors (JIK) is to first identify and dissect free the peroneal nerve on the lateral side. The biceps femoris and pes anserinus muscles and tendons are divided at the level of the knee joint. The two heads of the gastrocnemius muscles are detached as close to their origin on the femoral condyles as possible. Care must be taken not to disrupt the nerve supply to the gastrocnemius muscle because this muscle, together with the soleus, will become the reconstructed knee's primary extensor. This process allows for good visualization of the popliteal fossa neurovascular bundle. The patellar tendon is then divided, and complete capsulotomy of the knee joint is performed, carefully protecting the posterior neurovascular structures. The collateral and cruciate ligaments, if present, also are divided. The remaining muscular structures (semimembranosus and popliteus) are then identified and divided, which allows for good exposure of the popliteal artery and vein, which are further mobilized by dividing the geniculate branches. The distal femoral epiphysis

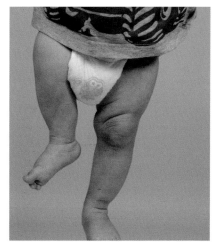

Figure 3 Clinical photograph of a young child with proximal femoral focal deficiency before rotationplasty.

and metaphysis and the proximal tibial epiphysis and portions of the metaphysis are thus exposed. The proximal tibial epiphysis together with the physis and a small portion of the metaphysis (approximately 5 mm) are excised with a saw. Likewise, the distal femoral epiphysis together with its physis and a portion of metaphysis are excised. The extent of the metaphyseal excision is guided by the ease of rotation of the distal part of the extremity. Complete 180° rotation must be achievable without vascular compromise. The previously marked peripheral pulses are carefully monitored with a sterile Doppler probe. Any compromise in circulation must be addressed by additional dissection and mobilization of the vessels and/or additional shortening of the femoral metaphysis.

The procedure is then completed by arthrodesis of the tibia, which is rotated 180° to the femur using intramedullary fixation of a Rush rod and securing the rotation alignment with either a cross pin or a small plate (**Figure 4**). Maintaining good vascular perfusion as monitored by Doppler is critical at this stage. Any compromise must be addressed immediately by further vessel decompression and mobilization. In very rare instances, the rotation can be controlled by cast immobilization

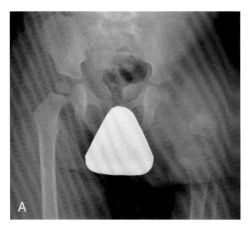
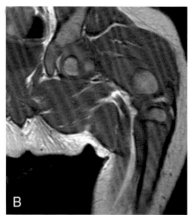
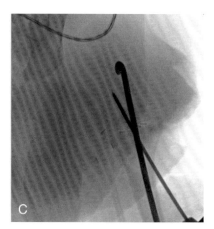

Figure 4 AP radiograph (**A**) and MRI (**B**) of a child with left-sided proximal femoral focal deficiency (Aitken type B). **C,** Intraoperative radiograph of the same child with a completed rotationplasty. A Rush rod and cross pin were used to control the rotation.

without an internal cross pin, allowing less-than-perfect rotation but obviating the need for implants. The final desired rotation can be achieved in 1 or 2 weeks during a cast change under anesthesia.

Before skin closure, the distal portion of the quadriceps is attached to the gastrocnemius to maximize knee extension power. Skin closure is sometimes facilitated with the trimming of excess skin.

Postoperative Care

The child's limb is immobilized in a hip spica-like dressing or a cast for 6 weeks, after which intensive rehabilitation with physical therapy is started (**Figure 5**). After both the arthrodesis and soft tissue are healed, the child is fitted with a rotationplasty prosthesis and begins physical therapy–guided gait training.

Alternative Technique

Brown[31] described a modification of the rotationplasty technique for patients with Aitken types C and D longitudinal deficiencies of the femur in an attempt to provide such patients with a stable hip. Arthrodesis of the distal femur to the side of the pelvis is performed with the leg rotated 180°, similar to the procedure described by Winkelmann[32] for tumors of the proximal femur and the hip (as described later in this chapter). Frequently, a very short femoral segment and an abnormal knee in these higher grade PFFDs limits the number of patients suitable for this procedural variant.[31,33]

Rotationplasty as a Limb Salvage Procedure

Rotationplasty has been used in limb salvage surgery for malignant tumors of the lower limb.[34] The procedure allows for wide margins in tumor resection similar to that accomplished by high transfemoral amputation if the sciatic nerve can be preserved without compromising tumor-free margins. The blood supply to the distal part of the limb can be spared by dissecting the femoral artery free (if tumor-free margins can be attained) or resecting the vessel together with the tumor and restoring circulation by anatomizing the proximal femoral artery and vein to the popliteal artery and vein.[6,34,35]

Surgical Technique

As with most tumor resection procedures, careful procedural planning is just as important as the actual surgical execution. Careful staging of the lesion with detailed MRIs showing the tumor extension, particularly near the neurovascular structure, is critical in determining which vessels to preserve or resect. One of this chapter's authors

(JIK) routinely obtains full-length radiographs of both lower limbs to plan the level of bone osteotomies in the proximal tibia and femur. The goal of the procedure is to have the thighs of equal (or very near equal) length at the end of the procedure.[36] The new rotationplasty thigh consists of the hip joint, the proximal femoral fragment, the tibia minus the proximal epiphysis, and portions of the metaphysis with the ankle joint. A relatively common mistake is to make the new thigh too long (not enough resection), which detracts from both cosmetic appearance and the functional result of the limb. To prevent these problems, the femur should be transected just below the lesser trochanter and the attachment of gluteus maximus muscles, and several centimeters of the proximal tibia also are resected.

In the operating room, the patient is placed on the operating table in the supine position, and the surgical limb is draped free from the toes to almost the umbilicus to ensure easy access to the proximal femoral and external iliac arteries.

Skin incisions are marked on the thigh, planning cylindroid resection of the skin of the mid and distal thigh (**Figure 6**). More obliquely oriented incisions are required distally to account for the relative diameter mismatch of the

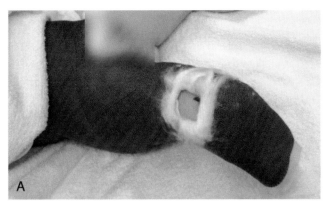 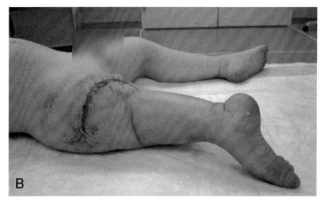

Figure 5   **A,** Clinical photograph of postoperative hip spica cast immobilization. **B,** Clinical photograph of early healing with postoperative appearance.

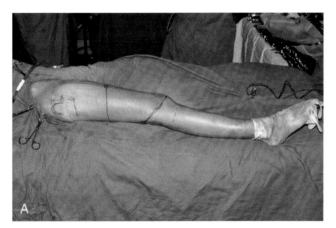 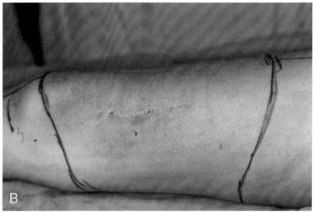

Figure 6   **A,** Intraoperative photograph of planned incision for rotationplasty in a patient with a lower limb tumor. **B,** Intraoperative photograph of the biopsy track, which is easily removed with the resected tumor.)

distal limb for all rotationplasty amputations. Incisions are extended vertically, proximally, and distally. Proximally, the extension is placed anterolaterally, allowing access to both the anterior vessels and lateral part of the proximal femur. Distally, the extension is medial, allowing for access to the medial part of the proximal tibia for ease of reconstruction. Additional skin incisions are made in the cylindroid portion (which will be resected) to gain easy access to the structure(s) to be preserved (the sciatic nerve and the femoral popliteal artery and veins).

The saphenous vein is frequently dissected and preserved to obtain additional venous drainage of the limb. All the muscles of the thigh are transected at the level of the planned proximal femoral osteotomy. The fascia lata

can be transected somewhat further distally so that it can be used for lateral thigh reconstruction in the future. Distally, the pes anserinus tendons are transected at the level of the tibial osteotomy, and the biceps femoris is detached from the fibular head. Care must be taken to protect and carefully mobilize the peroneal nerve at its entry into the anterior compartment of the leg. The heads of the gastrocnemius are transected near their origin on the femoral condyles. Maintaining appropriate tumor resection margins is critical at this stage and dictates the proximal extent of transection. Every care must be taken not to violate the tumor margin and preserve the nerve supply of the gastrocnemius because it exits the posterior tibial nerve. The patellar tendon is detached distally without entering the

knee joint proper. The sciatic nerve is dissected free posteriorly along its entire exposed length. The femoral popliteal artery and vein are dissected free if the tumor margins allow; if not, the vessels are isolated proximally and distally, and after the femoral and tibial osteotomies are completed, the vessels are divided to be reanastomosed. A portion of the thigh and the knee containing the tumor is removed after final transection of the soft tissue (popliteus muscle and periosteum at the tibial osteotomy site), while carefully protecting the trifurcation branches of the popliteal vessels.

The thigh is then reconstructed by bringing the leg portion proximally, internally rotating it 180°, and internally fixing the proximal femoral fragment to the proximal tibia (**Figure 7**). If the vessels were resected, vascular anastomosis

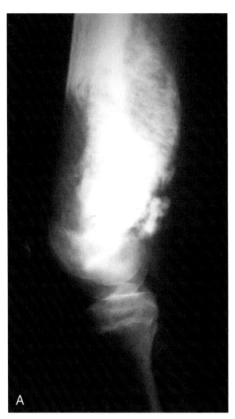
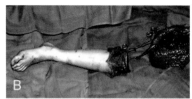
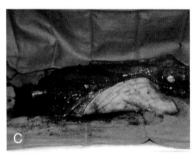
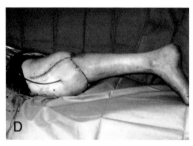

Figure 7 Preoperative and intraoperative images from a child with a diagnosis of osteosarcoma. **A,** Preoperative lateral radiograph shows distal femoral osteosarcoma. **B,** Intraoperative photograph of the distal part of the limb connected only by the sciatic nerve. The femoral artery and vein were resected with the tumor part, and the child will have vascular reanastomosis. **C,** Intraoperative photograph of the resected portion of the thigh, including the tumor. **D,** Intraoperative photograph of extremity appearance at the conclusion of the surgical procedure. Normal neurovascular function of the distal limb is checked before leaving the operating room.

is now performed to reestablish circulation to the limb. Relatively little is needed in terms of remaining muscle and soft-tissue reconstruction. The vessels, if preserved, and the sciatic nerve are gently coiled around the muscles, avoiding sharp kinks. The iliotibial band is anchored to the tibia to stabilize the lateral side, and the gastrocnemius heads are attached to the remaining proximal portion of the quadriceps. Skin flaps are trimmed for easy closure and closed in layers over a drain; a hip spica-like dressing is applied.[37]

For lesions arising in the proximal tibia, the procedure has been modified to allow for resection of most of the tibia, leaving only the distal metaphysis and the ankle joint (**Figure 8**). Proximally, the osteotomy is through the distal femoral metaphysis. The reconstruction is somewhat more complex because the new ankle/knee is powered by the thigh musculature. Good balance between the dorsiflexors (knee flexors) and the plantar flexors (quadriceps) must be achieved[38,39] (**Figure 9**). As a rule, patients with this reconstruction require a longer period of rehabilitation to maximize their new knee/ankle function compared with more commonly performed rotationplasty for distal femoral lesions. However, in the experience of one of the authors of this chapter (JIK), their eventual function is superior because

the powerful thigh muscles (quadriceps and hamstrings) power the new knee. Their gait in the prosthesis is indistinguishable from those who have a transtibial amputation.

Rotationplasty also has been adopted for reconstruction after tumor resection of lesions of the proximal femur involving the hip joint. In this situation, nearly the whole femur, including the femoral head and possibly the acetabulum, is resected together with the thigh soft tissues. The distal femoral metaphysis is then attached (via arthrodesis) to the pelvis after being rotated 180°. This allows the original knee to function as a uniplanar hip joint (flexion/extension), and the ankle again functions as a new knee joint (**Figure 10**). The gluteus maximus is reattached to the quadriceps tendon to provide hip extension, and the iliopsoas, the tensor fascia lata, and the sartorius are used for the new hip flexion.[32,40,41]

Most of these procedures are performed for malignant tumors requiring major resection to maximize a child's chances for survival. However, other etiologies, such as early or late failure of other limb-sparing reconstructions, including infection, tumor recurrence, the failure of endoprosthetic replacement, or a massive allograft replacement, can be salvaged with rotationplasty (**Figures 11** and **12**). Likewise, massive tissue loss of the proximal part of the limb because of trauma or infection can be salvaged by rotationplasty if the alternative is a high-level amputation.

Rehabilitation

As would be expected, regardless of etiology, these procedures require a substantial period of recovery and rehabilitation. Gradual progression from gentle range-of-motion exercises, gradual strengthening, and, finally, gait training with the new rotationplasty prosthesis require substantial time and care from the physiotherapy and prosthetic teams.

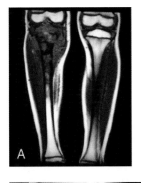
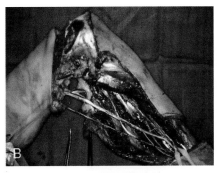
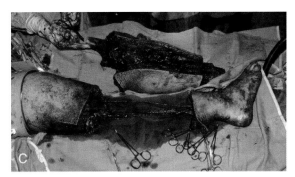

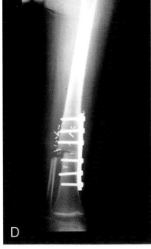
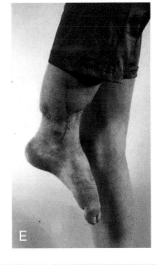

Figure 8 Images from a patient with osteosarcoma involving the proximal half of the tibia and the knee. **A,** Coronal cut MRI shows a large osteosarcoma with bone destruction and soft-tissue extension in the right proximal tibia. **B,** Intraoperative photograph of dissection that is isolating the neurovascular structures to be preserved. **C,** Intraoperative photograph of removal of the tumor. A wide margin is obtained throughout. **D,** AP radiograph at completion of the rotationplasty. **E,** Clinical photograph of the healed limb.

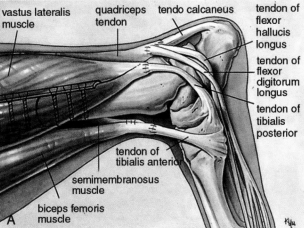
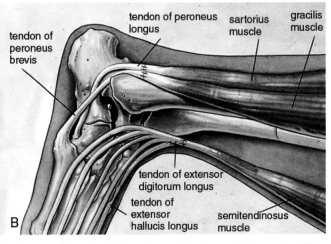

Figure 9 Illustrations of individual tendon-muscle reattachments in the case of rotationplasty performed for a tumor in the proximal tibia. **A,** Lateral view. **B,** Medial view.

Prosthetic Considerations

Advancements in limb salvage surgery have given the patient with a lower limb tumor more treatment options. In the past, children with a diagnosis of malignant tumors of the lower limbs usually faced amputation of the affected limb. Transfemoral amputation, hip disarticulation, or transpelvic amputation were the typical outcomes.[42]

Being a rare congenital deformity, PFFD is characterized by an incomplete or absent femur. It can be unilateral or bilateral. Fibular hemimelia is often associated with the condition, occurring in 70% to 80% of the PFFD population.[37] Surgery and prosthetic intervention are necessary for bipedal ambulation for a child with unilateral PFFD.[37]

Rotationplasty is an option for children with tumors of the distal or proximal third of the femur and the proximal

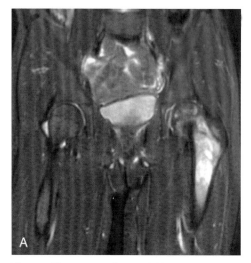
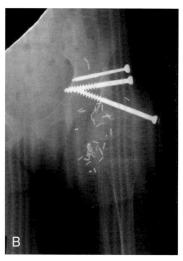

Figure 10 **A,** MRI from a child with Ewing sarcoma of the proximal femur. **B,** AP radiograph from a patient after rotationplasty. The patient had a distal femoral epiphysiodesis as a second procedure after chemotherapy was completed.

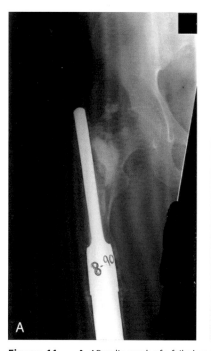
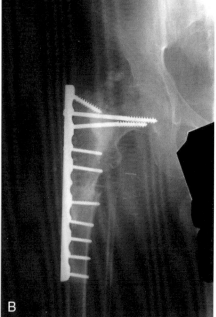

Figure 11 **A,** AP radiograph of a failed endoprosthesis in a patient with osteosarcoma. **B,** AP radiograph of the limb after being salvaged with rotationplasty.

tibia[42] and congenital PFFD. Clinically, the patient has a foot rotated 180° and an ankle that functions as a knee (**Figure 1**). The advantage of rotationplasty versus a Syme disarticulation in the child with PFFD—or proximal leg amputations for children with lower limb tumors—is the elimination of a mechanical prosthetic knee. Studies have reported more efficient energy-efficient ambulation after rotationplasty than with a mechanical knee.[7,11,12]

For children who have undergone rotationplasty because of tumor resection or PFFD, the prostheses are similar, but the design and the fit may differ. Because the population of patients with a rotationplasty is relatively small, only a limited number of prosthetists have experience in fitting rotationplasty prostheses. The collaboration of an experienced multidisciplinary team is paramount for a positive prosthetic outcome.

Prosthesis Molding

In preparation for molding the prosthesis, a pantaloon-style garment should be tailored to aid in the molding process and for the patient's modesty. With the patient standing, the residual limb is molded in a vertically extended position, with the foot in maximum hyper plantar flexion and the hips square to the body. If the patient is unable to stand, he or she should lie on his or her sound side, with the hips stacked, the limb in line with the torso, and the foot in maximum plantar flexion. On the pantaloon-style garment, the sulcus, the medial and lateral malleoli, the calcaneal tuberosity, the navicular, and the sustentaculum tali should be referenced. If a cut strip is used to remove the mold, it should be placed in a posterior position to avoid distorting bony prominences.

For the patient with PFFD, the shape of the thigh should be captured by wrapping one turn around the waist and then continuing to wrap the residual limb proximally to distally. Stability and flexibility of the hip are critical in the patient with Aitken types C and D deficiency.[18] The socket will resemble a ship's funnel shape,[42] having a high lateral wall to contain the residual tissue. The patient with a lower limb tumor may not require a thigh section as high as the ischial level. The wrap should be started above the level of the surgical site. While the molding material is still soft, the prosthetist places the web of his or her hand on the distal plantar calcaneus and his or her thumb in the sustentaculum tali.

The standing patient is then asked to bear weight moderately. If the patient is lying down, the prosthetist should apply pressure with the web of his or her hand to the distal plantar

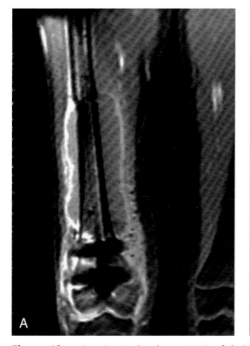
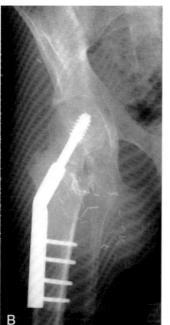
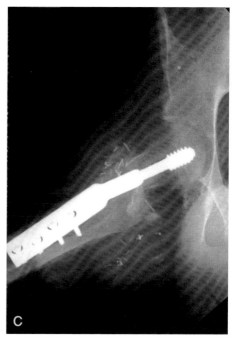

Figure 12   Imaging studies demonstrating failed primary treatment and reconstruction for sarcoma. **A,** MRI of a large tumor recurrence. AP (**B**) and frog-lateral (**C**) radiographs of a modified rotationplasty performed as a salvage procedure.

calcaneus, with his or her thumb in the sustentaculum tali. With the opposite hand, the sulcus is defined to create a weight-bearing shelf distal to the calcaneus. The sustentaculum tali groove will control mediolateral motion of the foot and provide navicular relief in the socket; the sulcus will aid in suspension. The mold is then removed.

Model Modification

Modifications to the positive model on the foot section will include the malleoli, navicular buildup, sulcus relief, sustentaculum tali groove relief, and extension of the distal toes by 0.50 to 0.75 inch. Reduction of the thigh section will depend on the amount of residual tissue.

Diagnostic Socket

A clear diagnostic socket is fabricated to determine fit, suspension, and joint placement. A mold of clear thermoplastic is draped over the modified mold. A vertical line is marked on the lateral and anterior foot and thigh sections to reference the relationship of the foot and thigh before removing the plastic from

the model. These sections are fit separately.[43] The foot section is checked for ease of donning, relief of bony prominences, and for adequate clearance over the malleoli with the ankle flexed and extended. Patients with PFFD and fibular hemimelia may use a combination of the subtalar joint for dorsiflexion and the talocrural joint for plantar flexion; this causes the calcaneus to be in hypereversion in dorsiflexion, thus affecting the placement of the mechanical knee joint.

The foot should slip easily through the ischial level thigh section. The residual thigh tissue and surgical site should be contained in the proximal socket or a thigh lacer. For the patient with PFFD, an intimate fit of the thigh section and a high lateral wall will control rotatory issues proximally and distally in the prosthesis.

The lateral malleolus is then marked on the diagnostic socket. Initial joint placement is at the apex of the lateral malleolus (anatomic medial malleolus) and slightly distal to the ankle with 5° of external rotation.[3] A squaring jig is used

to attach the medial joint to the foot section. The relationship of the foot socket to the thigh section is determined by using the vertical reference lines marked on the lateral side. The thigh section is attached perpendicular to the floor. The anatomic foot may not be perpendicular to the floor because of a lack of range of motion in plantar flexion.

With the patient bearing weight in the diagnostic socket, there should be sufficient clearance distally for the toes.[43] If adequate space distally is not available, ingrown toenails may develop. Appropriate suspension in the foot socket comes from the posterior dorsal strap, the heel shelf, and the sulcus depression.[44] Aitken types C and D deficiencies may require a hip joint and a pelvic band to prevent the thigh from sliding out of the proximal socket.[20] Trim lines are established with the patient both sitting and standing. A second check socket may be necessary to correct the fit of the socket.

The floor-to-socket height of the prosthesis is determined. The ankle will not be at the same height as the contralateral knee in the child who is skeletally immature.[42] The patient with Aitken type C or D PFFD may require the prosthetic side to be higher to compensate for the pelvis dropping at midstance during the gait cycle because of a dysplastic acetabulum or absence of the acetabulum and the bulk of the thigh tissue. A dynamic alignment jig is attached to the socket using transfemoral bench alignment.

Dynamic Alignment

Extensive physical therapy is critical for an acceptable prosthetic outcome for the patient with a newly acquired rotationplasty. The best outcome is achieved by dynamically aligning the prosthesis in a diagnostic socket. To accommodate socket and alignment changes as the patient progresses, physical therapy should occur with the patient using an unfinished, temporary prosthesis. The temporary prosthesis may be used for an undetermined amount of time, depending on the patient's status. A patient with a lower limb tumor who is simultaneously undergoing cancer treatment, physical therapy, and prosthetic fitting will need more time before being fit with a definitive prosthesis.

Dynamic alignment is similar to the thigh lacer and joint procedure.[1] Relative motion will exist in the socket because of the many axes of the ankle joint and the relationship of the single axis of the mechanical joint, but the relative motion should be minimal. Improper proximal or distal joint placement may cause pistoning in the socket. Joint placement for a patient with PFFD may not be in the line of progression because of derotation or subtalar/ankle motion.

During the gait cycle, a loading response may be absent after initial contact because of a decrease in knee extension in the swing phase.[7] Sliding the foot forward will aid knee extension at the loading response. Medial and lateral deviations can be corrected with foot placement beneath the socket or repositioning the joint placement in the transverse plane. During the prosthetic swing phase, vaulting on the sound side may be caused by insufficient knee flexion resulting from a lack of range of motion in the new anatomic knee. The cause of insufficient knee flexion may be a posterior strap that is too proximal, a long prosthesis, or a lack of proper suspension. At initial contact, the knee joints should be fully extended, and the patient will be able to feel the stop of the joints.

Weak adductors produce a Trendelenburg gait in the patient with PFFD. It may be reduced but not eliminated with an intimate fitting socket and a high lateral wall. Therapy will minimize or eliminate Trendelenburg gait in the patient with a lower limb tumor.

Components

The selection of pediatric-specific components is limited. The available space beneath the prosthesis for components will not only limit the prosthetist's selection but also affect durability and cosmesis for the prosthesis. As the child grows, a wider range of components becomes available. Distal component selection follows the traditional transtibial protocol. The child and his or her parents can choose between an endoskeletal prosthesis and an exoskeletal prosthesis.

The ankle has more planes of motion than the knee; therefore, the rotationplasty prosthesis needs mechanical joints to control medial and lateral motion of the foot and ankle.[44] It is critical that knee joints have extension stops and can withstand the activity level of the child. Stainless steel prosthetic joints are durable and preferred for the active child. Polycentric joints will replicate anatomic knee joint mechanics as the knee flexes and extends. Unfortunately, these joints are bulkier and not available in pediatric sizes. Adjustable extension stop joints may be needed if the child does not have full range of motion at the knee.

Finished Prosthesis

The definitive prosthesis should have a soft lining in the laminated foot section, which not only provides comfort but also aids in suspension. The distal and proximal sections are connected with medial and lateral knee joints. The proximal section of the prosthesis will differ in the patient with PFFD, in that it will have a laminated shell that extends to the ischial level to contain the proximal tissue and have a high lateral trim line. It will resemble a ship's funnel.

The patient with a lower limb tumor may need only a leather corset, but it should contain and be above the surgical site. If the contours of the thigh are unusual, the leather will have to be molded to the plaster model. A soft thermoplastic thigh section also is an option.

Special Considerations

Rotationplasty prostheses for the pediatric population have unique requirements and challenges. The patient must be frequently evaluated by the prosthetist for prosthetic changes, which will include growth adjustments, socket changes, and maintenance. The prosthetist must inform the multidisciplinary team of any pertinent changes. Loss of range of motion, strength, or derotation[31] will require reevaluation by other specialists on the team.

The ankle of the child who is skeletally immature will not be even with the contralateral side. For an integral part of a rotationplasty procedure, the surgeon will plan the length of the thigh so that the ankle is at the level of the contralateral knee when the patient is skeletally mature.[42]

Cosmesis can be compromised because of limited clearance between the floor and the socket, resulting in a bulky appearance to the lower section of the prosthesis. Limited plantar flexion range of motion places the foot under the anatomic heel, with the anatomic toes facing posteriorly instead of downward. Donning pants may be difficult, and they may have a bulky appearance in the sagittal plane.

Summary

Rotationplasty in all its variations allows for biologic reconstruction of the proximal joint (usually a knee) by a more distal joint (usually an ankle) in a variety of pathoetiologic situations. Fitting a prosthesis for a child who has undergone rotationplasty is challenging and requires considerable time. The availability of pediatric components and space confinements can limit prosthetic component selection. The patient's changing health and rehabilitation status may prolong the time before the fitting of a definitive prosthesis. A multidisciplinary team is required for positive surgical and prosthetic outcomes. With the careful selection of patients, attention to surgical details, and a dedicated rehabilitation and prosthetic team, excellent functional results with minimal long-term complications can be expected.

References

1. Borggreve J: Kniegelenksersatz durch das in der Beinlangaschse 180-Grad-gedrehte Fussgelenk. *Arch Orthop Unfallchir* 1930;28:175.

2. Van Nes CP: Rotationplasty for congenital defects of the femur: Making use of the ankle of the shortened limb to control the knee joint of a prosthesis. *J Bone Joint Surg* 1950;32:12.

3. Hall JE, Bochmann D: The surgical and prosthetic management of proximal femoral focal deficiency, in: *A Symposium: Proximal Femoral Focal Deficiency: A Congenital Anomaly.* Washington DC, National Academy of Sciences, 1969, pp 77-81.

4. Hall JE: Rotation of congenitally hypoplastic lower limbs to use the ankle joint as a knee. *InterClin Inform Bull* 1966;6(2):3.

5. Kostuik JP, Gillespie R, Hall JE, Hubbard S: Van Nes rotational osteotomy for treatment of proximal femoral focal deficiency and congenital short femur. *J Bone Joint Surg Am* 1975;57(8):1039-1046.

6. Salzer M, Knahr K, Kotz R, Kristen H: Treatment of osteosarcomata of the distal femur by rotation-plasty. *Arch Orthop Trauma Surg* 1981;99(2):131-136.

7. Ackman J, Altiok H, Flanagan A, et al: Long-term follow-up of Van Nes rotationplasty in patients with congenital proximal focal femoral deficiency. *Bone Joint J* 2013;95-B(2):192-198.

8. Hanlon M, Krajbich JI: Rotationplasty in skeletally immature patients: Long-term followup results. *Clin Orthop Relat Res* 1999;358:75-82.

9. Knahr K, Kotz R, Kristen H, et al: Clinical evaluation of patients with rotationplasty, in Enneking WE, ed: *Limb Salvage in Musculoskeletal Oncology.* London, England, Churchill Livingstone, 1987, pp 429-434.

10. Varni JW, Setoguchi Y: Correlates of perceived physical appearance in children with congenital/acquired limb deficiencies. *J Dev Behav Pediatr* 1991;12(3):171-176.

11. Alman BA, Krajbich JI, Hubbard S: Proximal femoral focal deficiency: Results of rotationplasty and Syme amputation. *J Bone Joint Surg Am* 1995;77(12):1876-1882.

12. Fatone S: Gait biomechanics and prosthetic management for children with PFFD. *ACPOC News* 2003;9(1):5-13.

13. Knahr K, Kristen H, Ritschl P, Sekera J, Salzer M: Prosthetic management and functional evaluation of patients with resection of the distal femur and rotationplasty. *Orthopedics* 1987;10(9):1241-1248.

14. McClenaghan BA, Krajbich JI, Pirone AM, Koheil R, Longmuir P: Comparative assessment of gait after limb-salvage procedures. *J Bone Joint Surg Am* 1989;71(8):1178-1182.

15. Murray MP, Jacobs PA, Gore DR, Gardner GM, Mollinger LA: Functional performance after tibial rotationplasty. *J Bone Joint Surg Am* 1985;67(3):392-399.

16. Aitken GT: Proximal femoral deficiency, in Swinyard CA, ed: *Limb Development and Deformity: Problems of Evaluation and Rehabilitation.* Springfield, IL, C. C. Thomas, 1969.

17. Amstutz HC: The morphology, natural history, and treatment of proximal femoral focal deficiency, in *A Symposium on Proximal Femoral Focal Deficiency: A Congenital Anomaly.* Washington DC, National Academy of Sciences, 1969, pp 50-76.

18. Crandal RC: Proximal femoral focal deficiency. *ACPOC News* 2007;13(1):5-25.

19. Fixsen JA, Lloyd-Roberts GC: The natural history and early treatment of proximal femoral dysplasia. *J Bone Joint Surg Br* 1974;56(1):86-95.

20. Krajbich JI: Proximal femoral focal deficiency, in Kalamchi A, ed: *Congenital Lower Limb Deficiencies.* New York, NY, Springer-Verlag, 1989, pp 108-127.

21. Gillespie R, Torode IP: Classification and management of congenital abnormalities of the femur. *J Bone Joint Surg Br* 1983;65(5):557-568.

22. Aitken GT: Proximal femoral deficiency: Definition, classification and management, in *A Symposium on Proximal Femoral Focal Deficiency: A Congenital Anomaly.* Washington DC, National Academy of Sciences, 1969.

23. Krajbich JI: Lower-limb deficiencies and amputations in children. *J Am Acad Orthop Surg* 1998;6(6):358-367.

24. Kritter AE: Tibial rotation-plasty for proximal femoral focal deficiency. *J Bone Joint Surg Am* 1977;59(7):927-934.

25. King RE, Marks TW: Follow-up findings on the skeletal lever in the surgical management of proximal femoral focal deficiency. *InterClin Inform Bull* 1971;11(3):1.

26. King RE: Providing a single skeletal lever in proximal femoral focal deficiency: A preliminary case report. *InterClin Inform Bull* 1966;6(2):23.

27. King RE: Some concepts of proximal femoral focal deficiency, in: *A Symposium: Proximal Femoral Focal Deficiency: A Congenial Anomaly*. Washington DC, National Academy of Sciences, 1969.

28. Gillespie R: Principles of amputation surgery in children with longitudinal deficiencies of the femur. *Clin Orthop Relat Res* 1990;256:29-38.

29. Torode IP, Gillespie R: Rotationplasty of the lower limb for congenital defects of the femur. *J Bone Joint Surg Br* 1983;65(5):569-573.

30. Friscia DA, Moseley CF, Oppenheim WL: Rotational osteotomy for proximal femoral focal deficiency. *J Bone Joint Surg Am* 1989;71(9):1386-1392.

31. Brown KL: Resection, rotationplasty, and femoropelvic arthrodesis in severe congenital femoral deficiency: A report of the surgical technique and three cases. *J Bone Joint Surg Am* 2001;83(1):78-85.

32. Winkelmann WW: Type-B-IIIa hip rotationplasty: An alternative operation for the treatment of malignant tumors of the femur in early childhood. *J Bone Joint Surg Am* 2000;82(6):814-828.

33. Steel HH, Lin PS, Betz RR, Kalamchi A, Clancy M: Iliofemoral fusion for proximal femoral focal deficiency. *J Bone Joint Surg Am* 1987;69(6):837-843.

34. Kotz R, Salzer M: Rotation-plasty for childhood osteosarcoma of the distal part of the femur. *J Bone Joint Surg Am* 1982;64(7):959-969.

35. Jacobs PA: Limb salvage and rotationplasty for osteosarcoma in children. *Clin Orthop Relat Res* 1984;188:217-222.

36. Krajbich JI: The method of predicting the level of the knee in the modified Van Nes rotationplasty, in *Program Book: Pediatric Orthopaedic Society of North America Annual Meeting, Toronto, Canada, May 19, 1987*. Park Ridge, IL, Pediatric Orthopaedic Society of North America, 1987.

37. Krajbich JI, Bochmann D: Van Nes rotationplasty in tumor surgery, in Bowker JH, Michael JW, eds: *Atlas of Limb Prosthetics: Surgical, Prosthetic, and Rehabilitation Principles,* ed 2. St Louis, MO, Mosby-Year Book, 1992, pp 885-899.

38. de Bari A, Krajbich JI, Langer F, Hamilton EL, Hubbard S: Modified Van Nes rotationplasty for osteosarcoma of the proximal tibia in children. *J Bone Joint Surg Br* 1990;72(6):1065-1069.

39. Hillmann A, Hoffmann C, Gosheger G, Krakau H, Winkelmann W: Malignant tumor of the distal part of the femur or the proximal part of the tibia: Endoprosthetic replacement or rotationplasty. Functional outcome and quality-of-life measurements. *J Bone Joint Surg Am* 1999;81(4):462-468.

40. Hillmann A, Rosenbaum D, Gosheger G, Hoffmann C, Rödl R, Winkelmann W: Rotationplasty type B IIIa according to Winkelmann: Electromyography and gait analysis. *Clin Orthop Relat Res* 2001;384:224-231

41. Shih C, Carroll NC: Modified Van Nes rotationplasty for the treatment of proximal femoral osteosarcoma in children. *J Bone Joint Surg Br* 1985;1:81-86.

42. Alexander I: *The Foot: Examination and Diagnosis*, ed 2. London, England, Churchill Livingstone, 1990, pp 29-40.

43. Banziger, E: Rotation plasty prostheses: A prosthetist's perspective. *ACPOC News* 2001;7(1):1-16.

44. Sinclair W, Maale G, Springfield D: Distal femur rotation-plasty prosthesis. *Orthot Prosthet* 1985;39(2):48-51.

Chapter 80

Lumbosacral Agenesis

Charles d'Amato, MD, FRCSC   Todd DeWees, BS, CPO   Joseph Ivan Krajbich, MD, FRCS(C)

Abstract

Lumbosacral agenesis is a rare congenital disorder resulting in the failure of formation of one or more vertebral segments and part or all of the sacrum. There is a wide spectrum of severity ranging from partial absence of the sacrum, with otherwise normal function, to absence of the lumbar and lower thoracic vertebrae and sacrum resulting in severe motor impairment and orthopaedic deformity. There are also frequent visceral abnormalities (such as imperforate anus, upper and lower urinary tract anomalies, and incontinence) and neural anomalies (such as tethered spinal cord, lipomeningocele, and diastematomyelia). When treating a patient with this condition, it is helpful to be familiar with the literature on the prevalence, etiology, and orthopaedic management of lumbosacral agenesis. An illustrative case is presented that describes the surgical and prosthetic management of a child with severe knee flexion contractures, absence of the lumbar vertebrae, and spinopelvic instability.

Keywords: lumbrosacral agenesis; severe knee flexion contracture; spinopelvic instability

Introduction

Lumbosacral deficiency is a disorder consisting of absence of one or more vertebral segments and partial or complete absence of the sacrum. Sacral agenesis and lumbosacral agenesis have been variably called vertebral agenesis, sacral-coccygeal agenesis, caudal regression syndrome, caudal dysplasia, caudal dysplasia sequence, and sacral regression.[1,2] The conditions described by these terms represent a rare, complex disorder with partial or complete absence of the sacrum and partial or complete absence of the lumbar spine. At one end of the spectrum, the condition may be mild and discovered as an incidental radiographic finding (**Figure 1**). At the extreme end of the severity spectrum, the sacrum and lumbar spine are completely absent, and the corresponding neural elements are also absent, causing weakness or complete paralysis of motor function, usually at the level of the last radiographically visible pedicles). In some instances, several more distal segments will be preserved or there will be asymmetric motor function. There is usually comparative sparing of sensation, which is preserved more distally or may even be normal.[3] Visceral deficiencies include renal anomalies, such as absent kidney, horseshoe kidney, and ectopic kidney, and anal-rectal abnormalities such as imperforate anus. Neurogenic bladder, urinary incontinence, and bowel incontinence are common and almost universally present in more severely affected patients. A substantial number of children have associated neurologic abnormalities such as myelodysplasia, tethered spinal cord, lipomeningocele, or diastematomyelia. Any of these abnormalities may affect neurologic function.[4] Fortunately, upper limb function and intelligence are usually normal.[5,6]

The management of more severely affected children presents substantial challenges to the treating orthopaedic surgeon, prosthetist, and rehabilitation team. The orthopaedic management of spinopelvic instability, hip dysplasia, hip dislocation, knee contractures, and foot deformities in more severely affected children has been controversial.

Children with partial sacral agenesis may have a normal appearance and motor function, although urinary incontinence or dribbling may occur. With total absence of the sacrum, dimpling of the buttocks may be present, and there is often substantial disproportion between the trunk and the lower limbs. When multiple lumbar spinal segments are absent, the trunk frequently has a funnel shape (**Figure 2**). Orthopaedic abnormalities include spinosacral instability, upper cervical instability, scoliosis, external rotation and flexion contractures of the hip, hip dislocation, and knee contractures. Severe popliteal webbing may occur in more severely affected patients with a higher-level neurologic abnormality. With weak or absent quadriceps power, the management of knee flexion contractures is difficult, and contracture recurrence is quite common. Foot deformities, such as clubfoot and congenital vertical talus, are frequently present.[3,6-8]

Dr. Krajbich or an immediate family member serves as a board member, owner, officer, or committee member of the Association of Children's Prosthetic and Orthotic Clinics and the Scoliosis Research Society and is a member of a speakers' bureau or has made paid presentations on behalf of K2m. Neither of the following authors nor any immediate family member has received anything of value from or has stock or stock options held in a commercial company or institution related directly or indirectly to the subject of this chapter: Dr. d'Amato and Dr. DeWees.

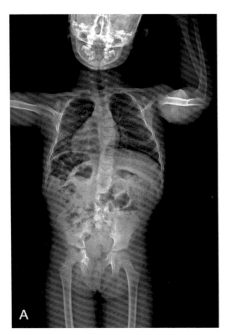
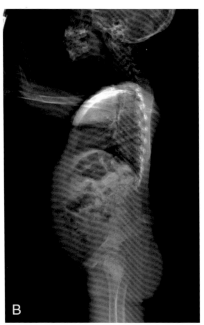

Figure 1 AP (**A**) and lateral (**B**) radiographs of a 10-year-old girl with partial sacral agenesis and normal motor, sensory, bladder and bowel function.

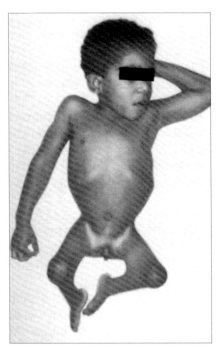

Figure 2 Photograph of a child with lumbar sacral deficiency shows the typical funnel-shaped trunk, knee flexion contractures, and popliteal webbing. (Reproduced with permission from Herring JA: Lower extremity injuries, in Herring JA: *Tachdijian's Pediatric Orthopaedics*, ed 5. Philadelphia, PA, Elsevier Saunders, 2013, vol 2, pp 1467-1472.)

Prevalence and Etiology

Sacral agenesis was first reported by Hohl in 1850.[9] In 1961, Duhamel[10] coined the term caudal regression to describe a spectrum of lumbosacral deficiencies. The incidence of caudal regression has been reported as 0.1 to 0.25 live births.[1] The etiology of this deficiency is likely multifactorial, but its association with diabetes has been recognized by many authors.[3,6,7,11] In a study of 22 patients with lumbosacral agenesis, Phillips et al[6] reported that mothers of 11 of the patients had diabetes. Banta and Nichols[3] reported insulin-dependent maternal diabetes in 5 of 7 patients with sacral agenesis, Guille et al[7] found a maternal history of diabetes in 6 of 18 patients and Andrish et al[11] in 2 of 17 patients. Women with insulin-dependent diabetes have a 200 to 400 times greater risk of giving birth to an infant with caudal regression syndrome than mothers without diabetes.[1] Although much work needs to be done to establish a causative effect, insulin injections are known to cause embryonic malformations in developing chickens.[12] Nonetheless, the large number of affected patients without a history of maternal diabetes makes the exact role of diabetes unclear.

A genetic cause of lumbosacral agenesis has been postulated. The autosomal dominant *HLXB9* homeobox gene located on chromosome 7q36 has been identified in Currarino Triad syndrome. This condition involves sacral agenesis, imperforate anus, perianal fistulas, and a presacral mass or abcess.[13] Postma et al[14] recently discovery a mutation in the *T* (brachyury) gene, a member of the T-box family of transcription factors, that causes a syndrome of sacral agenesis, abnormal ossification of vertebral bodies, and a persistent notochordal canal. In four patients from three consanguineous families, homozygosity mapping was used to find a common 4.1-Mb homozygous region on chromosome 6q27 containing the *T* (brachyury) homolog. Sequencing of the *T* gene in affected individuals led to the discovery of a missense mutation, pH171R. The mutation results in diminished DNA binding, increased cell growth, and interferes with the expression of genes involved in ossification and notochord and axial mesodermal development.

Classification

In 1978, Renshaw[8] recognized four consistent morphologic patterns of sacral deformity. Type I is partial or total unilateral sacral agenesis. Type II is partial sacral agenesis with a partial but bilaterally symmetrical defect and a stable articulation between the ilia. In type III, there is variable lumbar and total sacral agenesis. The ilia articulate with the sides of the lowest vertebra present. In type IV, there is variable lumbar and total sacral agenesis. The caudal end plate of the most distal vertebra rests above either fused ilia or an iliac amphiarthrosis.

More recently, Guille et al[7] proposed a classification that attempts to predict the potential for ambulation and identifies

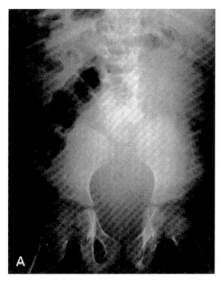 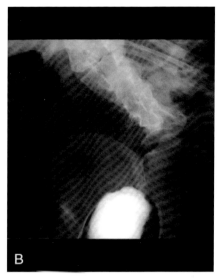 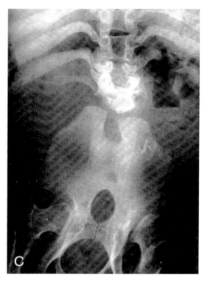

Figure 3   Radiographs demonstrating the Guille et al[7] classification of lumbosacral agenesis. This system correlates spinal deformIty witlı ambulatory function. **A,** The vertebral column articulates with the pelvis in the midline in a patient with a type A deformity. These patients have the best potential for ambulation. **B,** In type B deformity, the vertebral column articulates with one of the ilia shifted away from the midline. **C,** In type C deformity, the vertebral column does not articulate with the pelvis. (Reproduced with permission from Guille JT, Benevides R, DeAlba CC, Siriram V, Kumar SJ: Lumbosacral agenesis: A new classification correlating spinal deformity and ambulatory potential. *J Bone Joint Surg Am* 2002;84[1]:32-38.)

individuals who might benefit from treatment of their lower limb deformities. Guille et al[7] reviewed 18 patients, 13 with lumbosacral agenesis only (group I) and 5 who also had myelomeningocele (group II). The authors identified three types of spinal deformity (**Figure 3**). In the patients with a type A deformity, the ilia were fused in the midline or there was a slight gap between the ilia. The caudal spine articulated with the pelvis in the midline, and vertical alignment with the pelvis was maintained. One or more lumbar vertebrae were absent. Seven of eight patients in group I with a type A deformity were capable of community ambulation and, with one exception, had motor function below L3 or L4. In patients with a type B deformity, the pelvis was fused in the midline but the spinal articulation was not centered in the midline with respect to the pelvis and articulated with one of the ilia. One patient in group I with a type B deformity was a household ambulator. In patients with a type C deformity, there was agenesis of the lumbar spine and a gap was radiographically visible between the thoracic spine and

the pelvis, suggesting spinopelvic instability. All of the ambulatory patients had normal or near normal sensation. No patient with a type B or C deformity was a community ambulator. No group II patients with myelomeningocele were ambulatory.

Guille et al[7] recommend surgery for patients with type B and C deformities only if the lower extremity deformities interfered with sitting, footwear use, or bracing. None of the patients in in this study had been treated with spinal stabilization.

Orthopaedic Management

Most patients with an intact lumbar spine and complete or partial deficiency of the sacrum will be able to achieve independent community ambulation with minimal orthopaedic interventions because motor and sensory impairments are not severe.[3,6-8] However, in a patient with myelomeningocele or other untreated intraspinal anomalies, community ambulation may not be possible.[4,6,7]

Deformity in the lower extremity is related to the neurologic level, which often does not correspond to the anatomic

level. Phillips et al[6] reviewed 22 patients with lumbosacral agenesis, but with no myelomeningocele or congenital amputations, and focused on the level of neurologic impairment in those with more severe involvement. The patient's anatomic level of lumbosacral agenesis was classified based on the lowest radiographically visible lumbar pedicles. Detailed physical examinations were performed to record motor and sensory levels. Orthopaedic problems related to the level of spinal agenesis and neural levels included hip dislocation, hip flexion contractures, knee flexion contractures, and spinopelvic instability. However, foot abnormalities and scoliosis were not related to the functional neurologic level. The 12 patients with spinal agenesis at the T11, T12, or L1 levels (called the first-lumbar group), all had similar findings. This group exhibited the frequently described Buddha-like sitting posture, with abducted flexed hips and flexed knees. For patients in the first-lumbar group, treatment of substantial foot deformity was not needed. Ten of these 12 patients had such severe contractures and popliteal webbing that bilateral lower limb knee disarticulation was performed in 9 of the patients and subtrochanteric amputation in 1 patient. None of the patients with these neurologic levels had hip dislocations, although severe hip flexion contractures were often present.

In patients with lumbar agenesis at the second and third lumbar neurologic levels, hip dislocation occurs in most patients. In the foot, equinus, varus, equinovarus, and calcaneovarus deformities are seen. These patients may require manipulation, casting, or surgery to treat their foot deformities; however, these deformities seldom interfere with ambulation. Knee flexion deformities can be managed with simple bracing or surgery, and these patients do not require limb ablation.

In the study by Phillips et al,[6] scoliosis was identified in 11 of 21 patients for whom there were adequate spinal radiographs. Two of these patients had deformity associated with hemivertebrae. One patient had a 72° curve and back pain, and one had a gibbus deformity; these patients were surgically treated. The other patients with scoliosis had mild curvatures of less than 25°. In their study, Guille et al[7] reported atlantoaxial instability from odontoid hypoplasia and congenital fusions of the upper cervical spine.

The major orthopaedic controversies in the management of patients with lumbosacral agenesis are knee flexion contracture, spinopelvic instability, and, to a lesser extent, hip dislocation. The severity of knee flexion contracture is related to weakness of the quadriceps. In patients with neurologic involvement at the T11, T12, or L1 levels, attempts at reconstruction because of severe contractures associated with popliteal webbing are likely to fail and often result in multiple futile correction attempts and repeated surgeries and hospitalizations. For these patients, bilateral knee disarticulation facilitates sitting. Because the distal femoral growth plate remains

intact, normal femoral length occurs. This greatly facilitates prosthetic fitting. If spinopelvic stabilization is being considered, the tibiae can be used as structural bone graft.[15,16] Subtrochanteric osteotomy, which in the past was done to address this problem, is now of historical interest only.[8,17] This procedure sacrifices the distal femoral growth physis in the child, which leads to an extremely short femur, a disfigured body habitus, and requires a more complex and less efficient hip disarticulation prosthesis. It is worthwhile to preserve the lower limbs in patients with intact quadriceps function. When sensation and proprioception are preserved, successful ambulation is more likely.[3,11]

Surgery to treat bilateral hip dislocation may be worthwhile, but it can result in stiff, painful hips if complications such as osteonecrosis occur. In the past, aggressive management of hip dislocations had been recommended in the literature, with the aim of avoiding skin breakdown, pain, gait deterioration, and increased pelvic obliquity.[8] However, in the study by Phillips et al,[6] six patients with bilateral hip dislocation who were not treated were capable of community ambulation.

There are differing opinions on the need to surgically stabilize spinopelvic instability. Patients with complete absence of the sacrum sit on the posterior ilia, which are typically joined at the midline. The associated absence of several lumbar segments results in severe trunk flexion, with unphysiologic compression of the abdominal viscera and crowding of the diaphragm. This can potentially impair respiratory function. Spinopelvic instability also can lead to seating discomfort and positioning difficulties. However, some patients depend on the mobility between the spine and the pelvis to facilitate sitting and movement. This is particularly true when the hips are stiff and contracted. Thus, spinopelvic stabilization should be recommended only after careful functional

assessment of the adaptive needs of the individual patient.[18]

Perry et al[19] reported on four patients treated with Harrington rod fixation and grafting to fuse the vertebrae to the pelvis. Success was reported in enabling sitting without dependency on upper extremity support, along with relief of unphysiologic compression of the abdominal viscera. Winter[15] published a case report of spinopelvic stabilization in a girl aged 5 years and 11 months with absent vertebrae below T10 and complete absence of the sacrum. The child's lower limbs were drawn up and fixed under her buttocks, with severe flexion contractures of the hip and knees. There was no motor function in the lower limbs, but protective sensation was present. At the time of the spinopelvic stabilization surgery, bilateral knee disarticulation was performed. The patient was placed into halo femoral traction on the operating table to achieve trunk lengthening, and both tibiae were used as structural bone grafts along with Harrington compression instrumentation. Postoperatively, the patient was placed in a halo pantaloon spica cast for 5 months and then into a plastic orthosis for an additional 16 months to achieve solid fusion. To maintain spine and trunk lengthening during growth, lengthening was performed again twice—at age 10 years and 6 months and at age 12 years and 6 months. The lengthening and reinstrumentation was done because of crowding of the internal organs. After osteotomy and distraction through the fusion mass, a more robust modern segmental fixation was used; this eliminated the need for a brace or cast immobilization.

Dynamic compression plates, polysegmental fixation with Cotrel-Dubousset instrumentation, and modern transpedicular fixation are currently used for spinal fusion.[20] However, in patients without a sacrum, fixation with sacral screws, Dunn-McCarthy hooks, and Fackler transforaminal or Jackson intrasacral rods is not possible. In those patients, the ilia can be instrumented with Galveston or iliac screw fixation. Yazici et al[16] recently described their technique of using screws and rods anchored in the ilia, along with anterior tibial autograft and bone morphogenetic protein to achieve a solid connection between the trunk and the pelvis, with preservation of the limbs.

Orthotic and Prosthetic Treatment

Patient Evaluation

The orthotic and prosthetic treatment of sacral agenesis presents unique challenges and requires a comprehensive patient evaluation. Knowledge of the lowest intact vertebra alone is insufficient to fully understand a patient's motor, sensory, and proprioceptive limitations. This point is well illustrated by an example from a 2002 study by Guille et al.[7] In one of the patients in this study, the lowest vertebra was at the T12 level, and motor and sensory function was at the L5 level. This patient achieved community ambulation with the use of orthotic devices. In contrast, in another patient, the lowest vertebra was at the L1 level; however, this patient had no neurologic function in the lower limbs. Neither of these presentations would be expected based solely on knowledge of the lowest complete vertebral level. It is imperative to perform a thorough physical evaluation to assess range of motion, muscle strength, proprioception, and protective sensation before a treatment plan can be formulated. The stability of the spine in the region of the defect as well as the status of hip contractures also should be determined because these factors have a substantial effect on mobility potential.

Orthotic Management

Generally, the orthotic treatment of patients with sacral agenesis is similar to the orthotic treatment of any patient with loss of nervous innervation in the

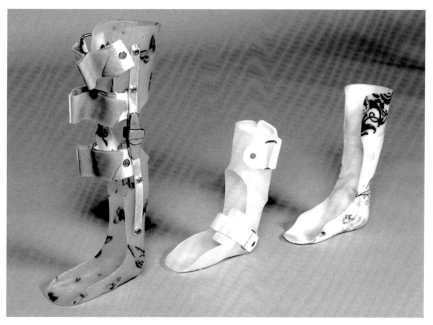

Figure 4   Photograph showing (left to right) a knee-ankle-foot orthosis, a ground-reaction ankle-foot orthosis, and an articulated ankle-foot orthosis.

lower extremity, such as those with myelomeningocele or spinal cord injury; however, a patient with sacral agenesis is likely to retain greater protective sensation and proprioception. The retention of protective sensation reduces the risk of unnoticed skin breakdown from an improperly fitting brace.

Orthotic intervention for patients with sacral agenesis can be broadly classified as functional or positional. Functional orthoses are used to aid in mobility and can include ankle-foot orthoses, ground-reaction ankle-foot orthoses, and knee-ankle-foot orthoses (**Figure 4**). Some patients can ambulate over short distances using an orthosis but will choose a wheelchair for longer distances to conserve energy. Positional orthoses, which are typically knee-ankle-foot or ankle-foot orthoses, are used at night and are important for maintaining range of motion to allow continued ambulation or for comfort in sitting. The loss of range of motion leads to the loss of functional ambulation, decreases the ability to sit comfortably, and causes difficulty with hygiene. The orthotic device is used to maximize the

functional independence of an individual, whether this means independent ambulation or wheelchair mobility. With proper orthopaedic and orthotic management, most patients can achieve a satisfactory functional status.[11] This highlights the need for an integrated team approach in the treatment of these highly complex patients.

Prosthetic Management

Nearly all patients with lumbosacral agenesis who undergo amputation have neurologic levels at T11, T12, or L1. Hip flexion contractures and severe knee flexion contractures associated with popliteal webbing can interfere with sitting and accomplishing the activities of daily living and should be treated with knee disarticulation and prosthetic fitting. In the past, amputation at the subtrochanteric level was primarily done to facilitate sitting balance. Although these patients technically had transfemoral amputations, the prosthetic fitting was performed as if they had a bilateral hip disarticulation because of the short femoral segments resulting from sacrifice of the distal femoral physis. Prosthetic management of patients with sacral agenesis who are treated with knee disarticulation is far more successful than subtrochanteric or transfemoral amputation because the longer resulting residual limb segment is easier to fit into a prosthesis and much more energy efficient. It should be noted that the prosthetic fitting can be complicated by limitations in hip range of motion.

Treatment Example

Although the treatment of patients with lumbosacral agenesis varies depending on the status of the individual patient, the following case example illustrates some of the problems, challenges, and potential treatments involved in caring for a patient with lumbosacral agenesis, spinal instability, and severe contractures of the knees and hips.

A male infant with myelomeningocele and Renshaw type IV sacral agenesis was first seen for orthopaedic treatment at the age of 9 months. Over the next 6 years, he was treated with serial casting, orthotic management, and physical therapy in an attempt to manage severe knee contractures. During this time, he also was treated with multiple medical and surgical procedures, including cephalad and peritoneal shunt revisions, bowel resection, cecostomy, bilateral hernia repair, and treatment for pathologic fractures of the femurs and tibiae. His mother reported that the contractures of the child's knees and feet prevented him from being placed in a car seat or in a sitting position on the school bus.

On physical examination, the child was able to ambulate on his hands while sliding his lower body along the floor. Substantial hyperextension of the elbows was present, and he had large callouses on the palmar aspects of both hands. He could ambulate with a walker, bearing all of his weight on his hands and using a swing-through gait. His trunk was short, and there

was marked spinopelvic instability. The right hip had no voluntary motion, and the left hip had a range of motion between 35° and 75° of flexion. Both hips were abducted 20° and externally rotated to 90°. Fixed knee flexion contractures, severe popliteal webbing, and fixed cavovarus deformities of both feet were present. Light touch sensation was preserved to the level of the knee. The child's spine collapsed when sitting because of the unstable connection of the spine and pelvis (**Figures 5 and 6**).

At the age of 7 years, after extensive discussion of the proposed treatment with the patient's family, the child underwent bilateral knee disarticulation with fusion of the spine from T12 to the ilium; the harvested tibia was used as a structural bone graft (**Figure 7**). A knee disarticulation prosthesis with a reciprocating gait system was fitted. The primary goal of the device was to provide standing stability, with the possibility of reciprocating gait. A substantial challenge with this approach was the limited range of motion of the hips as well as the fact that this patient had never taken steps and had previously only stood in a standing frame for limited periods of time. The device was fabricated with two-part sockets to allow the patient independent donning in the seated position (**Figure 8**). Manual locking knees were used for stability during stance. A posterior thoracic shell for trunk support incorporated a hooped-style cable reciprocating gait system. After the device was fabricated, the patient was allowed to stand and take his first steps with the use of a walker. The walker proved to be an impediment to the patient, who preferred to use forearm crutches (**Figure 9**). The attempts at ambulation were performed in a motion analysis laboratory so that a video of the patient's gait could be used to assist in optimizing balance and function. Within 30 minutes of transitioning to crutches as an assistive device, the patient was able to ambulate safely without the need

for close supervision. The patient preferred a reciprocating gait.

One obstacle to the patient's functional independence was getting in and out of his wheelchair while wearing the device. His excellent upper body strength allowed him to achieve this goal with relative ease, but his limited hip flexion tended to push him out of the wheelchair. This problem was resolved by tilting the seat and back of the wheelchair into a slightly more recumbent position. Within weeks of obtaining the device, he was using it as his primary means of mobility within his home and classroom environments, although he continued to use his wheelchair for traveling greater distances.

Summary

Independent function after skeletal maturity is the overarching treatment goal for patients with lumbosacral agenesis. Certain clinical features have an influence on patient outcomes. When motor function is preserved, especially with good quadriceps function, the management of knee flexion contractures is likely to be successful, and independent ambulation can often be achieved. With compromised quadriceps power, the management of contractures is more difficult. Without useful quadriceps function, the ability to achieve community ambulation is very unlikely. When knee contractures cannot be managed, knee disarticulation and prosthetic fitting are the best options, even if community ambulation is improbable after skeletal maturity. This treatment greatly facilitates sitting and accomplishing the activities of daily living. When knee contractures are not present or can be successfully treated, foot deformities can be managed with casting and surgery. Hip dislocation, especially bilateral hip dislocation, can remain untreated if contractures can be accommodated with prosthetic fitting. Spinopelvic stabilization with spinal instrumentation and structural grafts can be performed in selected patients.

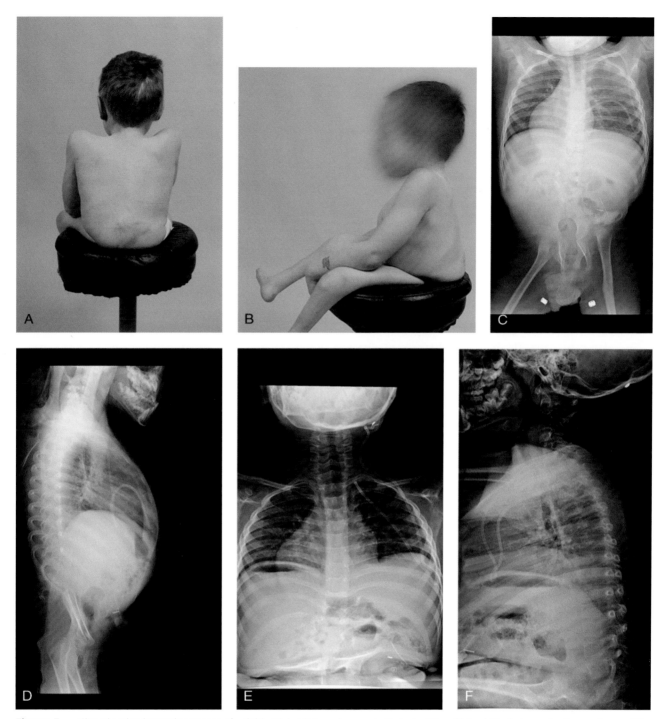

Figure 5 Clinical and radiographic images of a child with lumbosacral agenesis. Posterior (**A**) and lateral (**B**) photographs show collapse of the trunk onto the pelvis and thighs when sitting. **C,** Radiograph showing the L2 vertebra perched above the pelvis, with complete absence of the sacrum. **D,** Lateral radiograph showing the second lumbar vertebra posterior to the pelvis with an unstable articulation. AP (**E**) and lateral (**F**) radiographs show collapse of the trunk onto the pelvis. The patient is sitting on the posterior aspect of the pelvis.

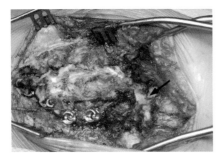

Figure 6 Intraoperative photograph of the patient in Figure 5 showing the unstable spinopelvic articulation (arrow).

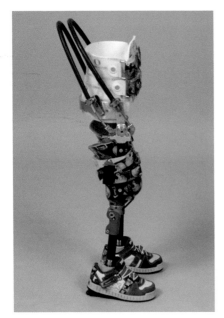

Figure 8 Photograph of a knee disarticulation prosthesis with an incorporate reciprocating gait orthosis.

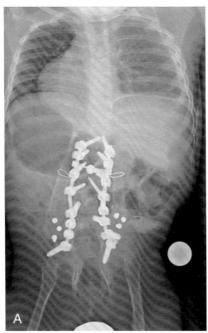 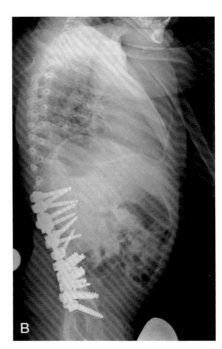

Figure 7 PA (**A**) and lateral (**B**) radiographs of the patient in Figure 5 after spinopelvic reconstruction using the patient's tibiae for structural bone graft.

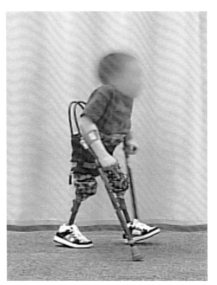

Figure 9 Photograph of the patient in Figure 5 using a knee disarticulation prosthesis and forearm crutches for ambulation.

References

1. Boulas MM: Recognition of caudal regression syndrome. *Adv Neonatal Care* 2009;9(2):61-69.

2. Chervenak F: Caudal regression syndrome. Available at: https://www.rarediseases.org/rare-disease-information/rare-diseases/byID/898/viewFullReport. Accessed June 10, 2015.

3. Banta JV, Nichols O: Sacral agenesis. *J Bone Joint Surg Am* 1969;51(4):693-703.

4. Emami-Naeini P, Rahbar Z, Nejat F, Kajbafzadeh A, El Khashab M: Neurological presentations, imaging, and associated anomalies in 50 patients with sacral agenesis. *Neurosurgery* 2010;67(4):894-900.

5. Caird MS, Hall JM, Bloom DA, Park JM, Farley FA: Outcome study of children, adolescents, and adults with sacral agenesis. *J Pediatr Orthop* 2007;27(6):682-685.

6. Phillips WA, Cooperman DR, Lindquist TC, Sullivan RC, Millar EA: Orthopaedic management of lumbosacral agenesis: Long-term follow-up. *J Bone Joint Surg Am* 1982;64(9):1282-1294.

7. Guille JT, Benevides R, DeAlba CC, Siriram V, Kumar SJ: Lumbosacral agenesis: A new classification correlating spinal deformity and ambulatory potential. *J Bone Joint Surg Am* 2002;84(1):32-38.

8. Renshaw TS: Sacral agenesis. *J Bone Joint Surg Am* 1978;60(3):373-383.

9. Blumel J, Evans EB, Eggers GW: Partial and complete agenesis or malformation of the sacrum with associated anomalies; etiologic and clinical study with special reference to heredity: A preliminary report. *J Bone Joint Surg Am* 1959;41(3):497-518.

10. Duhamel B: From the mermaid to anal imperforation: The syndrome of caudal regression. *Arch Dis Child* 1961;36(186):152-155.

11. Andrish J, Kalamchi A, MacEwen GD: Sacral agenesis: A clinical evaluation of its management, heredity, and associated anomalies. *Clin Orthop Relat Res* 1979;139:52-57.

12. Duraiswami PK: Insulin-induced skeletal abnormalities in developing chickens. *Br Med J* 1950;2(4675):384-390.

13. Horton WB, Steiner MA, Khan MA: Complete Currarino triad presenting with diarrhea in a 7-month-old girl. *South Med J* 2010;103(8):815-818.

14. Postma AV, Alders M, Sylva M, et al: Mutations in the T (brachyury) gene cause a novel syndrome consisting of sacral agenesis, abnormal ossification of the vertebral bodies and a persistent notochordal canal. *J Med Genet* 2014;51(2):90-97.

15. Winter RB: Congenital absence of the lumbar spine and sacrum: One-stage reconstruction with subsequent two-stage spine lengthening. *J Pediatr Orthop* 1991;11(5):666-670.

16. Yazici M, Akel I, Demirkiran HG: Lumbopelvic fusion with a new fixation technique in lumbosacral agenesis: Three cases. *J Child Orthop* 2011;5(1):55-61.

17. Russcll HE, Aitken GT: Congenital absence of the sacrum and lumbar vertebrae with prosthetic management. *J Bone Joint Surg Am* 1963;45(3):501-508.

18. Lubicky JP: Congenital absence of the lumbar spine and sacrum: One-stage reconstruction with subsequent two-stage spine lengthening. *J Pediatr Orthop* 1992;12(5):675.

19. Perry J, Bonnett CA, Hoffer MH: Vetebral pelvic fusions in the rehabilitation of patients with sacral agenesis. *J Bone Joint Surg Am* 1970;52(2):287-294.

20. Rieger MA, Hall JE, Dalury DF: Spinal fusion in a patient with lumbosacral agenesis. *Spine (Phila Pa 1976)* 1990;15(12):1382-1384.

Chapter 81

Partial Foot Deficiencies in Children

Robin C. Crandall, MD

Abstract

Childhood partial foot amputations are commonly seen and occur from a variety of etiologies. Treatment plans for congenital as well as acquired partial foot amputations may be both surgical and nonsurgical. To achieve the best possible patient outcomes, it is helpful to be aware of treatment options, possible complications, and prosthetic choices.

Keywords: children; congenital foot loss; partial foot deficiencies; pediatric partial foot amputation

Introduction

There has been a steady increase in the percentage of partial foot amputations seen in pediatric limb deficiency clinics. With improved limb salvage techniques, including wound vacuum-assisted closure, free flap techniques, and improved infection control, a higher percentage of trauma patients have successful partial foot amputations. Similarly, improved foot reconstruction techniques have yielded durable long-term partial foot survival in patients with congenital and neoplastic foot deficiencies.[1-5]

This chapter focuses on pediatric patients with congenital or acquired partial foot deficiencies and reviews etiology, nonsurgical and surgical treatment, and prosthetic management.

Etiology

The etiologies of partial foot deficiencies in children are broad reaching. Based on data gathered at multiple limb deficiency centers, approximately 60% of amputations in children are caused by congenital factors and 40% result from other causes.[6] The exact incidence of childhood partial foot loss in the United States from trauma or congenital causes is unknown.

Acquired Partial Foot Loss

Acquired partial foot loss can result from trauma and amputation related to reconstructive procedures for syndromes associated with limb deficiencies, infection, and congenital or in utero causes. Acquired partial foot amputations can result from vascular and ischemic causes secondary to cardiac or major vessel catheterization in young children or umbilical vessel catheterization in newborns.[7] Iatrogenic injury to blood vessels during foot reconstructive procedures in children can result in partial foot amputation. Traumatic foot amputations are usually caused by injuries from lawn mowers, farm equipment or animals, machinery, motor vehicle crashes, train-related trauma (such as falling from a moving train or injury during boarding), and thermal damage (burn or frostbite). Another class of partial foot deficiency includes loss related to reconstructive procedures for focal gigantism syndromes such as neurofibromatosis, Proteus syndrome, vascular arteriovenous malformation syndrome, Klippel-Trénaunay-Weber syndrome, and macrodystrophia lipomatosa. Infection-related causes of limb loss include purpura fulminans and insensate foot with chronic ulceration or osteomyelitis, which often occur in individuals with diabetes, spinal cord injury, or myelomeningocele. Congenital or in utero causes of partial foot deficiency include transverse deficiencies (mid to proximal tarsal loss), longitudinal (medial or lateral) deficiencies, split-hand/split-foot syndrome, and fetal alcohol syndrome.

General Principles of Treatment

Greene and Cary[8] reported that functional results of partial foot amputation are better than amputation at a higher level if a sensate plantigrade foot can be achieved. The authors showed that a Chopart amputation with equinus contracture is functionally inferior to an ankle disarticulation (Syme) procedure. The goal of surgery should be pain-free ambulation and the ability to wear durable, realistic footwear. A composite tissue free flap is an excellent method for covering massive foot wounds, but it is useless if the foot is in a fixed equinus position and the patient is unable to walk. Delicate, nondurable split-thickness skin grafts over weight-bearing areas can allow wound closure, but a lack of durability is an important issue that may require revision to a higher level. Without the expertise of a prosthetist capable of fitting complex partial foot prostheses, amputation at these levels can often result in prosthetic failure.

The perceived benefit of partial foot amputation can be lost if the patient requires a prosthesis that rigidly immobilizes the ankle.[9] Careful consideration must be used when planning how the remnant foot can be used functionally to prevent breakdown caused by pressure

---

Dr. Crandall or an immediate family member has stock or stock options held in Stryker.

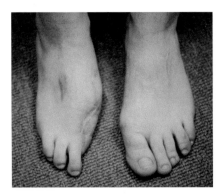

Figure 1 Photograph of the feet of a patient treated with a partial right foot amputation. Durable plantar skin is folded dorsally. Ray amputation was necessary in this patient to allow a smooth foot contour and easy fitting of a prosthetic shoe.

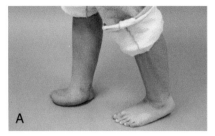 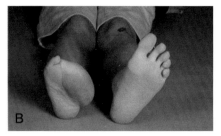

Figure 2 **A,** Photograph of the foot of a child with an injury caused by a lawn mower that necessitated a partial amputation of the right foot, with latissimus dorsi free flap coverage. **B,** Photograph showing the increase in the bulk of the latissimus dorsi free flap, which occurs with the child's growth and weight gain. Further revision surgery was needed.

or shear stresses. Because children are usually very active, reinjury is a possibility. A team approach to care by surgeons and prosthetists is often required.

Traumatic Injuries
Lawn Mower Injuries
Many partial foot amputations result from injuries caused by a lawn mower. In a multicenter review of 144 children with traumatic injuries caused by a lawn mower, Loder et al[10] reported that the toes were the most often injured part of the foot (63%), with most of the injured children being bystanders or passengers on riding mowers. The injury resulted in an amputation present on admission in 59 children, with an additional 8 children requiring an amputation before hospital discharge. Of the 67 amputations, 51 were partial foot amputations (40 at the toe level, 5 at the transmetatarsal level, and 6 at the Chopart level). Children injured by riding mowers were generally younger than those injured by push mowers (mean, 5.4 versus 11.0 years, respectively). Adult operators of riding or push mowers often use hearing and eye protection and are unaware of the presence and impending danger to a nearby child. Loder et al[10] reported that 85% of foot injuries in children could be prevented if children younger than 14 years were not permitted to operate

a push or riding lawn mower or be present in the immediate mowing area. The Amputee Coalition of America has compiled a checklist of precautions to prevent lawn mower trauma.[11]

Complications and unsatisfactory results are common after a lawn mower injury. Nearly 10% of the patients in the Loder et al[10] study had residual infection or osteomyelitis, and a 50% complication rate was reported. Infection from lawn mower trauma commonly involves multiple organisms, including bacteria, fungi, and mycobacteria.[12] Daley and McIntyre[13] reported that infecting organisms such as Stenotrophomonas maltophilia are common in lawn mower injuries, making it difficult to use empiric antibiotic therapies. Repeated surgical débridement is usually needed. Skin breakdown and amputation at a higher level occur at high rates.[14,15]

The surgical team should evaluate the injured foot to determine the options for skin coverage and plan the final shape and functionality of the residual limb. Durable plantar skin should be saved whenever feasible (**Figure 1**). Physeal damage should be objectively assessed. Dormans et al[16] proposed a simple classification system of lower limb lawn mower injuries. Type I is a shredding-type injury, and type II is a paucilaceration. All of the shredding-type injuries required amputation because of the difficulty of limb salvage. In the group with a paucilaceration injury, excellent results were achieved

with more minimalistic procedures. In all groups, 4.9 procedures per patient were required.

Microvascular free flap reconstruction and composite tissue grafting has been successfully used in the distal lower limbs; however, these procedures have a complication rate of at least 62%.[1] Children treated with reconstruction involving free flaps within 2 days of injury had lower complication rates.[1] Partial foot amputation with free flap reconstruction in pediatric patients is problematic because children have small blood vessels. It is important to recognize that donor-site composite grafts may increase in bulk as the child ages, creating a residual limb that cannot be placed in a shoe (**Figure 2**).

Negative-pressure wound therapy has been shown to be valuable in treating large, soft-tissue injuries to the foot and ankle.[2,3] Shilt et al[3] specifically showed its effectiveness in lawn mower injuries in children. However, shredding-type foot and ankle injuries should be treated with a high degree of caution. Families should be advised of the high complication rates and the possibility that revision at a higher amputation level may be needed.

Attempting to salvage a foot that will not allow plantigrade ambulation is a substantial problem in reconstruction of traumatic partial foot injuries. If the foot is in severe equinus, painful, and unusable after a successful composite free flap procedure, amputation at a higher

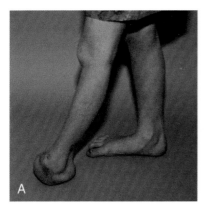
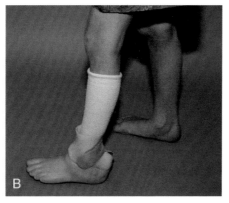

Figure 3 Photographs of the foot of a child who has undergone a partial foot amputation at the Chopart level. **A,** Equinus contracture developed in the postoperative interval. **B,** Because equinus contracture makes it difficult to obtain a good prosthetic fit, the perceived benefit of a Chopart-level partial foot amputation may be inferior to the functionality that could be obtained with amputation at a higher level.

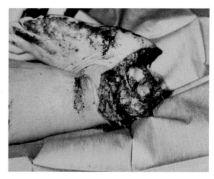

Figure 4 Photograph of the lower limb of an adolescent with massive shredding hindfoot trauma. This type of injury can occasionally be managed with calcanectomy and intercalary bone excision, but multiple débridements and a high complication rate should be expected.

level may be needed. This scenario is particularly common with traumatic lawn mower injuries. With loss of dorsiflexors, the need to immobilize the residual limb in a weight-bearing position is important. This becomes increasingly difficult in more-proximal foot amputations, such as those at the Lisfranc (tarsometatarsal) or Chopart (midtarsal) levels. If functional ankle dorsiflexion cannot be achieved, a Boyd amputation or Syme ankle disarticulation may be preferable at the initial surgery as opposed to later when additional subjective issues may play a role. A limb that heals in equinus can be one of the most difficult limbs to fit with a prosthesis (**Figure 3**).

A massive, shredding traumatic injury to the hindfoot can be a particularly difficult injury to treat when caused by a lawn mower or other machinery (**Figure 4**). Extensive hindfoot and intercalary loss can be managed successfully with a calcanectomy and a subsequent ankle-foot orthosis with a spacer block to substitute for heel loss.[17] Failure of a calcanectomy with an intact forefoot may require a Syme disarticulation with an anterior flap.

Farm-Related Injuries

Partial foot amputation in children frequently results from injuries sustained on a farm. In a series of farm-related injuries analyzed by Cogbill et al,[18] 46% of the injuries were related to machinery and tractors, with the remaining injuries caused by animals or falls. In a study by McClure and Shaughnessy[19] of farm injuries in children requiring amputation, all the injuries were open type IIIC Gustilo fractures and had polymicrobial contamination. In a 3-year study of farm injuries in 292 children, Lubicky and Feinberg[20] noted that most of the injuries occurred in the lower limbs and that the average age of the injured children was 11.9 years. Although the authors did not specify how many of the children required a partial foot amputation, they noted that 41 of 127 open fractures (32%) occurred in the tarsal or metatarsal toe areas.

The general principles of treating foot injury from farm-related causes are similar to those used in managing lawn mower trauma. The wounds are often infected with multiple contaminants, and multiple procedures are needed to achieve a successful residual limb. It is important to achieve durable skin coverage. For farming families with limited financial resources, those who live in

ethnic communities, and those with limited access to tertiary care centers, the ability to wear normal footwear is of utmost importance.[21]

Motor Vehicle and Train-Related Injuries

In a study by Loder[22] of 256 traumatic amputations in children, the third and fourth most common injuries involved motor vehicle and train-related trauma. Train-related injuries often occur in the process of boarding or jumping from a moving train. Although Loder[22] did not specify the incidence of partial foot amputations from train-related trauma, 10 of 24 train-related injuries in his study occurred in the lower limbs. Because wounds from train-related injuries tend to be sharper and cleaner than injuries from lawn mower and farm-related trauma, fewer débridements may be needed and wound closure may be easier.

Jawadi[23] recently reported on 21 cases of partial foot amputation in young children related to all-terrain vehicle injuries. These children often had bare or sandaled feet, which offered little protection from injury. Loder[22] reported substantial seasonal variation in pediatric amputations caused by motor vehicle injuries, with more amputations occurring in June and July and many involving young drivers. Specific data and follow-up regarding partial foot amputations from motor vehicle trauma in children are unknown, but skin breakdown and traumatic partial foot amputation have been reported in the adult population after motor vehicle injuries.[14,15]

Thermal Injuries

Frostbite injuries can result in partial foot amputation in children because they are particularly vulnerable to these injuries, along with elderly people, individuals with alcoholism, and drug users. Very young children often cannot or do not communicate that they are very cold, do not recognize the symptoms of impending frostbite, and may stay outside for long periods with improper footwear for protection from the cold.

In a review by Miller and Chasmar[24] of 101 patients admitted to hospitals with frostbite injuries in Canada, it was found that rapid rewarming and adequate delay before conservative débridement or surgical amputation were important treatment principles. The authors reported on the need to allow demarcation to occur to clearly show the location of the full-thickness injury. Other studies have indicated that after 5 days, scintigraphy and MRI may be useful in determining viable tissue.[25,26] Golant et al[27] recommended rewarming of the affected limb at 104° to 107.6° for 15 to 30 minutes and avoidance of rewarming until definitive medical care is involved.

Sharp demarcation between viable and nonviable tissue may indicate that a partial foot amputation is necessary. Imray et al[28] believed that the unwillingness to delay surgery was a major cause of avoidable morbidity. The authors suggested that no surgical intervention should occur without a waiting period of 6 to 12 weeks after injury.

It is important to carefully follow the pediatric patient for possible evidence of physeal damage that can occur with thermal injury. Frostbite injuries in the foot can look similar to injuries from purpura fulminans. The physician should wait at least several weeks before débridement and amputation. The management of acute frostbite injury to prevent possible amputation includes thrombolytic agents, hyperbaric oxygen, and prostacyclin.[29-32] Databases are needed to extract the exact incidence of partial foot amputations caused by frostbite injuries in children.[33]

Burns from either electrical or thermal sources also can result in severe tissue damage necessitating partial foot amputation. A partial foot amputation was reported in a patient with neurologic loss caused by a third-degree burn from a laptop computer.[34]

Nontraumatic Partial Foot Amputation

Focal Gigantism Syndromes

Focal gigantism syndromes involving portions of the foot and the toes can necessitate partial foot amputation. In children, these syndromes include vascular arteriovenous malformation syndrome, neurofibromatosis, Proteus syndrome, Klippel-Trénaunay-Weber syndrome, and macrodystrophia lipomatosa. It is important that all abnormal tissue be removed in a soft-tissue or bony reduction to prevent the growth of residual abnormal tissue as the child grows. Central ray partial foot amputation is often needed in patients with these syndromes (**Figure 5**). Khan et al[35] reported on four cases of macrodystrophia lipomatosa, which is characterized by enlargement of the second or third digits of the hands or feet. MRI is useful in the diagnosis of this syndrome because it shows adipose tissue in subcutaneous areas without encapsulation. A diagnosis of macrodystrophia lipomatosa can be difficult to make because the symptoms are similar to those of Proteus syndrome.[36-38] The visual manifestations of any of the focal gigantism syndromes can be nearly identical.

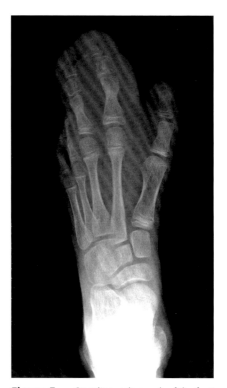

Figure 5 Standing radiograph of the foot of a patient with classic macrodystrophia lipomatosa. The second and third toes are enlarged and the remainder of foot is normal. A distal toe amputation with physeal ablation of metatarsal heads 2 and 3 can allow successful shoe wear. Central ray partial foot amputation may become necessary.

Treatments of focal gigantism syndromes involving the foot are similar to each other. Often, inequalities occur that require physeal manipulation at a later time as the child ages. Physeal growth arrest of metatarsals and even phalanges are sometimes used together with distal phalangeal amputation to maintain a reasonable foot size. The child will need a shoe of similar size to the contralateral unaffected side. Tissue debulking with segmental ray resection or partial foot amputation is frequently required. In children with Proteus syndrome, tissues that initially appear relatively normal may enlarge, and amputation at a higher level may be required. In focal gigantism syndromes, it is important to carefully evaluate the child's limb length to allow planning for physeal manipulation as needed.

Infection

Purpura fulminans represents an important cause of partial foot amputation in children. Many children with this infection have quadrimembral involvement. Purpura fulminans generally occurs in children younger than 5 years after an acute bacterial or a viral infection; the rate of amputation is 60%.[39] Risk factors for purpura fulminans include age younger than 5 years and the presence of factor V G1691A mutation. Gürgey et al[39] suggest that all patients with purpura fulminans be screened for this mutation and receive anticoagulation therapy to prevent further necrosis. Purpura fulminans has been associated with Meningococcus, Streptococcus, Pneumococcus, Staphylococcus aureus, and varicella and rubella viral diseases. The thrombosis that occurs in purpura fulminans is widespread and microvascular. Large amounts of tissue necrosis and loss are common.

The orthopaedic surgeon is often consulted when the child has severely swollen limbs. This clinical appearance can suggest that a transtibial amputation may be needed; however, at this stage of the disease the problem is not the infection but the associated underlying tissue necrosis and substantial swelling. Viable tissue is often present despite the swelling and edema. Waiting for demarcation to occur is critically important. A child who appears to need a transtibial amputation may eventually require only a partial foot amputation (**Figure 6**). Amputation at a higher level may be needed, but it should be performed only after a minimum of 4 to 6 weeks of observation. The skin and subcutaneous tissues of residual limbs after purpura fulminans are generally thin, somewhat dystrophic, and often have multiple split-thickness skin grafts. Consultation with an experienced prosthetist is important for achieving the best functional outcome for the child.

Partial foot amputation in a child can occur because of infections involving

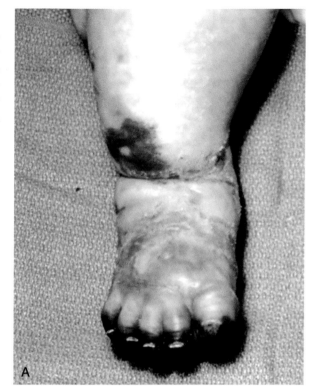 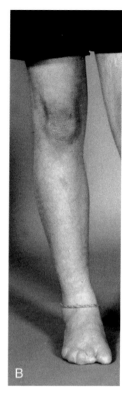

Figure 6 **A,** Photograph of the distal lower limb of a child with purpura fulminans. In the early stages of the disease, it may appear that a transtibial amputation is necessary. **B,** Photograph of the limb at a later age. By waiting for full demarcation before choosing the definitive amputation level, the child was treated with a partial foot amputation and had only minimal functional loss.

failed foot reconstruction; insensate feet, as seen in spinal cord injury; and myelomeningocele. Deep heel ulcers in patients with spinal cord injury and myelomeningocele may require hindfoot amputation and calcanectomy.[2] In a study of 36 ambulatory patients with sacral-level myelomeningocele, 11 of the patients required a total of 14 amputation procedures.[40] Nine of these procedures were partial foot amputations. In this particular population, ambulation on insensate feet can be a significant problem. Although this study involved adult patients, the treatment principles also apply to pediatric patients who are active community ambulators.

Neoplasms

Neoplasms involving the soft tissue or bone of the foot are rare. The most common neoplasm is rhabdomyosarcoma, which occurs more often in boys than girls. In younger children, rhabdomyosarcoma more commonly occurs in the head, the neck, and the pelvis. In adolescents, tumors are most commonly seen in the limbs. Synovial sarcoma can occur in teenagers, with lower-grade lesions generally found around the hands and feet. Chou et al[41] reported that in 2,660 surgically treated musculoskeletal tumors in children and adults, only 5.7% involved the foot or ankle.

Local radiation therapy with surgical resection of the lesion to retain function of the foot has been recommended rather than primary amputation at a higher level.[4] Local radiation, however, is controversial because of complications and adverse side effects seen at long-term follow-ups. Its use in children's feet largely has been abandoned in favor of wider surgical excision. It is important to note that surgical resection with adequate margins in the foot can be difficult to obtain without underlying ray or combined ray amputation.

Children with a neoplastic foot lesion should have a thorough evaluation at a tertiary oncology care center and should be referred to an oncology center for treatment. A diagnosis of rhabdomyosarcoma is made in approximately 250 pediatric patients each year, with 65% of the tumors occurring in children younger than 6 years.[42]

Many types of malignant osseous tumors have been reported in the foot. Treatment of pediatric and adolescent bone tumors in the foot has greatly evolved. Long-term survivability has increased, with amputation and limb salvage having similar long-term outcomes.[5] Partial foot salvage in these individuals may fail, however, if a plantigrade, sensate residual foot cannot be achieved.

Congenital Causes of Partial Foot Deficiencies

Transverse Deficiencies of the Foot

Transverse deficiencies of the foot not associated with constriction band syndrome are decidedly more rare than transverse defects in the upper limb. The most common transverse deficiency occurs in the forearm. The International Organization for Standardization describes limb deficiencies by stating the missing elements. For example, a transverse deficiency of the foot is described as phalanges all, metatarsals 1 through 5 incomplete. Because this method is somewhat cumbersome, this deficiency also may be described as a transverse partial foot deficiency. Deficiency can occur at the phalangeal, tarsal, or metatarsal level.

The skin covering the partial foot in children tends to be robust, and prosthetic intervention often is not needed. Limb length inequality should be evaluated. Children with transverse deficiencies may have dysplasia of the entire lower limb; failure to address the difference in limb length can result in an

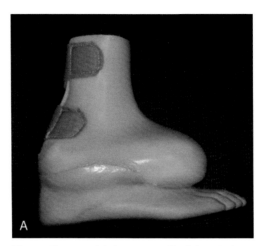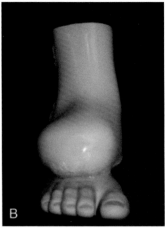

Figure 7 Careful observation of limb-length discrepancy is important in children to prevent the necessity for a cosmetically displeasing prosthesis. Lateral (**A**) and AP (**B**) views of a foot prosthesis for a patient with a limb-length discrepancy.

awkward and cosmetically displeasing partial foot prosthesis (**Figure 7**).

In a small study, Jain and Lakhtakia[43] found that hindfoot transverse defects were less common than forefoot transverse defects. Transverse deficiencies are sporadic in nature and not generally associated with other visceral defects. Transverse deficiencies of the foot can occur if the apical ectodermal ridge is removed during embryogenesis.[44] This ridge is one of the three signaling centers that affect limb development. These limb defects are thought to be caused by mechanical and vascular factors, with no specific heritability patterning. Partial foot deficiency can be seen with coagulation deficiency and sometimes after prenatal sampling of chorionic villi.[45,46] As with many congenital limb defects, these deficiencies can often be detected prenatally with fetal ultrasonography.[47]

The exact incidence of transverse foot defects not associated with constriction band or chorionic villi sampling is unknown. Drugs that may create vascular-related partial foot defects include ergotamine and misoprostol. In a study by McGuirk et al[48] of 161,252 births in the Boston area, the prevalence rate of limb reduction defects as a result of presumed vascular disruption was 0.22 per 1,000 births.

In this large series, eight children had partial foot deficiencies; three of these children had constriction band syndromes and one had split-hand/split-foot syndrome.

Longitudinal Deficiencies of the Foot

Longitudinal deficiencies of the foot are generally associated with longitudinal long bone deficiency. This is particularly true with all types of fibular deficiencies with associated lateral ray loss. Some of these patients are considered to have partial foot deficiencies because of minimal limb-length discrepancy and the use of leg lengthening procedures; however, most of these patients are treated with foot ablation if leg length is projected to be short. An exception is a child with bilateral plantigrade feet and similar leg lengths (**Figure 8**). Medial longitudinal deficiencies of the foot that are not associated with long bone deficiency are extremely rare and may be associated with constriction band syndromes. It is important to carefully examine hindfoot function in any longitudinal foot deficiency to evaluate for limb-length discrepancies and tarsal coalitions. Some isolated longitudinal medial foot deficiencies can be seen with Goltz syndrome and fetal alcohol syndrome.[48-50]

Bilateral longitudinal fibular deficiency often is associated with lateral partial foot amputation. Because the feet are plantigrade, no higher amputation level is needed, and the patient is fitted with a partial foot prosthesis.

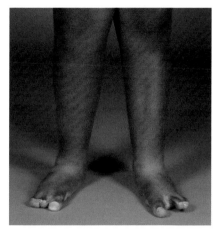

Figure 8 Clinical photograph of the lower limbs of a child with a bilateral longitudinal fibular deficiency and lateral ray loss. Because the child has plantigrade feet, amputation at a higher level is not necessary.

Amniotic Band Syndrome

Amniotic band syndrome is a relatively common cause of partial foot amputation. This syndrome occurs in 1 in 10,000 births.[51] These patients may have numerous other organ system involvements, and all four limbs often are affected. Although each manifestation of the syndrome is essentially different, involvement of the lower limbs is common. Digital ring constrictions, distal atrophy, intrauterine transverse or longitudinal deficiencies, syndactyly, and clubfoot can occur in the lower limbs.[52] Digital amputation is frequently necessary in these patients. Constriction band release, however, may salvage a foot or a partial foot.[53] Although not generally considered an inherited condition, many predisposing factors, including maternal smoking, drug use, hyperglycemia, hypertension, amniocentesis, and first-degree relatives with the syndrome, have been identified in patients with constriction band syndrome.[54] Some theories suggest that amniotic band syndrome is the result of a vascular insult early in embryogenesis.[54]

Split-Hand/Split-Foot Syndrome

Split-hand/split-foot syndrome, also known as ectrodactyly-ectodermal dysplasia, is believed to be an autosomal dominant condition in which a variety of systems can be involved.[55] If the degree of foot involvement allows the use of normal footwear, surgical intervention may be unnecessary. Often, however, one limb may be more involved than the other, creating the need for reconstruction and possible partial foot amputation. The goal is to allow the patient to use normal footwear (**Figure 9**).

Prosthetic Choices

Prosthetic choices for children with a partial foot amputation or deficiency have evolved considerably over the past two decades. Custom-made leather, lacing-type prostheses have been replaced with sophisticated, lifelike molded synthetic constructs. In children with

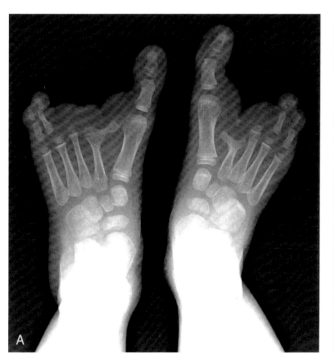
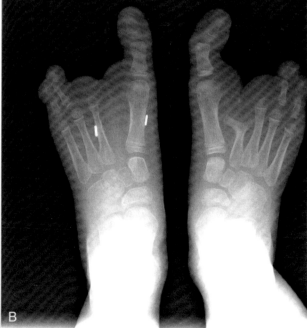

Figure 9 **A,** Standing preoperative radiograph of the feet of a patient with split-hand/split-foot syndrome. The left foot is wider than the right foot. **B,** Postoperative radiograph taken after intercalary resection of the second metatarsal of the foot, with use of a cross metatarsal suture anchor. The procedure narrowed the left foot, allowing easier shoe wear.

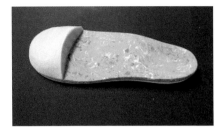

Figure 10 Photograph of a simple foam filler, which can be attached to an orthotic device in a patient with partial foot loss.

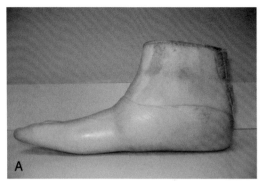
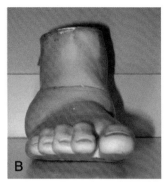

Figure 11 Lateral (**A**) and AP (**B**) views of a prosthetic foamer foot, which is used in midlevel to proximal level partial foot amputations.

simple metatarsophalangeal loss, toe spacers and foam shoe fillers may suffice (**Figure 10**). Most children with simple toe loss or even multiple toe loss can ambulate with no observable gait abnormalities.[9] Dillon and Fatone[56] reported that after metatarsal heads are compromised, foot length becomes an issue, and the center of pressure remains behind the residual limb until after contralateral heel contact. Patients with very short partial foot amputation levels may benefit from ankle immobilization with a relatively stiff forefoot prosthesis.

At the institution of this chapter's author (Twin Cities Shriners Hospital, Minneapolis, MN), success has been reported with a "foamer foot" construct, using a prosthetic foot shell alone without rigid ankle immobilization[57] (**Figure 11**). Impregnation of fabric within the plastic foot shell has markedly increased its durability. In this construct, the residual limb is placed in an alginate mold in a semi–weight-bearing seated position with the knee in 90° of flexion. The plaster impression is then modified by building up plaster over bony prominences and removing plaster around the ankle circumference. This results in more space over bony prominences, with less space around the ankle to accommodate stretching of the prosthesis. The final prosthesis has proven extremely durable in 12 pediatric patients fitted with a "foamer foot" construct after partial foot amputation.[57] This prosthesis is less expensive than typical prostheses used for ankle disarticulation or Chopart-level amputations and offers excellent cosmesis and function. In an analysis of 141 clinical visits, only two patients required a visit more than once per year.[57] More objective data are needed regarding different prosthetic models for partial foot amputation.

Summary

Various etiologies, such as traumatic, syndrome-related, congenital, infectious, and vascular etiologies, are often the reason for partial foot amputation in children. Durable skin coverage and obtaining a plantigrade foot are essential for a successful partial foot amputation. In patients with congenital deficiency or gigantism syndrome, leg-length inequality must be assessed. An experienced prosthetist is needed to fabricate pediatric prosthetic devices for amputations and deficiencies at more proximal levels of the lower limb.

References

1. Rinker B, Valerio IL, Stewart DH, Pu LL, Vasconez HC: Microvascular free flap reconstruction in pediatric lower extremity trauma: A 10-year review. *Plast Reconstr Surg* 2005;115(6):1618-1624.

2. Lee HJ, Kim JW, Oh CW, et al: Negative pressure wound therapy for soft tissue injuries around the foot and ankle. *J Orthop Surg Res* 2009;4:14.

3. Shilt JS, Yoder JS, Manuck TA, Jacks L, Rushing J, Smith BP: Role of vacuum-assisted closure in the treatment of pediatric lawn-mower injuries. *J Pediatr Orthop* 2004;24(5):482-487.

4. La TH, Wolden SL, Su Z, et al: Local therapy for rhabdomyosarcoma of the hands and feet: Is amputation necessary? A report from the Children's Oncology Group. *Int J Radiat Oncol Biol Phys* 2011;80(1):206-212.

5. Nagarajan R, Neglia JP, Clohisy DR, Robison LL: Limb salvage and amputation in survivors of pediatric lower-extremity bone tumors: What are the long-term implications? *J Clin Oncol* 2002;20(22):4493-4501.

6. Tooms RE: Acquired amputations in children, in Bowker JH, Michael JW, eds: *Atlas of Limb Prosthetics: Surgical, Prosthetic, and Rehabilitation Principles*, ed 2. St. Louis, MO, Mosby–Year Book, 1992, pp 735-742.

7. Alpert J, O'Donnell JA, Parsonnet V, Brief DK, Brener BJ, Goldenkranz RJ: Clinically recognized limb ischemia in the neonate after umbilical artery catheterization. *Am J Surg* 1980;140(3):413-418.

8. Greene WB, Cary JM: Partial foot amputations in children: A comparison of the several types with the Syme amputation. *J Bone Joint Surg Am* 1982;64(3):438-443.

9. Dillon MP, Barker TM: Comparison of gait of persons with partial foot amputation wearing prosthesis

to matched control group: Observational study. *J Rehabil Res Dev* 2008;45(9):1317-1334.

10. Loder RT, Brown KL, Zaleske DJ, Jones ET: Extremity lawn-mower injuries in children: Report by the Research Committee of the Pediatric Orthopaedic Society of North America. *J Pediatr Orthop* 1997;17(3):360-369.

11. Lawn Mower Accidents are the Leading Cause of Major Amputations for Children Under 10. Available at: http://www.cirsop.com/news/lawn-mower-accidents-are-leading-cause-major-amputations-children-under-10. Accessed April 7, 2015.

12. Harkness B, Andresen D, Kesson A, Isaacs D: Infections following lawnmower and farm machinery-related injuries in children. *J Paediatr Child Health* 2009;45(9):525-528.

13. Daley AJ, McIntyre PB: Stenotrophomonas maltophilia and lawn mower injuries in children. *J Trauma* 2000;48(3):536-537.

14. Lange TA, Nasca RJ: Traumatic partial foot amputation. *Clin Orthop Relat Res* 1984;185:137-141.

15. Mueller MJ, Allen BT, Sinacore DR: Incidence of skin breakdown and higher amputation after transmetatarsal amputation: Implications for rehabilitation. *Arch Phys Med Rehabil* 1995;76(1):50-54.

16. Dormans JP, Azzoni M, Davidson RS, Drummond DS: Major lower extremity lawn mower injuries in children. *J Pediatr Orthop* 1995;15(1):78-82.

17. Crandall RC, Wagner FW Jr: Partial and total calcanectomy: A review of thirty-one consecutive cases over a ten-year period. *J Bone Joint Surg Am* 1981;63(1):152-155.

18. Cogbill TH, Busch HM Jr, Stiers GR: Farm accidents in children. *Pediatrics* 1985;76(4):562-566.

19. McClure SK, Shaughnessy WJ: Farm-related limb amputations in children. *J Pediatr Orthop* 2005;25(2):133-137.

20. Lubicky JP, Feinberg JR: Fractures and amputations in children and adolescents requiring hospitalization after farm equipment injuries. *J Pediatr Orthop* 2009;29(5):435-438.

21. Land M: Ethical Dilemmas in the Health Care of the Pediatric Amish Population. Available at: https://med.uth.edu/mcgovern/files/2014/10/land.pdf. Accessed April 7, 2015.

22. Loder RT: Demographics of traumatic amputations in children: Implications for prevention strategies. *J Bone Joint Surg Am* 2004;86(5):923-928.

23. Jawadi AH: Traumatic foot amputation in young children secondary to all-terrain vehicles: A case series. *Injury* 2011;42(11):1380-1383.

24. Miller BJ, Chasmar LR: Frostbite in Saskatoon: A review of 10 winters. *Can J Surg* 1980;23(5):423-426.

25. Bhatnagar A, Sarker BB, Sawroop K, Chopra MK, Sinha N, Kashyap R: Diagnosis, characterisation and evaluation of treatment response of frostbite using pertechnetate scintigraphy: A prospective study. *Eur J Nucl Med Mol Imaging* 2002;29(2):170-175.

26. Barker JR, Haws MJ, Brown RE, Kucan JO, Moore WD: Magnetic resonance imaging of severe frostbite injuries. *Ann Plast Surg* 1997;38(3):275-279.

27. Golant A, Nord RM, Paksima N, Posner MA: Cold exposure injuries to the extremities. *J Am Acad Orthop Surg* 2008;16(12):704-715.

28. Imray C, Grieve A, Dhillon S; Caudwell Xtreme Everest Research Group: Cold damage to the extremities: Frostbite and non-freezing cold injuries. *Postgrad Med J* 2009;85(1007):481-488.

29. Cauchy E, Cheguillaume B, Chetaille E: A controlled trial of a prostacyclin and rt-PA in the treatment of severe frostbite. *N Engl J Med* 2011;364(2):189-190.

30. Bruen KJ, Ballard JR, Morris SE, Cochran A, Edelman LS, Saffle JR: Reduction of the incidence of amputation in frostbite injury with thrombolytic therapy. *Arch Surg* 2007;142(6):546-551, discussion 551-553.

31. Twomey JA, Peltier GL, Zera RT: An open-label study to evaluate the safety and efficacy of tissue plasminogen activator in treatment of severe frostbite. *J Trauma* 2005;59(6):1350-1354, discussion 1354-1355.

32. Cauchy E, Chetaille E, Marchand V, Marsigny B: Retrospective study of 70 cases of severe frostbite lesions: A proposed new classification scheme. *Wilderness Environ Med* 2001;12(4):248-255.

33. Cochran A: Coming in from the cold: Management of frostbite. University of Utah Grand Rounds. March 16, 2011. Available at: http://www.slideshare.net/amaliacochran/frostbite-grand-rounds-2011. Accessed March 4, 2015.

34. Paprottka FJ, Machens HG, Lohmeyer JA: Third-degree burn leading to partial foot amputation: Why a notebook is no laptop. *J Plast Reconstr Aesthet Surg* 2012;65(8):1119-1122.

35. Khan RA, Wahab S, Ahmad I, Chana RS: Macrodystrophia lipomatosa: Four case reports. *Ital J Pediatr* 2010;36:69.

36. Kwon JH, Lim SY, Lim HS: Macrodystrophia lipomatosa. *Arch Plast Surg* 2013;40(3):270-272.

37. Blacksin M, Barnes FJ, Lyons MM: MR diagnosis of macrodystrophia lipomatosa. *AJR Am J Roentgenol* 1992;158(6):1295-1297.

38. Biesecker L: The challenges of Proteus syndrome: Diagnosis and management. *Eur J Hum Genet* 2006;14(11):1151-1157.

39. Gürgey A, Aytac S, Kanra G, Secmeer G, Ceyhan M, Altay C: Outcome in children with purpura fulminans: Report on 16 patients. *Am J Hematol* 2005;80(1):20-25.

40. Brinker MR, Rosenfeld SR, Feiwell E, Granger SP, Mitchell DC, Rice JC: Myelomeningocele at the sacral level: Long-term outcomes in adults. *J Bone Joint Surg Am* 1994;76(9):1293-1300.

41. Chou LB, Ho YY, Malawer MM: Tumors of the foot and ankle: Experience with 153 cases. *Foot Ankle Int* 2009;30(9):836-841.

42. Dagher R, Helman L: Rhabdomyosarcoma: An overview. *Oncologist* 1999;4(1):34-44.

43. Jain S, Lakhtakia PK: Profile of congenital transverse deficiencies among cases of congenital orthopaedic anomalies. *J Orthop Surg (Hong Kong)* 2002;10(1):45-52.

44. Kozin SH: Upper-extremity congenital anomalies. *J Bone Joint Surg Am* 2003;85(8):1564-1576.

45. Hunter AG: A pilot study of the possible role of familial defects in anticoagulation as a cause for terminal limb reduction malformations. *Clin Genet* 2000;57(3):197-204.

46. Chitayat D, Silver MM, O'Brien K, et al: Limb defects in homozygous alpha-thalassemia: Report of three cases. *Am J Med Genet* 1997;68(2):162-167.

47. Ermito S, Dinatale A, Carrara S, Cavaliere A, Imbruglia L, Recupero S: Prenatal diagnosis of limb abnormalities: Role of fetal ultrasonography. *J Prenat Med* 2009;3(2):18-22.

48. McGuirk CK, Westgate M-N, Holmes LB: Limb deficiencies in newborn infants. *Pediatrics* 2001;108(4):E64.

49. Pauli RM, Feldman PF: Major limb malformations following intrauterine exposure to ethanol: Two additional cases and literature review. *Teratology* 1986;33(3):273-280.

50. van Rensburg LJ: Major skeletal defects in the fetal alcohol syndrome: A case report. *S Afr Med J* 1981;59(19):687-688.

51. Orioli IM, Ribeiro MG, Castilla EE: Clinical and epidemiological studies of amniotic deformity, adhesion, and mutilation (ADAM) sequence in a South American (ECLAMC) population. *Am J Med Genet A* 2003;118A(2):135-145.

52. Walter JH Jr, Goss LR, Lazzara AT: Amniotic band syndrome. *J Foot Ankle Surg* 1998;37(4):325-333.

53. Gabos PG: Modified technique for the surgical treatment of congenital constriction bands of the arms and legs of infants and children. *Orthopedics* 2006;29(5):401-404.

54. Cignini P, Giorlandino C, Padula F, Dugo N, Cafà EV, Spata A: Epidemiology and risk factors of amniotic band syndrome, or ADAM sequence. *J Prenat Med* 2012;6(4):59-63.

55. Buss PW, Hughes HE, Clarke A: Twenty-four cases of the EEC syndrome: Clinical presentation and management. *J Med Genet* 1995;32(9):716-723.

56. Dillon MP, Fatone S: Deliberations about the functional benefits and complications of partial foot amputation: Do we pay heed to the purported benefits at the expense of minimizing complications? *Arch Phys Med Rehabil* 2013;94(8):1429-1435.

Chapter 82

The Child With Multiple Limb Deficiencies

Anna Cuomo, MD   Hugh G. Watts, MD

Abstract

A child with multiple limb deficiencies requires special consideration. A complete physical examination with careful attention to other organ systems is warranted. Most children are extremely adaptive and can be psychologically well adjusted when they are provided with a supportive environment. Treatment should be pursued at centers dedicated to the challenges of integrating occupational therapy, physical therapy, and individualized prosthetic components throughout the child's intellectual and physical development. Because of the increased size and weight of multiple prostheses and associated issues of heat retention and difficulty with donning and doffing equipment, the child with multiple limb deficiencies may achieve optimal functioning using assistive devices, such as a wheelchair with a lift and adaptive computers. Technological advances such as computerized devices with voice recognition systems hold great promise for improving functional independence.

Keywords: acquired limb amputation; congenital limb amputation; multimembral limb deficiency; multiple limb deficiency; pediatric; prosthesis

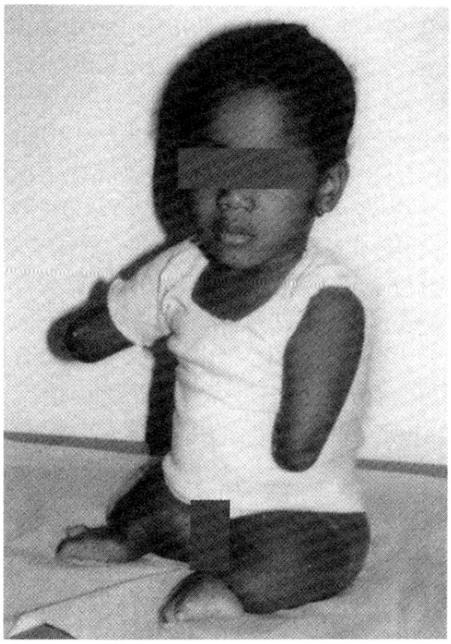

Figure 1 Photograph of a child with multiple limb deficiencies.

Introduction

Children with limb deficiencies have special problems not shared by adult amputees, and the difficulties increase exponentially for children with multiple limb involvement (**Figure 1**). These children should be cared for in special treatment facilities.

The term multiple limb deficiencies covers many possibilities, ranging from a child missing two minor toes and a single finger on the nondominant hand to a child born with no arms or legs. Children may have multiple limb deficiencies, either because they were born with the deficiencies or as a result of an accident or illness. Common sense and a creative team approach are needed to recognize and appropriately treat the varied needs of these children.

Congenital Multiple Limb Deficiencies

The incidence of congenital limb deficiencies is approximately 1 in 2,000 births. In the United States, approximately 1,500 infants annually are born with upper limb reductions and approximately 750 have lower limb reductions.[1] Reports in the literature from British Columbia range from 0.31% per 1,000 to 0.79% per 1,000 births. The variability in incidence likely results from differences in gene pools and reporting methods in different locations.[2-4] Approximately 30% of these infants have deficits in more than one limb (15% with two limbs, 5% with three limbs, and 10% with all four limbs).[5-7] The most common deficit for all congenital deficiencies is digital reductions, which account for approximately 50% of all reported cases. In approximately one-third to one-half of patients, other organs systems also are involved.

Etiology and Presentation

The most common apparent cause of all congenital limb deficiencies is vascular disruptions, such as amniotic band–related limb deficiency, which accounts for approximately 35% of cases. Other congenital causes include gene mutation, familial occurrence, and known syndromes (24%); chromosome abnormalities (6%); teratogenic causes (4%); and unknown causes (32%).[8] In

Dr. Cuomo or an immediate family member serves as a board member, owner, officer, or committee member of the Pediatric Orthopaedic Society of North America. Neither Dr. Watts nor any immediate family member has received anything of value from or has stock or stock options held in a commercial company or institution related directly or indirectly to the subject of this chapter. This chapter is adapted from Watts H: Multiple limb deficiencies, in Smith DG, Michael JW, Bowker JH, eds: Atlas of Amputations and Limb Deficiencies: Surgical, Prosthetic, and Rehabilitation Principles, ed 3. Rosemont, IL, American Academy of Orthopaedic Surgeons, 2004, pp 923-929.

general, digits are more often affected than long bones, longitudinal defects are more common than transverse defects, intercalary deficits are rare, and upper limb deficits are either reported slightly more frequently or occur at an equal frequency as lower limb deficits. Both the upper and the lower limbs are affected in approximately 8% of infants.[8,9] Amelia is reported to be 1.41 in 100,000, and phocomelia is 0.62 per 100,000 births.[10,11]

Limb deficiency can refer to the absence of a limb as well as to limb anomalies that might require a prosthesis or modified prosthesis for one or more of the involved limbs. For example, a child with the most severe form of thrombocytopenia–absent radius (TAR) syndrome may have phocomelic upper limbs and fusion of both knees caused by congenital synchondroses. These children cannot effectively use their feet to replace limited hand function because their knees do not bend sufficiently to allow the foot to reach the mouth. If bilateral knee disarticulations are performed, the child would be able to sit in a chair more easily but would be unable to rise from the floor after a fall because his or her short arms could not provide adequate assistance.

Approximately 60% of children treated in amputee clinics have congenital conditions.[6,12] In addition, 10% of children with acquired amputations have a loss of more than one limb, although underreporting may occur because these children are generally treated in the community and not in pediatric amputee centers. This is particularly true of children with lower limb amputations, which are easier to manage in a less-specialized facility than are upper limb amputations.[13] Among children who have acquired amputations, 40% involve the upper limb; however, in children treated at amputee clinics, congenital upper limb involvement is twice as likely as lower limb involvement.[6]

Associated Anomalies

The limbs form at 4 to 7 weeks of gestation, as do organs such as the kidneys and heart. Therefore, a thorough examination for associated anomalies is mandatory in a child with one congenital anomaly. The clinician should begin the examination at the head and work downward, checking the cranial nerves (especially cranial nerve VII) to test for associated Möbius syndrome, the palates (soft and hard), and the eyes and ears for placement and formation. The chest should be checked for the proper number and location of nipples, and the pectoral muscles should be examined. The heart should be examined for heart murmur, the anus for normal formation, and the spine for curvature and sacral dimples. The other limbs should be carefully evaluated for the presence of even minor abnormalities that could change the diagnostic (and possibly prognostic) category from single-limb to multiple-limb involvement. The presence of petechiae or bruises can suggest TAR syndrome. The infant's mother and his or her nurses should be questioned regarding the infant's sucking and swallowing to assess for tracheoesophageal abnormalities. If the infant's urine is abnormal, renal anomalies should be considered.

Additional studies may be indicated. Renal ultrasonography and radiography should be used to evaluate the spine and heart for all infants with a limb deficiency. A complete blood count and differential, including a platelet count, should be obtained for a child with a radial deficiency. Because upper limb deficiency syndromes, such as Holt-Oram syndrome, can have a particularly high association with cardiac defects, echocardiography should be strongly considered. Currently, there are no recommendations for a screening echocardiogram specifically for a child with multiple limb reductions or anomalies; however, the most recent disease-based guideline from the American Society of Echocardiography lists clinically suspected syndrome or extracardiac congenital anomaly know to be associated with congenital heart disease as an appropriate indication for a newborn screening echocardiogram.[14]

Anomalies in the central nervous system or one of the receptive senses (vision or hearing) are of particular importance. Children are generally extremely adaptable, but if the central nervous system is involved, the child's adaptive capacity may be compromised.

Acquired Multiple Limb Deficiencies

Not all multiple limb loss results from congenital causes. Purpura fulminans, commonly caused by meningococcal disease, results in disseminated intravascular clotting. This condition can occur after other bacteremias (for example, pneumococci) or a viremia (for example, chicken pox) and can necessitate the amputation of multiple limbs.[15] Incidents involving trains are another cause of multiple limb loss. A common scenario is that of a child trying to hop a train at the after-end ladder, losing his or her grip, and being spun around the back end of the railway car and thrown on the tracks in front of the following car. This commonly results in the loss of two or more limbs. Lawnmower injuries, automobile collisions, electrical burns, and injuries caused by explosive devices are other traumatic causes of multiple limb loss.

Special Needs

Children with multiple limb loss present special challenges to the professionals who work with them, and each patient has unique needs and abilities. The knowledge gained by treating one child may not be applicable to another child with limb loss.

Prosthetic Components

Children with multiple limb deficiencies have a greater need for specialized prosthetic components than do those with single limb deficiencies. Several characteristics of prosthetic components should be considered in relation to the special needs of the child with multiple deficiencies.

Size and Weight

Prosthetic components for adults are usually available in large, medium, and small sizes, with perhaps an extra small size that is appropriate for smaller women. Children, however, need an array of sizes, ranging from those that can fit a tiny 1-year-old toddler up to devices for a teenager of nearly adult proportions. Although competition has encouraged many manufacturers to address this niche market, it is not economically feasible for manufacturers of prosthetic components to fabricate and store large stocks of multiple-sized items because of the relatively low demand. Therefore, some components may need to be individually crafted. The weight of prosthetic components is an issue not only because of the smaller muscle mass available to move the prostheses but also because children with multiple limb deficiencies find that minor difficulties with one prosthesis can adversely affect the functioning of another.

Heat Retention

Wearing a prosthesis can be hot, especially in warm climates. The limbs provide an increase in total surface area of the skin, which is the primary source of cooling the core body temperature.[16] Children who wear two, three, or even four prostheses may not have enough bare skin to disperse heat adequately. In addition, prostheses for higher levels of limb deficiency demand greater energy expenditure by the child, compounding the heat problem. This is a particular problem if the child has a hip or shoulder disarticulation requiring a prosthesis that covers a considerable area of the trunk. Body temperature may become

substantially elevated. Reasonable, normal activities may be prohibitive in any season but especially in the summer, and the child may understandably refuse to wear the prostheses as a result.

Integration of Prosthetic Components

Children with multiple limb deficiencies frequently require custom-designed components, which often require custom fabrication. For example, an 8-year-old boy who was born with bilateral hip disarticulations and an absent left hand was able to walk on bilateral lower limb prostheses by using a regular forearm crutch with his normal right arm and using a custom-made crutch as the terminal device of the left upper limb prosthesis. When the boy was not walking, the left arm prosthesis included a quick-disconnect wrist that allowed him to easily exchange the crutch for a hook. Fabrication of such special items is labor intensive and expensive; however, the challenge of helping these complex patients stimulates creative solutions and provides satisfaction to both the patient and the treatment team.

Donning and Doffing

The design of the prostheses must allow independent donning and doffing. The child with multiple limb deficiencies may wear such an array of devices that it can be difficult for a parent, let alone the child, to apply them. If the child is to become an independent adult, this aspect must be considered. The need to achieve independence depends on the child's age and psychosocial development and the relationships within the family. Many parents are reluctant to relinquish their own need to assist the child and must be encouraged by the clinical staff to allow the child to gain independence. Prostheses appropriately designed for easy donning and doffing may be helpful. For example, pull tabs with a fabric hook and loop fastener system can be used on belts and harnesses to allow easy grasping with a prosthetic

hook for donning a suction socket or a total elastic suspension belt.

Wheelchair Use

Various factors need to be considered if wheelchair use is required. If a powered wheelchair is not necessary, a standard chair is preferable because the exercise it requires can help with the common problem of obesity. If a powered chair is necessary, its size and weight must be considered. It will usually be necessary for the parents to have a van modified with a lift or ramp to accept the chair because power chairs are heavy. For adolescents of driving age, a van will need to be modified to allow the wheelchair user to operate the vehicle.

For the most severely involved children, such as those missing both arms and both legs, the wheelchair may need to be adjustable to almost floor level. This allows the child to crawl or roll onto the seat, and then raise the seat to a level more functional for table activities. Such wheelchairs are individually fabricated and often are expensive.

Gadget Tolerance

Members of the rehabilitation team or the family may devise a complicated mix of equipment, especially electronics, to allow the child to perform an array of activities. Often, these devices outstrip the child's needs and desires. Despite their adaptability, children often will not tolerate having a large number of highly technical mechanical devices applied to them. This is commonly called poor gadget tolerance (**Figure 2**). Children often function much better without highly sophisticated equipment. An electronic replacement for an upper limb often does not have long-term acceptance by a child with multiple limb deficiencies. Many reasons have been given for this lack of acceptance, but factual information is lacking. Many children find it difficult to articulate why they prefer not to wear upper limb prostheses. It has been speculated that the excessive

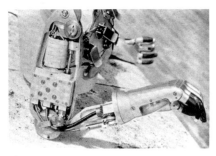

Figure 2 Photograph of a prosthesis developed for a bilateral high-level upper limb amputee. This type of prosthesis is unlikely to be worn by a child born with the absence of both upper limbs because it will be hot, heavy, and provide little sensory feedback. It also exceeds a child's gadget tolerance.

heat buildup, high energy consumption, discomfort, and, most importantly, the lack of sensory feedback are important factors in prosthesis rejection. Other clinicians have speculated that children born with a limb deficiency may lack an appropriate representation in the brain for the absent limb. This theory has been supported in recent brain mapping studies comparing individuals with congenital and traumatic upper limb loss.[17] The lack of willingness among children to wear upper limb prostheses provides a difficult challenge for those working to develop and improve upper limb prosthetic components for this population.

Economic Implications
Given the need for multiple prostheses, a special wheelchair, and a customized van for the child's transportation, the major limitation experienced by the family of a child with multiple limb deficiencies is likely to be the ability to pay for the ancillary equipment. Some financial help may be available from government agencies and charitable organizations. Accessibility to the classroom and assistants to help these children (especially with toileting while they are at school) are more commonly available since the passage of legislation ensuring educational opportunities for all children in many countries.

Developmental Capabilities
As is true of able-bodied children, the developmental capabilities of children with limb deficiencies are constantly changing. Unlike able-bodied children, however, those with multiple limb deficiencies face greater challenges, and the adaptation required may be overwhelming. Although there have been reports of successful fittings of toddlers with a unilateral prosthesis incorporating an articulated knee, the child with multiple limb loss faces a greater challenge. Mastering two articulated lower limb prostheses is very difficult, and, if upper limb deficiency is present, the child's ability to avoid injury in a fall is compromised. It is much simpler for these children to learn to use nonarticulated limbs. The child's intellectual development as well as physical coordination and strength are important in planning the prosthetic program. A 5-year-old child cannot be expected to manage myoelectrically controlled hands with the same dexterity as a 13-year-old adolescent. Prosthetic components for children should be appropriate for the developmental age of the child and for the degree of multiple challenges faced by a particular child.

Age of First Fitting
The child with multiple limb deficiencies may be limited in his or her ability to fulfill experiences important for normal intellectual and motor development, such as mobility to explore surroundings, the ability to manipulate objects, and obtaining tactile and proprioceptive feedback. However, most children will naturally seek to substitute other methods for gaining these experiences, and this should be encouraged. It has been proposed that directional sense, such as up and down, left and right, and rotation, is impaired in children with limb deficiencies because they cannot easily explore their surroundings. However, a study by French and Clarke[18] found no difference in directionality test scores between congenital and traumatic

amputees, who presumably had the opportunity and ability for normal development before limb loss. There was a trend, however, toward poorer scores with increased severity of the pattern of deficiency. Every effort should be made to help children with multiple limb deficiencies reach appropriate milestones to aid their intellectual and motor development.

Some care providers have advocated fitting children younger than 6 months of age with upper limb prostheses so the children can be trained to develop bimanual eye-hand coordination. Current practice, however, is to wait until a child is beginning to develop sitting balance, usually at approximately 5 to 6 months of age. The first fitting may occur later in a child with multiple limb loss, however, developmental delay or other health needs may intervene.

Age of Activation of Terminal Devices
The age at which the terminal devices in a child's prostheses should be activated will depend on the child's psychomotor development. Ordinarily, the terminal device is mounted at the time the prosthesis is first applied. At first, the therapists and parents open the device and place objects in it so that the child can understand the principle of the device. If a myoelectric prosthesis is to be used, some clinics will fit the child very early (at age 12 to 24 months) with a simpler single-electrode system, which alternately controls opening and closing. If a body-powered prosthesis is to be used, the activating cable is usually connected at approximately 18 to 24 months of age, when the child is more developmentally ready. The major factor in the timing of these decisions is the child's developmental readiness. In children with multiple limb deficiencies, the timetable may need to be extended.

Sports and Recreational Activities
As is the case with able-bodied children, those with multiple limb

deficiencies learn by playing. These children may have an even greater psychological and physical need for active play than able-bodied children because they have few activities to help them burn calories and because food is often offered to these children in sympathy by parents and siblings. This is especially true for children with multiple high-level deficiencies, in whom the propensity for obesity should be counteracted with exercise and caloric limitation. Children with distal deficiencies who wear prostheses and are very active may burn calories at a high rate and need additional calories to maintain a normal weight.

Although parents may worry that swimming is not safe for children with multiple limb deficiencies, swimming is a good sport for amputees, and it can be readily done by those with no legs. Even children with missing arms and legs can perform a porpoise-like trunk motion that will propel them through the water. Although supervision is imperative, many groups welcome the challenge of helping these children learn to swim.

Skiing is also a favorite sport among many amputees because it gives them an opportunity to experience the exhilaration of speed. The child will need help, and prostheses may need to be modified. An extra socket may be needed to protect the residual limb and keep it warm when no prosthesis is worn. For ski poles, modified forearm crutches are fitted with small ski tips (outriggers). Instruction is important to teach the child how to use new equipment. If tritrack or three-track skiing is unrealistic, a child with multiple limb deficiencies can learn to ski seated in a special frame mounted over a single ski.

Special centers are available at which amputees can learn to participate in a variety of sports. Parents should be encouraged to allow their children to participate because it is natural for them to be overprotective. This may require an active effort on the part of the clinical

team to reassure parents. A referral to a recreational therapist may be beneficial.

Sexuality

Children with multiple limb deficiencies will undergo normal sexual maturation and have normal concerns about sex. These children face many of the same issues as their able-bodied peers, but their sexual development is often complicated by added concerns about their altered body image and how they will be accepted by a potential partner. Adult amputees discuss issues of sexuality among themselves. Clinic team members are often reluctant to discuss sexuality, but they must provide the developing child with appropriate information and/or counseling. Adult men without arms or legs have fathered children, limbless women have given birth to children, and limb-deficient parents have successfully raised children.

Adolescents with congenital deficiencies commonly worry about passing their condition on to potential offspring. Such worries are generally unfounded, but a referral to a genetic counselor may provide valuable insight and, in most cases, will relieve anxiety.

Psychological Needs of the Child and Family

It might be expected that multiple limb deficiency would exact a heavy toll on a child's psyche, but studies have shown that these children do well psychologically.[19-23] These studies have found that the effect of perceived physical appearance on psychological distress is mediated by general self-esteem, not by the severity of the physical involvement. There is also empiric evidence that coping mechanisms are tied to perceived social support from parents, teacher, and classmates and to the level of family/marital conflict and organization. In essence, the child's self-perception is a reflection of the attitudes of those with whom he or she interacts. This is an important point for parents and

caregivers to learn early in the process of caring for their child, because they will have a great influence on the child's self-esteem.

A long-term prosthetic treatment plan may be easier to accomplish in a child than in an adult who is employed and cannot miss work. However, intervening during childhood means that more people (the patient, the parents, and sometimes grandparents) are involved with prosthetic management decisions. To ensure the best care for the child, all concerned parties should be informed of their rights, and treatment options should be explained and discussed. If a conversion amputation is being considered, there is usually no need to rush into an elective conversion amputation until everyone is comfortable with the need to proceed.

The need for cultural sensitivity has assumed more importance in recent decades. Some cultures are much more resistant to conversion amputation, although the clinical team may see the need as obvious. These cultural differences can be compounded because of misunderstandings caused by language translation. Putting the child's family in contact with other families who share the same cultural traditions can often be very beneficial.

Special Aspects of Upper Limb Absence
Scoliosis

Children with upper limb deficiencies have an increased chance for the development of scoliosis, either congenital or idiopathic.[24-28] If the scoliosis becomes progressive, the curves are very resistant to bracing, if for no other reason than braces are difficult to wear for a child with upper limb absence. If spinal fusion is being considered, the possible effects on the child's ability to reach the mouth with the feet should be carefully considered, because most of these children choose to use their feet rather than prostheses. Decisions should be made

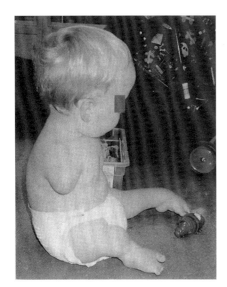

Figure 3 Photograph of a child with bilateral upper limb loss using his feet to replace hand function.

based on advantages and disadvantages to the child's lifetime functioning rather than on the basis of radiographic findings alone.

Use of Upper Limb Prostheses

Children born without one or both upper limbs can have extraordinary functional capability. James et al[29] concluded children with unilateral transradial transverse deficiencies have nearly normal function and quality of life regardless of whether they wear a prosthesis. The effect of an upper limb prosthesis on quality of life and function in children with multiple limb deficiencies is not well studied; however, it is acknowledged that they can readily be taught to feed themselves and perform many tasks using their feet and toes (**Figure 3**). Objects can be grasped between the chin and shoulder or between a very short residual humerus and the chest wall.[30] The sensory feedback provided by using feet or residual limbs is advantageous over prostheses use. The increased energy consumption required to manipulate a prosthesis can be problematic for a child with a multiple limb deficiency. The recent focus on highly technical components for adults has not

had a substantial effect in the field of prosthetic devices for children because of the high costs. These factors can lead to difficulty when trying to convince a child to wear an upper limb prosthesis because the child may be more facile, especially initially, without the prosthesis. Most children who are born without arms will not wear prostheses throughout their lifetime.[31-33] The percentage of such children who use prostheses may depend on the enthusiasm of the clinic team for fitting such children and the age at which such children are first fitted.[34]

Although there are notable exceptions, many children born with upper limb deficiency function better without prosthetic help. By the time they reach adulthood, they are able to do almost everything for themselves, including driving an automobile with their feet. In contrast, children who lose their arms because of trauma are much more likely to struggle with the limb loss.

No prosthesis may be prescribed for a child because of common sense concerns and a need to carefully husband the limited financial resources of the child's family. Other factors, however, should be considered. For example, at some point in the patient's life, especially during adolescence, an individual born without arms may request simple cosmetic arms to be used for special occasions.

Initially, most parents want their child to be fitted with prosthetic arms. As a consequence, a trial of prosthetic fitting may be a necessary stage that a family must go through so that they can personally experience the rejection of the prostheses by the child. Consequently, the prescription of a set of arm prostheses with expensive myoelectric components may not be a practical decision. There may be a temporary need, however, to provide lifelike passive hands for an infant so that a parent will not reject the child.

Because these children will probably not use prosthetic arms and will

function by using the feet in place of the hands, it is important to know the status of the motion and muscle control of the hips, knees, ankles, and toes. Careful examination is essential, because congenital anomalies are frequently associated with other anomalies.

The skill of the occupational therapist in upper limb prosthetic training may play only a limited role in the child's care if the child rejects long-term prosthesis use. The therapist's most important role may be to teach the child how best to substitute the feet for the missing arms and how to use adaptive equipment creatively. The ability to shrug the shoulders can be useful for grasping objects between the side of the neck and the upper scapula. The use of assistive devices (for example, a mouth stick for typing) can help the older child interact with the world. Toileting is a major problem for the child without arms, especially if the child wants to use public restrooms.

Computers may change the lives of children with upper limb absence. Computers can be used as controllers to activate remote switches (for example, turning lights on and off or answering a telephone), although control of a computer keyboard is still a problem. There are mouth-controlled stick devices available for keyboards as well as touch-screen devices.

Voice-controlled software has not yet proved to be as effective for children as it is for adults, although this technology holds great future promise for limb-deficient children. Voice recognition systems for adults have improved dramatically over the past decade because of larger databases of training data, which result in more accurate models of human speech. Faster computers and improved algorithms have resulted in better accuracy of speech-to-text systems and have improved overall accuracy for all users. However, quantification of the speech of children still lags behind adult speech because of the lack of training data specifically applicable to children. Children speak differently than adults in a few key dimensions, including higher pitch (fundamental frequency), more irregular prosody (the "tune" of how someone talks), uneven loudness (including shouting-type speech that itself has different characteristics), uneven or unusual durations of words and syllables (both too long or too short), as well as unusual word choice (covering both mispronunciations such as "aminal" and ungrammatical utterances such as "I goed there") (Brian Langer, PhD, Senior Speech Scientist, Toy Talk, San Francisco, CA, personal communication, 2015). Although voice recognition technology has great potential to augment the use of assistive devices in general, there are currently no commercially available prosthetics or medical devices for patients with limb deficiencies.

In the future, children are likely to embrace more technology as computer interfaces become more playful and devices become more like toys. However, the devices must not detract from the child's own agility or sensation and must provide immediate positive feedback to maintain the child's interest. Small devices that are playful, durable, and have responsive voice-recognition software will likely revolutionize the world for a child with multiple limb deficiencies.

Summary

Multiple limb deficiency is rare in children, but those affected often require care at a specialized center that is equipped with a creative team to assist the child in gaining independent function. The needs of children change over the course of their intellectual and physical development. Because congenital limb reductions are often associated with other organ system anomalies, a through physical examination and strong consideration of other specialized tests are required. Care providers must resist the temptation to simply replace the multiple limb deficits with multiple prostheses, which may result in problems with decreased agility, heat retention, and difficulty with component integration. Instead, there should be a focus on optimizing function and independence. For children with profound deficits, this is often achieved with assistive devices, such as wheelchairs with an elevator platform and computers with a mouth-controlled stick for typing. Voice recognition systems may play an important role in the future. As technology improves, there may be an increasing role for assistive devices at earlier ages if the interfaces are playful and provide immediate positive feedback.

References

1. Canfield MA, Honein MA, Yuskiv N, et al: National estimates and race/ethnic-specific variation of selected birth defects in the United States, 1999-2001. *Birth Defects Res A Clin Mol Teratol* 2006;76(11):747-756.

2. Froster-Iskenius UG, Baird PA: Limb reduction defects in over one million consecutive livebirths. *Teratology* 1989;39(2):127-135.

3. Froster UG, Baird PA: Upper limb deficiencies and associated malformations: A population-based study. *Am J Med Genet* 1992;44(6):767-781.

4. Froster UG, Baird PA: Congenital defects of lower limbs and associated malformations: A population based study. *Am J Med Genet* 1993;45(1):60-64.

5. Tooms RE: Congenital amputee, in Morrissy RT, ed: *Lovell and Winter's Pediatric Orthopedics*, ed 3. Philadelphia, PA, JB Lippincott, 1990, pp 1023-1070.

6. Krebs DE, Fishman S: Characteristics of the child amputee population. *J Pediatr Orthop* 1984;4(1):89-95.

7. Wilson JG, Brent RL: Are female sex hormones teratogenic? *Am J Obstet Gynecol* 1981;141(5):567-580.

8. Gold NB, Westgate MN, Holmes LB: Anatomic and etiological classification of congenital limb deficiencies. *Am J Med Genet A* 2011;155A(6):1225-1235.

9. Makhoul IR, Goldstein I, Smolkin T, Avrahami R, Sujov P: Congenital limb deficiencies in newborn infants: Prevalence, characteristics and prenatal diagnosis. *Prenat Diagn* 2003;23(3):198-200.

10. Bermejo-Sánchez E, Cuevas L, Amar E, et al: Amelia: A multi-center descriptive epidemiologic study in a large dataset from the International Clearinghouse for Birth Defects Surveillance and Research, and overview of the literature. *Am J Med Genet C Semin Med Genet* 2011;157C(4):288-304.

11. Bermejo-Sánchez E, Cuevas L, Amar E, et al: Phocomelia: A worldwide descriptive epidemiologic study in a large series of cases from the International Clearinghouse for Birth Defects Surveillance and Research, and overview of the literature. *Am J Med Genet C Semin Med Genet* 2011;157C(4):305-320.

12. Kay HW, Fishman S: *1018 Children With Skeletal Limb Deficiencies*. New York, NY, New York University Post-Graduate Medical School, Orthotics and Prosthetics, 1967.

13. Davies EF, BR, Clippinger FJ: Children with amputations. *Inter-Clin Info Bull* 1969;9:6-19.

14. Campbell RM, Douglas PS, Eidem BW, Lai WW, Lopez L, Sachdeva R: ACC/AAP/AHA/ASE/HRS/SCAI/SCCT/SCMR/SOPE 2014 appropriate use criteria for initial transthoracic echocardiography in outpatient pediatric cardiology: A report of the American College of Cardiology Appropriate Use Criteria Task Force, American Academy of Pediatrics, American Heart Association, American Society of Echocardiography, Heart Rhythm Society, Society for Cardiovascular Angiography and

Interventions, Society of Cardiovascular Computed Tomography, Society for Cardiovascular Magnetic Resonance, and Society of Pediatric Echocardiography. *J Am Coll Cardiol* 2014;64(19):2039-2060.

15. Canavese F, Krajbich JI, LaFleur BJ: Orthopaedic sequelae of childhood meningococcemia: Management considerations and outcome. *J Bone Joint Surg Am* 2010;92(12):2196-2203.

16. González-Alonso J: Human thermoregulation and the cardiovascular system. *Exp Physiol* 2012;97(3):340-346.

17. Reilly KT, Sirigu A: Motor cortex representation of the upper-limb in individuals born without a hand. *PLoS One* 2011;6(4):e18100.

18. French R, Clarke S: The directional senses of the child amputee. *ICIB* 1975;14(7):9-13.

19. Pruitt SD, Varni JW, Seid M, Setoguchi Y: Prosthesis satisfaction outcome measurement in pediatric limb deficiency. *Arch Phys Med Rehabil* 1997;78(7):750-754.

20. Varni J, Setoguchi Y: Perceived physical appearance and adjustment of adolescents with congenital/acquired limb deficiencies: A path-analytic model. *J Clin Child Psychol* 1996;25:201-208.

21. Varni JW, Rubenfeld LA, Talbot D, Setoguchi Y: Determinants of self-esteem in children with congenital/acquired limb deficiencies. *J Dev Behav Pediatr* 1989;10(1):13-16.

22. Tyc V: Psychological adaptation of children and adolescents with limb deficiencies: A review. *Clin Psychol Rev* 1992;12:275-291.

23. Bryant PR, Pandian G: Acquired limb deficiencies: 1. Acquired limb deficiencies in children and young adults. *Arch Phys Med Rehabil* 2001;82(3, suppl 1):S3-S8.

24. Makley JT, Heiple KG: Scoliosis associated with congenital deficiencies of the upper extremity. *J Bone Joint Surg Am* 1970;52(2):279-287.

25. Heyman HJ, Ivankovich AD, Shulman M, Millar E, Choudhry YA: Intraoperative monitoring and anesthetic management for spinal fusion in an amelic patient. *J Pediatr Orthop* 1982;2(3):299-301.

26. Herring JA, Goldberg MJ: Amelia and scoliosis. *J Pediatr Orthop* 1985;5(5):605-609.

27. Lester DK, Painter GL, Berman AT, Skinner SR: "Idiopathic" scoliosis associated with congenital upper-limb deficiency. *Clin Orthop Relat Res* 1986;202:205-210.

28. Samuelsson L, Hermansson LL, Norén L: Scoliosis and trunk asymmetry in upper limb transverse dysmelia. *J Pediatr Orthop* 1997;17(6):769-772.

29. James MA, Bagley AM, Brasington K, Lutz C, McConnell S, Molitor F: Impact of prostheses on function and quality of life for children with unilateral congenital below-the-elbow deficiency. *J Bone Joint Surg Am* 2006;88(11):2356-2365.

30. Herring JA: Functional assessment and management of multilimb deficiency, in Herring JA, Birch JG, eds: *The Child With a Limb Deficiency*. Rosemont, IL, American Academy of Orthopaedic Surgeons, 1998, pp 437-445.

31. Crandall RC, Tomhave W: Pediatric unilateral below-elbow amputees: Retrospective analysis of 34 patients given multiple prosthetic options. *J Pediatr Orthop* 2002;22(3):380-383.

32. Davidson J: A survey of the satisfaction of upper limb amputees with their prostheses, their lifestyles, and their abilities. *J Hand Ther* 2002;15(1):62-70.

33. Kruger LM, Fishman S: Myoelectric and body-powered prostheses. *J Pediatr Orthop* 1993;13(1):68-75.

34. Scotland TR, Galway HR: A long-term review of children with congenital and acquired upper limb deficiency. *J Bone Joint Surg Br* 1983;65(3):346-349.

Index